CLINICAL MANUAL OF
MEDICAL-SURGICAL NURSING

Prepared by

JUDITH K. SANDS, R.N., Ed.D.
Associate Professor of Nursing,
University of Virginia School of Nursing, Charlottesville, Virginia

Based on material from

MEDICAL-SURGICAL NURSING

CONCEPTS AND CLINICAL PRACTICE

FOURTH EDITION

BY

WILMA J. PHIPPS, R.N., Ph.D., F.A.A.N.

Professor Emerita of Medical-Surgical Nursing,
Frances Payne Bolton School of Nursing,
Case Western Reserve University, Cleveland, Ohio

BARBARA C. LONG, R.N., M.S.N.

Associate Professor Emerita of Medical-Surgical Nursing,
Frances Payne Bolton School of Nursing,
Case Western Reserve University, Cleveland, Ohio

NANCY F. WOODS, R.N., Ph.D., F.A.A.N.

Professor and Chairperson,
Department of Parent and Child Nursing,
University of Washington, Seattle, Washington

VIRGINIA L. CASSMEYER, Ph.D., R.N.

Associate Professor of Medical-Surgical Nursing,
University of Kansas College of Health Sciences, Kansas City, Missouri

Clinical Manual of
MEDICAL-
SURGICAL
NURSING

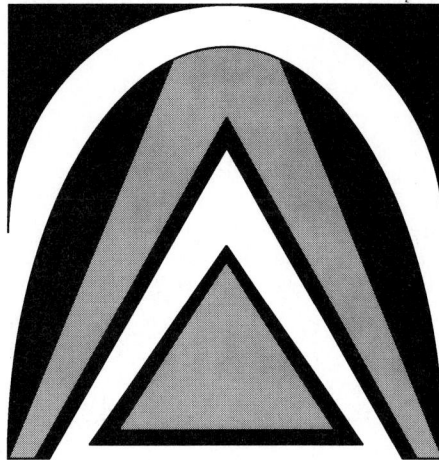

SECOND EDITION

Mosby
Year Book

St. Louis Baltimore Boston Chicago London Philadelphia Sydney Toronto

Mosby
Year Book
Dedicated to Publishing Excellence

Editor: Linda L. Duncan
Project Supervisor: Barbara Merritt
Editing and Production: University Graphics, Inc.
Design: Gail Morey Hudson

Copyright © 1991 by Mosby–Year Book, Inc.

A Mosby Imprint of Mosby–Year Book, Inc.

Printed in the United States of America

Mosby–Year Book, Inc.
11830 Westline Industrial Drive, St. Louis, Missouri 63146

Library of Congress Cataloging in Publication Data

Sands, Judith K.
   Clinical manual of medical-surgical nursing.—2nd ed. / prepared
by Judith K. Sands.
      p.   cm.
   Based on material from: Medical-surgical nursing / edited by Wilma
J. Phipps . . . [et al.]. 4th ed. 1990.
   Rev. ed. of: Clinical handbook of medical-surgical nursing / Wilma
J. Phipps, Barbara C. Long, Nancy F. Woods. 1987.
   Includes bibliographical references and index.
   ISBN 0-8016-4107-1 (spiral)
   1. Nursing—Handbooks, manuals, etc. 2. Surgical nursing—
Handbooks, manuals, etc. I. Phipps, Wilma J., 1925-   Clinical
handbook of medical-surgical nursing. II. Medical-surgical nursing.
III. Title.
   [DNLM: 1. Nursing—handbooks. 2. Surgical Nursing—handbooks.
WY 39 S221c]
RT51.P46 1991
610.73—dc20
DNLM/DLC
for Library of Congress   90-13690
                                              CIP

CL/VH 9 8 7 6 5 4 3 2 1

Preface

The second edition of the *Clinical Manual of Medical-Surgical Nursing* has been revised and expanded, but still is designed to meet its original purposes. It is a concise yet thorough clinical resource book that presents the essential nursing care involved in most common medical and surgical conditions. It is designed to serve as a reference book for nursing students, new graduates, part-time and returning nurses, and active practitioners in multiple practice settings.

The *Clinical Manual* is not designed to be a full textbook or a specialist reference. It is instead a concise and easy to use reference guide to the broad field of medical-surgical nursing. Practice settings in both acute and long-term care today force nurses to become specialists in a relatively narrow area of practice. It is virtually impossible to remain current with the trends and changes occurring outside of the specialty. At the same time, the realities of day to day practice include being "floated" to different units and caring for a wide variety of "boarder" patients in virtually any setting. And the multisystem nature of many admissions means that diabetes complicates psychiatric admissions, hypertension affects joint surgery, and pulmonary disease alters the approach to trauma care. To be able to provide safe care, practicing nurses need ready access to concise, up to date information on common conditions.

The *Clinical Manual of Medical-Surgical Nursing* can fill that need.

The book is organized in a modified outline format to present the most comprehensive information possible in a minimum of space. For the most commonly occurring conditions, the full nursing process is covered. Less common conditions are summarized in boxes or tables. The *Manual* makes liberal use of boxes and tables to highlight the content, present additional related material, and provide the reader easy access to relevant information. The approach is practical and practice oriented, making the *Manual* a useful resource for both care planning and care delivery.

To help the reader find material quickly and easily, the *Manual* is organized by body systems. Chapters are also included on commonly occurring clinical situations such as fluid and electrolyte disorders and oncology. This second edition also contains a chapter on pain. Nursing care is presented in a nursing process framework to assist in development of the care plan. This style should also assist students in preparing patient-related assignments and new graduates in reviewing for the NCLEX licensure exam. The nursing diagnoses have been modified to incorporate the Ninth NANDA Conference list and wording. Medication and treatment approaches have been significantly updated, particularly in the areas of cardiovascular nursing. The coverage of reproductive problems has been expanded, and a significant section on the management of AIDS has been added.

It is my hope that the *Clinical Manual of Medical-Surgical Nursing* will serve as a practical day-to-day resource for students and practicing nurses as they cope with the fast-paced changes and challenges of nursing in the nineties. I want to thank the editorial staff at Mosby–Year Book for their support and assistance in preparing the second edition and the wonderful secretarial staff at the University of Virginia School of Nursing for their tireless efforts. Lastly, my thanks to my boys for their patience through another summer of deadlines. You guys are my pride and joy.

Judith K. Sands

Contents

CLINICAL MANUAL OF
MEDICAL-SURGICAL NURSING

CHAPTER 1

Fluid and Electrolyte Imbalance

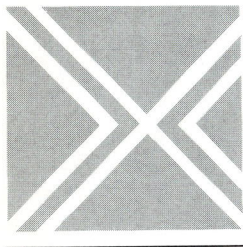

The monitoring of fluid and electrolyte balance is a major nursing responsibility since this homeostatic balance may be threatened by virtually any medical or surgical disorder. It is also threatened by many common medical therapies. The nurse must be able to do the following:

1. Recognize situations likely to cause imbalances
2. Identify patients at risk for developing imbalances
3. Initiate measures to prevent imbalances from occurring
4. Recognize the signs and symptoms of common imbalances
5. Carry out therapeutic measures prescribed by the physician
6. Monitor patient responses to the interventions

Fluid and electrolyte imbalances are commonly categorized for discussion as specific excesses or deficits, although more than one may, and commonly does, exist in any clinical situation. Table 1-1 lists normal serum values for the body's major electrolytes and fluid osmolality.

PRIMARY FLUID IMBALANCES

Although sodium and water imbalances are frequently encountered together, it is important to differentiate between them. The treatments used for disturbances in sodium or fluid vary substantially depending on the specific cause. Table 1-2 summarizes the normal daily fluid intake and output of an adult.

EXTRACELLULAR WATER DEFICIT (HYPEROSMOLAR IMBALANCE): DEHYDRATION

An extracellular water deficit occurs when the amount of water is decreased in proportion to the amount of solute in the water, causing the osmolality to exceed 300 mOsm/L. It may result from an inadequate intake of fluid, an increased solute intake, or an accumulation of solutes related to a disease condition.

PATHOPHYSIOLOGY

Hyperosmolality causes water to move from the cells to the vascular compartment to help maintain the circulating blood volume. Osmotic diuresis occurs as the kidneys attempt to excrete the excess solute. Dehydration worsens as a result of the loss of fluid used to flush out solutes in the urine.

TABLE 1-1 Normal serum electrolyte and fluid osmolality values

Electrolyte or Fluid	Serum Value
Sodium (Na^+)	135-145 mEq/L
Potassium (K^+)	3.5-5.0 mEq/L
Chloride (Cl^-)	100-106 mEq/L
Phosphate (PO_4^{2-})	2.8-4.5 mEq/L
Calcium (Ca^{2+})	4.5-5.8 mEq/L
Bicarbonate (HCO_3^-)	20-30 mEq/L
Body fluid osmolality	275-295 mOsm/L

TABLE 1-2 Approximate daily fluid intake and output for an adult eating 2500 calories

Intake		Output	
Method	Amount (ml)	Method	Amount (ml)
Water in food	1000	Skin	500
Water from oxidation	300	Lungs	350
Water as liquid	1200	Feces	150
		Kidneys	1500
TOTAL	2500	TOTAL	2500

RISK FACTORS LEADING TO EXTRACELLULAR WATER DEFICIT

Inability to recognize thirst:
    Confusion
    Altered consciousness
Inability to obtain fluids:
    Aphasia (person cannot request fluids)
    Paralysis, either general or restricted to swallowing
Inability to conserve fluids:
    Profuse sweating
    Vomiting, diarrhea, or gastrointestinal suctioning
    Profuse diuresis, as in diabetes insipidus
Hyperosmolar dietary intake:
    Tube feedings with concentrated protein, electrolytes, or glucose
Buildup of solutes secondary to a disease process:
    Renal failure
    Diabetic ketoacidosis
    Other endocrine and metabolic disorders

TABLE 1-3 Signs and symptoms of extracellular water deficit

Body System	Signs and Symptoms
Skin	Flushed, dry, poor turgor
Mouth	Dry, sticky mucous membranes
Eyes	Decrease in tears
	Soft, sunken eyeballs
Cardiovascular	Orthostatic hypotension
	Tachycardia
Central nervous	Apprehension, restlessness, weakness
Blood (values)	Increased Na$^+$ and Hct (hematocrit), higher osmolality
Urine	Decreased output, higher osmolality, increased specific gravity
Other	Thirst, weight loss

Failure to intervene has the following consequences:

The intracellular fluid compartment becomes depleted, markedly impairing cell function. NOTE: Brain cells are particularly sensitive, and mental status changes may be among the first signs.

Extracellular fluid losses impair circulation, further interrupting cellular metabolism and possibly leading to vascular collapse.

Water deficit is not usually a problem for an alert individual who has sufficient fluid available and is able to swallow. The box above lists risk factors that can lead to extracellular water deficit. Table 1-3 presents common signs and symptoms.

MEDICAL MANAGEMENT

Medical management consists of replacing lost fluids plus supplying current daily needs. The amount of fluid loss can be estimated from weight loss: 1 kg of body weight equals 1 L of fluid. The method of fluid delivery may be oral, IV, or both. Initial fluid replacement is frequently glucose and water, supplemented by electrolyte solutions once the patient's renal function is ensured. Replacement may take place over several days to avoid overtaxing the heart.

EXTRACELLULAR WATER EXCESS (HYPOSMOLAR IMBALANCE): WATER INTOXICATION

An extracellular water excess occurs when the amount of water is increased in proportion to the amount of solute in the water, causing the osmolality to fall below 275 mOsm/L. This imbalance is uncommon but can occur when intake of water exceeds the ability of the kidneys to excrete it.

PATHOPHYSIOLOGY

Extracellular water excess rapidly becomes intracellular water excess as fluid moves into the cells to equalize the solute concentration, causing the cells to swell. NOTE: Brain cells are particularly sensitive to water increases, and the most common symptoms are changes in the patient's mental status.

Water excess rarely occurs under normal conditions since a falling osmolality usually suppresses the antidiuretic hormone (ADH), allowing the excess water to be excreted by the kidney. The box below lists risk factors and conditions that can lead to extracellular water excess. Table 1-4 presents common signs and symptoms.

RISK FACTORS AND CONDITIONS LEADING TO EXTRACELLULAR WATER EXCESS

Excessive water intake:
    Instillation of a hyposmolar solution into a body cavity from which it is absorbed through mucous membrane, such as multiple tap water enemas, or continuous irrigation of bladder after prostatic surgery
    Psychiatric disorder characterized by excessive drinking of water or other hyposmolar fluids
    Excessive administration of hyposmolar fluids
Excessive water retention:
    Increase in antidiuretic hormone (ADH) in response to stress, drugs, anesthesia, inflammatory conditions, or tumors of brain or other organs
    Renal disease

TABLE 1-4 Signs and symptoms of extracellular water excess

Body System	Signs and Symptoms
Skin	Warm, moist, good turgor
	Slight peripheral edema
Cardiovascular	Bounding pulse, widened pulse pressure
Central nervous	Lethargy, confusion, convulsions
Gastrointestinal	Anorexia, nausea, vomiting
Blood (values)	Decreased Na^+ and Hct, lower osmolality
Urine	Increased output and lower osmolality, decreased specific gravity
Other	Sudden weight gain

MEDICAL MANAGEMENT

Most patients respond well to simple water restriction. If severe symptoms are present, the patient may be treated with the infusion of hypertonic saline IV plus the administration of furosemide (Lasix) in addition to fluid restriction.

ISOTONIC VOLUME DEFICIT

An isotonic volume deficit occurs in conditions in which both extracellular water and electrolytes are lost from the body. Volume is decreased, but the osmolality remains in the normal range.

PATHOPHYSIOLOGY

An isotonic volume loss does not disturb serum osmolality, and the deficit is therefore restricted to the extracellular compartment. Severe losses can deplete the extracellular volume rapidly, leading to vascular collapse. The box on this page lists risk factors and conditions that can lead to isotonic volume deficit. Table 1-5 presents common signs and symptoms.

MEDICAL MANAGEMENT

Treatment consists of identifying and correcting the underlying cause of fluid loss and then replacing the fluids and electrolytes that have been lost with appropriate isotonic fluids or blood products. See Table 1-6 for the osmolality of common IV solutions.

ISOTONIC VOLUME EXCESS

An isotonic volume excess occurs in conditions in which both extracellular water and electrolytes are retained by the body. Volume is increased, but the osmolality remains in the normal range. Edema results when fluid accumulates in the interstitial space.

RISK FACTORS AND CONDITIONS LEADING TO ISOTONIC VOLUME DEFICIT

Hemorrhage
Profuse sweating
Excessive gastrointestinal losses resulting from
  Vomiting or diarrhea
  Ileostomy drainage or gastrointestinal fistulas
  Nasogastric suctioning
Systemic infection

TABLE 1-5 Signs and symptoms of isotonic volume deficit

Body System	Signs and Symptoms
Skin	Cool, poor turgor
Mouth	Dry mucous membranes
Cardiovascular	Postural hypotension (early sign): Blood pressure of client when sitting or standing is more than 10 mm Hg lower than when client is lying down
	Low blood pressure, tachycardia, decreased vein filling
Respiratory	Increased respiratory rate
Urine	Low output, increased specific gravity
Other	Weight loss, weakness, fatigue

TABLE 1-6 Osmolality of common IV solutions

Type of Solution	Osmolality	Use
5% Dextrose in water (D_5W)	Hyposmolar	Replacement of water losses
Normal saline (0.9% NaCl)	Isotonic	Hyponatremia (sodium deficit)
Lactated Ringers' solution	Isotonic	Extracellular volume deficit
5% Dextrose in 0.45% saline ($D_5\frac{1}{2}NS$)	Hyperosmolar	Maintenance of fluid levels

PATHOPHYSIOLOGY

Isotonic volume excess involves the extracellular fluid compartment. Osmotic fluid movement does not occur across cell walls, and the fluid accumulates in the vascular and interstitial spaces. Interstitial fluid overload (edema) results from hydrostatic and osmotic pressures that move fluid from the vascular compartment to the interstitial spaces. The box on the next page lists common causes of edema by their physiologic mechanism.

CAUSES OF EDEMA ACCORDING TO UNDERLYING PHYSIOLOGIC MECHANISM

FLUID PRESSURE

Increased capillary fluid pressure

Increased venous pressure

Vein obstruction
  Varicose veins
  Thrombophlebitis
  Pressure on veins from casts, tight bandages, or garters
Increased total volume with decreased cardiac output
  Congestive heart failure
Fluid overloading: too rapid infusion of IV fluids, especially in the elderly

Sodium and water retention, increased aldosterone from:

Decreased renal blood flow
  Congestive heart failure
  Renal failure
Increased production of aldosterone
  Cushing's syndrome
Aldosterone added to system
  Corticosteroid therapy
Inability to destroy aldosterone
  Cirrhosis of liver

ONCOTIC PRESSURE

Decreased capillary oncotic pressure

Loss of serum protein

Burns, draining wounds, fistulas
Hemorrhage
Nephrotic syndrome
Chronic diarrhea

Decreased intake of protein

Malnutrition
Kwashiorkor

Decreased production of albumin

Liver disease

Increased interstitial oncotic pressure

Increased capillary permeability to protein

Burns
Inflammatory reactions
  Trauma
  Infections
Allergic reactions (hives)

Blocked lymphatics: decreased removal of tissue fluid and protein

Malignant diseases
Surgical removal of lymph nodes
Elephantiasis

From Phipps, WJ, Long, BC, and Woods, NF: Medical-surgical nursing: concepts and clinical practice, ed 4, St Louis, 1990, Mosby–Year Book, Inc.

TABLE 1-7 Signs and symptoms of isotonic volume excess

Body System	Signs and Symptoms
Skin and superficial tissues	Edema, especially dependent edema; skin may be tight, smooth, and shiny, or cool, and pale
Cardiovascular	Neck vein engorgement (vein distention even in upright position)
Respiratory	Rales; dyspnea, frothy cough, and cyanosis indicate pulmonary edema, a medical emergency
Other	Weight gain is the best early sign of volume excess, since several liters of fluid may be retained without visible evidence of edema

Table 1-7 presents common signs and symptoms of isotonic volume excess.

MEDICAL MANAGEMENT

The treatment of isotonic volume excess depends on the underlying condition. The management of congestive heart failure, cirrhosis, renal failure, and other conditions that result in isotonic volume excess is dealt with in depth in other portions of the book.

NURSING MANAGEMENT OF PRIMARY FLUID IMBALANCES

Assessment

Factors to be assessed include the following:
  Risk factors as presented in tables
  Vital signs—orthostatic blood pressures
  Weight
  Skin turgor
  Urine output—fluid intake and output balance
  Urine specific gravity
  Edema
  Level of consciousness—changes in mental status

Nursing Diagnoses

Fluid volume deficit related to disturbances in intake or failure of regulatory mechanisms

Fluid volume excess related to excessive fluid intake or failure of regulatory mechanisms

Potential for injury related to altered mental status

Altered cerebral and peripheral tissue perfusion related to fluid loss

Potential impairment of skin integrity related to interstitial edema

Expected Outcomes

Patient will return to a normal hydration status as evidenced by the alleviation of symptoms and restoration of normal laboratory values.

Patient will not experience injury during the period of altered mental status.

Patient will maintain intact skin.

Nursing Interventions

Prevention and monitoring

Monitor IV fluid rates closely.

Monitor daily AM weights.

Monitor urine output, intake and output (I & O) balance, and urine specific gravity.

Assess vital signs, mental status, skin turgor, and mucous membranes.

Treatment

Administer drugs as prescribed by physician.

Give or restrict oral and IV fluids as prescribed by physician.

Comfort and safety

Provide frequent mouth care.

Provide skin care; turn and position patient frequently, particularly if edema is present; avoid immobility.

Elevate dependent body parts to promote venous return.

Use side rails; supervise ambulation.

Orient patient to surroundings and treatment.

Patient teaching to prevent recurrence

Discuss fluid needs during exercise and in hot weather.

Explain prescribed medications: diuretics.

Explain sodium restrictions in diet. Teach patients to read food ingredient labels carefully.

Evaluation

Electrolytes, intake and output, and serum osmolality are within normal ranges.

Patient maintains a stable weight.

Patient is free of accidental injury and skin breakdown.

Patient and family can describe medications and diet to be followed and can describe preventive measures to avoid recurrence of fluid imbalance.

RISK FACTORS AND CONDITIONS LEADING TO SODIUM DEFICIT

Sodium loss from gastrointestinal tract:
  Vomiting or diarrhea
  Gastrointestinal suction
  Gastrointestinal drainage: fistulas, biliary, ileostomy
Profuse perspiration:
  Fever
  Exercise
Excess diuretic effect
Shift of body fluids:
  Massive edema—ascites
  Burns
  Small bowel obstruction

ELECTROLYTE IMBALANCE

No single electrolyte can be out of balance without other electrolytes also being out of balance. Sodium, potassium, and calcium are all essential for the passage of nerve impulses. Whenever the balance of any of these electrolytes is disrupted, the imbalance is reflected in the nervous stimulation of muscles.

SODIUM IMBALANCE

Sodium is the primary extracellular cation and controls the osmotic pressure of the extracellular fluid compartment. Sodium is essential for neuromuscular functioning, for many intracellular chemical reactions, and for helping to maintain acid-base balance in the body. Sodium balance is largely controlled by aldosterone.

SODIUM DEFICIT (HYPONATREMIA)

Pathophysiology

A serum sodium level below 138 mEq/L can result from either a sodium loss or a water excess. As the sodium level in the extracellular fluid decreases, potassium moves out of the intracellular fluid, causing subsequent disturbances in potassium balance. Even if there is no excess of body water, the decreasing osmolality creates a condition similar to water excess; water moves into the cell by osmosis, leaving the extracellular compartment depleted. Both circulatory and cellular functioning are impaired. The box above lists risk factors and conditions that result in sodium deficit. Table 1-8 presents common signs and symptoms of both sodium deficit and sodium excess.

Medical Management

Lost sodium and water are replaced by the rapid administration of saline solution (0.9% NaCl) plus plasma expanders if the patient is in shock. Other electrolytes are

TABLE 1-8 Signs and symptoms of sodium imbalance

Body System	Signs of Sodium Deficit	Signs of Sodium Excess
Skin	Poor turgor; may be cool and clammy if shock is incipient	Flushed, warm; dry, sticky mucous membranes; rubbery skin turgor
Cardiovascular	Orthostatic hypotension (severe cases lead to circulatory collapse, shock)	Hypotension, tachycardia
Central nervous system	Headache, apathy (severe cases lead to confusion and coma)	Irritability
Gastrointestinal	Anorexia, nausea, cramps	Thirst
Muscular	Muscle weakness, fatigue	Muscle weakness

RISK FACTORS AND CONDITIONS LEADING TO SODIUM EXCESS

Excessive ingestion of sodium:
  Normal saline infusions
  Oral intake of salt tablets
Loss of body water without proportional sodium loss
Inability to excrete sodium properly:
  Renal failure
  Increased aldosterone production
  Congestive heart failure

RISK FACTORS AND CONDITIONS LEADING TO POTASSIUM DEFICIT

Decreased potassium intake:
  NPO
  Severe dieting
  Failure to adequately replace losses
Increased potassium loss:
  Gastrointestinal losses
  Vomiting or diarrhea
  Draining fistulas
  Potassium wasting diuretics (thiazide diuretics)
  Losses from cellular trauma, such as burns
Cellular shifts of potassium:
  Acidosis
  Alkalosis

replaced as need is established by blood values. Treatment is aimed at correcting the underlying cause. Salt or salty foods may be added to the diet.

SODIUM EXCESS (HYPERNATREMIA)

Pathophysiology
A serum sodium level greater than 145 mEq/L exists when there is an excess of sodium in relation to water in the extracellular fluid. Osmolality increases and water leaves the cells by osmosis to dilute the extracellular fluid, leaving the cells water-depleted and disrupting their function. The box above lists risk factors and conditions that result in sodium excess. Signs and symptoms were presented in Table 1-8.

Medical Management
A sodium excess is treated with the liberal administration of water alone if cardiac and renal function are adequate. The patient may be given D_5W intravenously or water by mouth. Diuretics may be used to facilitate sodium excretion.

POTASSIUM IMBALANCE

Potassium is the primary intracellular cation. It has a direct effect on muscle and nerve excitability, maintains intracellular osmotic pressure, and helps maintain acid-base balance. Potassium enters the cells during anabolism and glucose conversion to glycogen; potassium leaves the cell during cellular breakdown resulting from either trauma or catabolism. The body conserves potassium less effectively than it conserves sodium, excreting potassium through the kidneys even when the body needs it.

POTASSIUM DEFICIT (HYPOKALEMIA)

Pathophysiology
A serum potassium below 3.5 mEq/L alters the polarization of cells, causing them to be less excitable. This loss of excitability can be life threatening when it occurs in cardiac muscle. The box above lists risk factors and conditions that result in potassium deficit. Table 1-9 presents common signs and symptoms of both potassium deficit and potassium excess.

Medical Management
Medical management consists of prompt administration of potassium either orally or by IV infusion. Oral admin-

TABLE 1-9 Signs and symptoms of potassium excess or deficit

Body System	Signs of Potassium Deficit	Signs of Potassium Excess
Cardiovascular	Arrhythmias ECG changes (flattened T waves) Cardiac arrest	Arrhythmias ECG changes (elevated T waves) Fibrillation/arrest
Gastrointestinal	Anorexia, nausea, vomiting Paralytic ileus	Nausea, vomiting Diarrhea
Central nervous	Lethargy, diminished deep tendon reflexes Mental depression	Numbness and tingling Irritability
Muscular	Muscle weakness Flaccid paralysis, respiratory arrest	Muscle irritability and spasticity Muscle weakness (late) Flaccid paralysis

FOODS RICH IN POTASSIUM

FRUITS	VEGETABLES*	PROTEIN FOODS	BEVERAGES
Apricots	Asparagus	Beef	Cocoa
Bananas	Dried beans	Chicken	Cola drinks
Grapefruit	Broccoli	Liver	Dry instant tea and coffee
Melon	Cabbage	Pork	Milk
Honeydew	Carrots	Veal	
Canteloupe	Celery	Turkey	
Dried fruits	Mushrooms	Nuts	
Figs, dates, raisins	Dried peas	Peanut butter	
Oranges	Potatoes, white and sweet		
	Spinach		
	Squash		

*Most raw vegetables contain potassium, but it is frequently lost in cooking.

istration may be by foods rich in potassium (see box above), or by oral potassium preparations. Intravenous infusions of potassium ideally should not exceed 20 mEq per hour and should be extremely diluted (40 mEq/L) to control peripheral vein irritation.

POTASSIUM EXCESS (HYPERKALEMIA)

Pathophysiology

A serum potassium above 5.5 mEq/L rarely occurs in the presence of normal renal function. Excess potassium decreases the membrane potential of cells, causing them to become more excitable. Moderate excess causes nerve and muscle irritability, but severe hyperkalemia leads to weakness and flaccid paralysis. The box at the right lists risk factors and conditions that result in potassium excess. Signs and symptoms are presented in Table 1-9.

RISK FACTORS AND CONDITIONS LEADING TO POTASSIUM EXCESS

Decreased potassium loss
  Renal failure
  Adrenal insufficiency
  Potassium-sparing diuretics
Cellular shifts of potassium
  Trauma
  Metabolic acidosis
Excess potassium intake
  Dietary excess (in presence of renal insufficiency)
  Excessive IV administration

Medical Management

Medical management includes the following:

Administration of cation exchange resins (sodium polystyrene sulfonate; Kayexalate) orally or by enema to bind the potassium in exchange for other cations; administration of sorbitol enhances bowel motility to increase excretion of potassium

Administration of 10% glucose with insulin to stimulate the movement of potassium into the cell

Bed rest with no oral food or fluid

Administration of IV calcium to antagonize the effect of excess potassium on the cardiac muscle

Correction of underlying acidosis

CALCIUM IMBALANCE

Calcium is present in the blood in two forms: ionized and bound to plasma proteins. Only the ionized calcium is physiologically active. It functions to support blood clotting; smooth, skeletal, and cardiac muscle function; and nerve function. Both parathyroid hormone and vitamin D are necessary for normal absorption of calcium from the GI tract.

CALCIUM DEFICIT (HYPOCALCEMIA)

Pathophysiology

A serum calcium level below 4.5 mEq/L affects cell membrane chemistry. In hypocalcemia, depolarization takes place more easily, producing increased excitability of the nervous system and the skeletal, smooth, and cardiac muscles. It can lead to muscle spasms, tingling sensations, and even tetany if severe. The box on this page lists risk factors and conditions that result in calcium deficit. Table 1-10 presents common signs and symptoms of both calcium deficit and calcium excess.

RISK FACTORS AND CONDITIONS LEADING TO CALCIUM DEFICIT

Inadequate calcium intake
  Dietary deficiency
Excess loss of calcium
  Kidney disease
  Draining intestinal fistula
Decreased absorption from GI tract
  Insufficient vitamin D
  Insufficient parathyroid hormone
  Pancreatic or intestinal disease—malabsorption
Excess binding of ionized calcium
  Transfusion with citrated blood
  Alkalosis

Medical Management

Medical management includes administration of oral calcium salts and a high calcium diet. Slow administration of IV calcium gluconate may be ordered for severe deficits. Parathyroid hormone or vitamin D also may be administered if there are deficiencies in these substances.

CALCIUM EXCESS (HYPERCALCEMIA)

Pathophysiology

A serum calcium level above 5.8 mEq/L affects cell membrane chemistry by inhibiting depolarization and depressing the function of nerves and skeletal, smooth, and cardiac muscles. Any condition causing immobility results in calcium leaving the bone and concentrating in the extracellular fluid. Excess calcium passing through the kidneys can cause precipitation and stone formation, especially in the presence of urine alkalinity.

TABLE 1-10 Signs and symptoms of calcium imbalance

Body System	Signs of Calcium Deficit	Signs of Calcium Excess
Cardiovascular	Arrhythmias Cardiac arrest	Depressed activity Arrhythmias Cardiac arrest
Central nervous	Numbness, tingling, especially in fingertips, toes, and lips Twitching and convulsions in severe cases	Decreased deep tendon reflexes Lethargy, coma in severe cases
Muscular	Painful muscle spasm—tetany Positive Trousseau's and Chvostek's signs	Muscle fatigue and decreased tone
Gastrointestinal	Increased peristalsis—nausea, vomiting, diarrhea	Decreased gastrointestinal motility, anorexia, constipation
Skeletal	Osteoporosis and fractures	Bone pain Osteoporosis and fractures
Other	Abnormal calcium deposits in body tissue	Kidney stones Thirst, polyuria

RISK FACTORS AND CONDITIONS LEADING TO CALCIUM EXCESS

Calcium loss from bones
  Immobilization
  Carcinoma with bone metastasis
  Multiple myeloma
Excessive dietary intake
  High calcium diet, especially milk products
  Antacids containing calcium
Increased absorption or mobilization from bones
  Vitamin D therapy
  Increased parathyroid hormone
  Steroid therapy

The box above lists risk factors and conditions that result in calcium excess. Common signs and symptoms are presented in Table 1-10.

Medical Management

The only definitive treatment of calcium excess is the removal of the cause. Administration of IV saline (physiologic flushing) followed by a thiazide diuretic promotes calcium excretion with the sodium. Administration of inorganic phosphate, mithramycin (Mithracin), or glucocorticoids increases calcium excretion. Acidification of the urine through an acid ash diet and increased fluid intake (3 to 4 L) may be ordered to prevent formation of calcium stones by the kidney.

NURSING MANAGEMENT OF ELECTROLYTE IMBALANCES

Assessment

Factors to be assessed include the following:
  Risk factors as presented in tables
  Vital signs
    Orthostatic blood pressures
    ECG changes
  Weight changes
  Medication history and use
  Skin turgor and mucous membranes
  Urine
    Intake and output balance
    Specific gravity and pH
  Edema
  Level of consciousness—changes in mental status
  Subjective complaints
    Headache
    Muscle weakness
    Fatigue
    Anorexia, nausea
    Numbness or tingling
  Hyperreflexia
  Tetany—positive Chvostek's/Trousseau's signs
  Vomiting

Diarrhea
Dietary intake

Nursing Diagnoses

Fluid volume deficit related to disturbances in intake of electrolytes or failure of regulatory mechanisms
Fluid volume excess related to disturbances in intake of electrolytes or failure of regulatory mechanisms
Activity intolerance related to muscular weakness and fatigue
Pain related to neuromuscular and gastrointestinal symptoms
Potential for injury related to weakness and decreased mental status
Decreased cardiac output related to conduction disorders

Expected Outcomes

Patient will return to a normal fluid and electrolyte balance as evidenced by alleviation of symptoms and restoration of normal laboratory values.
Patient will not experience injury during periods of altered mental status.
Patient will have sufficient energy and muscular strength to complete normal activities of daily living.
Patient will experience relief of symptoms of thirst, nausea, and diarrhea.
Patient will maintain an intake of nutrients adequate to meet body's need.

Nursing Interventions

Record accurate intake and output.
  Evaluate dietary intake.
  Evaluate balance of intake and output.
Assess vital signs frequently: skin turgor, status of mucous membranes, and level of consciousness.
Monitor laboratory values.
Check daily AM weights.
Administer IV fluids and medications as prescribed.
Provide comfort and safety measures.
  Administer mouth and skin care frequently.
  Use side rails; supervise ambulation.
Adjust patient activity level to energy level and tolerance.
Assist with activities of daily living as required.
Provide frequent position changes and skin massage.
Adjust meal content and schedule to include patient preferences.
Patient and family teaching (to prevent recurrence):
  Describe correct use of and compliance with medications.
  Explain diet restrictions or supplements if ordered—Na^+, K^+, Ca^{++}.
  Explain signs and symptoms indicative of imbalance.
  Describe measures to prevent imbalances during gastrointestinal illnesses.

Evaluation

Electrolytes, intake and output, serum osmolality, urine specific gravity, and vital signs are within normal ranges.

Patient maintains a stable weight.

Patient is able to complete self-care and participate in usual activities of daily living.

Patient eats and digests a normal diet without occurrence of gastrointestinal symptoms.

Patient does not experience injury.

Patient and family can describe medications and diet to be followed at home and can describe preventive measures to avoid recurrence of electrolyte imbalance, if appropriate.

ACID-BASE IMBALANCES

The regulation of body pH is vital because even slight deviations from the normal range will cause significant changes in the rate of cellular chemical reactions. The following values indicate normal acid-base parameters:

pH   7.35-7.45
P_{CO_2} 35-43 mm Hg
HCO_3 21-28 mEq/L

The body's three major mechanisms for controlling acid-base balance are chemical buffers in the cells and extracellular fluid, respiratory retention or excretion of CO_2, and kidney regulation of the quantity of sodium bicarbonate. The chemical buffers work continuously and instantaneously. Respiratory adjustments require minutes to hours, and kidney adjustments require hours to days. Together these mechanisms maintain the normal ratio of 20 parts of bicarbonate to 1 part of carbonic acid. In a disease state in which normal acid-base balance is upset, the lungs and kidneys attempt to compensate for the imbalance by initiating appropriate changes in blood CO_2 and bicarbonate levels.

PATHOPHYSIOLOGY

Table 1-11 discusses the four major acid-base imbalances with their causative features, signs and symptoms, and method of compensation.

TABLE 1-11 Common acid-base imbalances: causes, signs and symptoms, and mechanisms of compensation

Imbalance	Physiologic Causes	Signs and Symptoms	Mechanism of Compensation
Respiratory acidosis pH < 7.35 P_{CO_2} > 45 HCO_3 normal	Hypoventilation (lungs not removing sufficient amounts of CO_2), caused by: Respiratory infections CNS depression Paralysis of respiratory muscles Poor thoracic excursion—atelectasis Abdominal distention	Hypoventilation Decreased chest excursion Cyanosis Drowsiness Tachycardia	Kidneys retain and manufacture more bicarbonate. Hydrogen ions excreted in urine. Compensated values: pH 7.40 P_{CO_2} > 45 HCO_3 > 28

Respiratory alkalosis
pH > 7.45
P_{CO_2} < 35
HCO_3 normal
	Hyperventilation (lungs removing too much CO_2), caused by:
	Emotions—fear, hysteria
	Fever
	O_2 lack
	CNS stimulation
		Hyperventilation
		  Dizziness
		  Light-headedness
		  Tingling face and hands
		Convulsions
			Kidneys excrete large amounts of bicarbonate.
			Compensated values:
			pH 7.40
			P_{CO_2} < 35
			HCO_3 < 21

Metabolic acidosis pH < 7.35 P_{CO_2} normal HCO_3 < 21	Bicarbonate loss Diarrhea Fistula drainage Acid gain or retention, caused by: Diabetic ketoacidosis Lactic acidosis Renal failure K^+ excess Salicylate poisoning	Headache, dizziness Kussmaul respiration Fruity breath odor Disorientation, coma Weakness High serum K^+	Lungs hyperventilate to excrete CO_2 and reduce serum carbonic acid levels. Compensated values: pH 7.40 P_{CO_2} < 35 HCO_3 < 21
Metabolic alkalosis pH > 7.45 P_{CO_2} normal HCO_3 > 28	Acid loss, caused by: Vomiting/GI suction Potassium depletion Steroids Bicarbonate retention, caused by: Excessive intake of baking soda Transfusion of citrated blood	Hypoventilation Numbness and tingling in extremities Bradycardia Confusion	Lungs hypoventilate to retain CO_2 and increase serum carbonic acid levels. Compensated values: pH 7.40 P_{CO_2} > 45 HCO_3 > 28

MEDICAL MANAGEMENT

Treatment depends on the specific imbalance:

Respiratory acidosis—improve alveolar exchange of O_2 and CO_2 by deep breathing, chest physical therapy, and bronchodilators.

Respiratory alkalosis—treat underlying condition; reduce respiratory rate; counter tetany with calcium gluconate.

Metabolic acidosis—treat underlying cause; if acidosis is severe, cautiously administer sodium bicarbonate IV; monitor fluid and potassium levels as condition resolves.

Metabolic alkalosis—treat underlying condition; administer sodium, potassium, and ammonium chloride either orally or IV as indicated by laboratory values.

NURSING MANAGEMENT

Assessment

Both subjective and objective factors should be assessed.

Subjective complaints

Numbness and tingling in face and extremities

Dizziness, light-headedness

Headache, weakness

Objective signs

Rate and depth of respiration

Vital signs

Changes in mental status

Nursing Diagnoses

Impaired gas exchange related to hyperventilation or hypoventilation

Pain related to neuromuscular symptoms

Expected Outcomes

Patient will return to an effective respiratory pattern.

Patient will experience relief of symptoms such as weakness, dizziness, numbness, and tingling.

Patient will return to a normal acid-base balance as evidenced by relief of symptoms and normal blood gas values.

Nursing Interventions

Have the patient turn, cough, and deep breathe every hour.

Clear airway—suction if needed, position in semi-Fowler's position.

Administer O_2 and medications as ordered.

Calm patient.

Use rebreather if needed to slow hyperventilation.

Monitor patient's vital signs and intake and output carefully.

Monitor blood gases and electrolyte values.

Assess effectiveness of prescribed interventions.

Evaluation

Patient is breathing room air with a respiratory rate of 12 to 18 breaths per minute. Lungs are clear to auscultation.

Patient's blood gases, electrolytes, and vital signs are within the normal range.

Patient is able to resume activity level and self-care activities.

BIBLIOGRAPHY

Ahrens T and Rutherford K: The new pulmonary math, Am J Nurs **87**:106-110, 1987.

Barta M: Correcting electrolyte imbalances, RN **50**(2):30-34, 1987.

Chenevy B: Overview of fluids and electrolytes, Nurs Clin North Am **22**:749-760, 1987.

Folk-Lighty M: Solving the puzzles of patients fluid imbalance, Nursing 84 **14**(2):34-41, 1984.

Goldberger E: A primer of water, electrolytes and acid base syndromes, ed 7, Philadelphia, 1986, Lea & Febiger.

Kee J: Fluids and electrolytes with clinical applications: a programmed approach, ed 4, New York, 1986, John Wiley & Sons, Inc.

Lancaster L: Renal and endocrine regulation of water and electrolyte balance, Nurs Clin North Am **22**:761-772, 1987.

Mathewson M: Intravenous therapy, Crit Care Nurse **9**(2):21-23, 26-28, 30-36, 1989.

Mathewson M and Mathewson R: Establishing acid base balance. Crit Care Nurse **7**(5):77-86, 1987.

Methany NM: Fluid and electrolyte balance: nursing considerations, ed 3, Philadelphia, 1987, JB Lippincott.

CHAPTER 2

Cancer

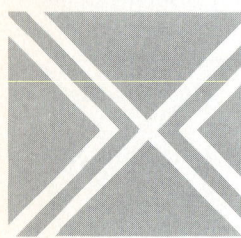

Few diseases evoke greater feelings of anxiety and fear than cancer. Its physiologic and psychologic impact on patients and families is profound. Despite significant progress in cancer care and control, the diagnosis still signifies pain, mutilation, and death to many. Nurses are products of their society and may share many of its negative attitudes toward the disease. Cancer nursing challenges every aspect of a nurse's creativity, skill, and commitment.

Despite significant advances in treatment, cancer remains the second leading cause of death in the United States. It is estimated that one out of every four Americans develops some form of cancer during their lifetime. Cancer occurs in all age groups, both sexes, and all races, although the incidence statistics vary among the groups. The incidence of all forms of cancer increases with age, and 52% of all cancers occur in persons over age 65. Figure 2-1 shows the incidence by involved organ for both cancer and cancer deaths for males and females. Current research indicates that the development of cancer is multicausal, involving an interplay of heredity; environment; exposure to viruses, pollutants, or radiation; and the individual's own immune competency. The box below lists the major risk or predisposing factors for the development of cancer. Early detection through mass cancer-screening programs plays an integral role in the successful treatment of the disease.

EARLY DETECTION AND PREVENTION

Primary prevention through the identification and control of carcinogens in the environment coupled with early detection of cancers offers the best approach to the reduction of the incidence of cancer deaths.

Table 2-1 lists the American Cancer Society's guidelines for cancer-related checkups. Educating the public about the seven warning signs of cancer (*CAUTION*) is essential:

C hange in usual bowel or bladder function
A sore that does not heal
U nusual bleeding or discharge
T hickening or lump in the breast or elsewhere
I ndigestion or dysphagia
O bvious change in a wart or mole
N agging cough or hoarseness

Education programs for cancer prevention focus on the major strategies of eliminating tobacco use, reducing alcohol consumption, modifying the diet to increase fiber and reduce fat intake, and reducing sun exposure. The identification of specific occupational risks is another major focus.

PREDISPOSING OR RISK FACTORS

LIFESTYLE FACTORS	ENVIRONMENTAL FACTORS	GENETIC FACTORS
Diet	Air and water pollution	Racial and sexual factors
Use of tobacco	Chemical pollutants	Immunologic deficiency
Excessive alcohol use	Ionizing radiation	Family history
Excessive sun exposure	Cultural and geographic factors	
Physiologic and psychologic stress and coping patterns	Use of exogenous hormones	
Occupational exposure to carcinogens		

CANCER INCIDENCE BY SITE AND SEX†

	Male		Female	
SKIN	2%		2%	SKIN
ORAL	4%		2%	ORAL
			28%	BREAST
LUNG	20%		11%	LUNG
COLON & RECTUM	14%		15%	COLON & RECTUM
PANCREAS	3%		3%	PANCREAS
			4%	OVARY
PROSTATE	21%		9%	UTERUS
URINARY	10%		4%	URINARY
LEUKEMIA & LYMPHOMAS	8%		7%	LEUKEMIA & LYMPHOMAS
ALL OTHER	18%		15%	ALL OTHER

CANCER DEATHS BY SITE AND SEX

	Male		Female	
SKIN	2%		1%	SKIN
ORAL	3%		1%	ORAL
			18%	BREAST
LUNG	35%		21%	LUNG
COLON & RECTUM	11%		13%	COLON & RECTUM
PANCREAS	4%		5%	PANCREAS
			5%	OVARY
PROSTATE	11%		4%	UTERUS
URINARY	4%		3%	URINARY
LEUKEMIA & LYMPHOMAS	9%		9%	LEUKEMIA & LYMPHOMAS
ALL OTHER	20%		20%	ALL OTHER

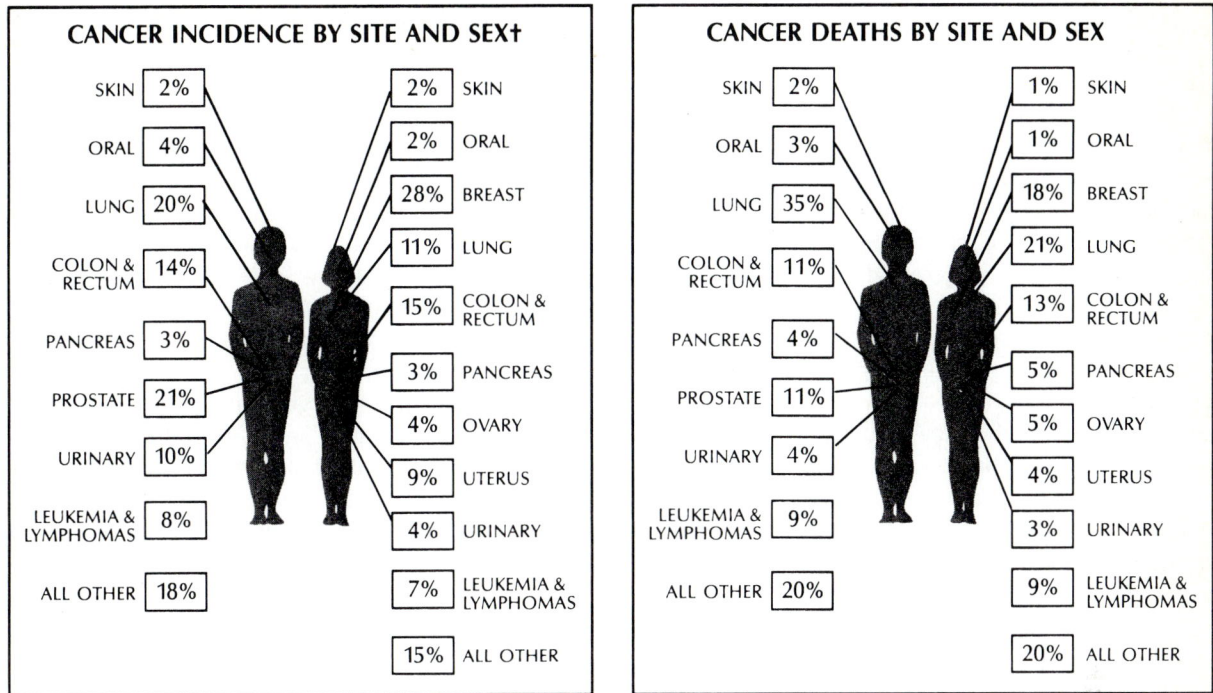

†Excluding non-melanoma skin cancer and carcinoma in situ.

FIGURE 2-1 Comparison of cancer incidence and deaths by site and sex. (From American Cancer Society: 1988 Cancer facts and figures, New York, 1988, The Society.)

TABLE 2-1 Guidelines for cancer-related checkups (American Cancer Society Guidelines)

Test or Examination	Sex	Age (yr)	Testing Intervals
Papanicolaou test (Pap test)	Female	Over 20; under 20 if sexually active	q 3 yr after two initial negative tests 1 yr apart
Pelvic examination	Female	20-40 Over 40 or at menopause	q 3 yr Yearly
Endometrial tissue sample	Female	At menopause if high risk	High risk: history of infertility, obesity, failure of ovulation, abnormal uterine bleeding, estrogen therapy
Breast self-examination	Female	Over 20	Monthly
Breast physical examination	Female	20-40 Over 40	q 3 yr Yearly
Mammogram	Female	35-40 Over 50	One baseline mammogram Yearly
Stool guaiac slide test	Male and female	Over 50	Yearly
Digital rectal examination	Male and female	Over 40	Yearly
Sigmoidoscopic examination or colonoscopy	Male and female	Over 50	q 3-5 yr after two initial negative examinations 1 yr apart

From Phipps WJ, Long BC, and Woods NF: Medical-surgical nursing: concepts and clinical practice, ed 4, St Louis, 1990, Mosby–Year Book, Inc.

PATHOPHYSIOLOGY OF CANCER

Cancer cells differ from normal cells in a variety of ways. The underlying process is believed to involve a disturbance in the regulatory functions of cell DNA. Characteristics of cancer cells include the following:

Anaplasia—succeeding generations of cells increasingly lose their similarity to the parent tissue

Uncontrolled growth pattern—diminished or absent resting phase of the cell cycle

Metastasis—ability to spread via blood or lymph system or directly extend into new locations and begin new growth

Larger and irregularly shaped nuclei

Disorderly growth—tumors are not encapsulated and may be necrotic at core because of poor vascular supply

Cancers produce symptoms in patients when they cause the following:

Obstruction of function

Pressure on surrounding tissue

Infiltration and destruction of surrounding tissue

Hemorrhage

Infection and ulceration

Pain

Cachexia syndrome—anorexia, weight loss, tissue wasting, hypermetabolism

TUMOR CLASSIFICATION SYSTEM

The extent of disease in each individual cancer patient is classifiable by the TNM (Tumor, Node, Metastases) quantification system shown in the box below. This

---

TNM STAGING CLASSIFICATION SYSTEM

TUMOR

TO	No evidence of primary tumor
TIS	Carcinoma in situ
T1, T2, T3, T4	Ascending degrees of tumor size and involvement

NODES

NO	No regional nodes demonstrably abnormal
N1a, N2a	Demonstrable regional lymph nodes; metastasis not suspected
N1b, N2b, N3	Demonstrable regional lymph nodes; metastasis suspected
Nx	Regional nodes cannot be assessed clinically

METASTASIS

MO	No evidence of distant metastasis
M1, M2, M3	Ascending degrees of metastatic involvement of host including distant nodes

From Phipps WJ, Long BC, and Woods NF: Medical-surgical nursing: concepts and clinical practice, ed 4, St Louis, 1990, Mosby–Year Book, Inc.

---

classification system is used to provide a common basis for describing the extent of illness, to develop treatment protocols, and to identify prognosis.

MEDICAL MANAGEMENT OF CANCER

Research concerning the most appropriate and effective medical management for cancer is ongoing but revolves around four major forms of intervention. These therapies are usually employed in combination to reduce the associated toxic effects and increase the chances of destroying the malignant cells.

Surgery is the oldest and still most common form of treatment. Surgery may be used for diagnosis and staging, palliation, pain control, and reconstruction. Its most common use, however, is in the attempt to cure through the removal of all cancerous tissue before it metasta-

---

PRINCIPLES OF RADIATION THERAPY AND PROTECTION OF STAFF

- Radiation applied externally can cause injury only during the time the treatment is being administered. NOTE: Patient is never radioactive.
- Radiation with alpha or beta rays applied internally creates no hazard to staff, since these rays cannot pass through the patient's skin. Substances emitting gamma rays cause the patient to transmit gamma radiation.
- Each radiation substance has its own half-life: the period of time in which half its radioactivity is dissipated and the dangers of radiation are reduced.

To protect staff from the effects of radiation, the following factors should be considered:

Amount of exposure to radiation sources

Radiation doses are cumulative. Limit interactions with patients with internal radiation therapy to 15 minutes per visit; group activities to maximize use of time.

Each nurse must wear his or her own film badge when in contact with source to monitor cumulative exposure levels.

Strength of radiation substance

Radiation safety officer can and should provide data about substance—its half-life, nature of rays, and ways it may be excreted from the body, for example, in urine, sweat, saliva, and so on.

Distance from radiation source

Rays are more numerous and concentrated at close range. Exposure risks decrease sharply with distance.

Type and degree of shielding in use

Lead-lined container and long-handled forceps must always be in room to contain source if dislodged.

Proper receptacles for linens and excreta should be used if needed (necessary only when source is not sealed).

Lead aprons should be used by nursing staff if indicated.

Risk to staff

Rotate nursing care among nurses who are at least risk from radiation hazard; pregnant nurses should not provide care. Follow restrictions on time at bedside carefully.

sizes. Cancer surgery attempts to ensure a margin of healthy tissue and frequently results in significant loss of function as well as body image disturbance.

Radiotherapy is the use of ionizing radiation to cause damage and destruction to cancerous cells during their replicative cycles. Radiotherapy can be delivered externally, by exposing the patient to rays generated by machines, or internally, by placing radioactive material within the tissues or a body cavity.

Radiotherapy may be given as primary or adjuvant

therapy after surgical removal of all identifiable cancer tissue. It works at the cellular level and is aimed at the control of micrometastases. All body tissue is affected to some degree, and rapidly dividing cells are affected first. Some degree of skin reaction and bone marrow suppression are expected from external therapy. In addition most patients experience some degree of radiation syndrome, which includes fatigue, headache, anorexia, nausea, and vomiting. Specific reactions unique to the tissue being treated may also occur. The box on p. 14

TABLE 2-2 Drugs used in cancer chemotherapy

Agent	Mechanism of Action	Major Toxic Manifestations
Alkylating Agents		
Chlorambucil (Leukeran) Melphalan (Alkeran) Cyclophosphamide (Cytoxan) Myleran (Busulfan) Triethylenethiophosphoramide (Thiotepa) Mechlorethamine (nitrogen mustard)	Interfere with DNA replication by attacking DNA synthesis throughout cell cycle (cell cycle nonspecific)	Bone marrow depression with leukopenia, thrombocytopenia, and bleeding; cyclophosphamide may cause alopecia and hemorrhagic cystitis
Antimetabolites		
Methotrexate (MTX) 6-Mercaptopurine (6-MP) 5-Fluorouracil (5-FU) Arabinosylcytosine (Cytosar, Ara-C) 6-Thioguanine (Thioguan)	Structural analogs of essential metabolites and therefore interfere with synthesis of these metabolites (cell cycle specific)	Bone marrow depression; oral and gastrointestinal ulceration
Antibiotics		
Doxorubicin (Adriamycin) Bleomycin (Blenoxane) Dactinomycin (Cosmegen) Daunorubicin (Cerubidine) Mithramycin (Mithracin) Mitomycin (Mutamycin)	Interfere with DNA or RNA synthesis, varying with the drug (cell cycle nonspecific)	Stomatitis, gastrointestinal disturbances, and bone marrow depression Doxorubicin and daunorubicin cause cardiac toxicity at cumulative doses over 500 mg/m^2 Bleomycin can cause alopecia and pulmonary fibrosis, but only minimal bone marrow depression
Plant Alkaloids		
Vinblastine (Velban)	Interfere with mitosis (cell cycle specific)	Alopecia, areflexia, bone marrow depression
Vincristine (Oncovin)		Neurotoxicity with ataxia and impaired fine motor skills, constipation and paralytic ileus
Steroid Hormones		
Androgens (Neo-Hombreol) Estrogens (DES) Progestins (Depoprovera) Adrenocorticosteroids (Prednisone)	Alter the host environment for cell growth (cell cycle nonspecific)	Specific for the actions of the hormone
Other		
L-Asparaginase	Inhibits protein synthesis	Fever and hypersensitivity
Cisplatin	Inhibits DNA, RNA, and protein synthesis	Renal damage
Procarbazine	Inhibits DNA, RNA, and protein synthesis	CNS depression reaction

Adapted from Porth C: Pathophysiology: concepts of altered health states, ed 2, Philadelphia, 1986, JB Lippincott Co.

TABLE 2-3 Immunotherapy for cancer

Specificity	Active	Passive
Specific	Inactivated tumor vaccines (autologous, allogenic) Human tumor hybrids	Monoclonal antibodies Human heterologous antiserum T lymphocytes Monoclonal lymphocytes Bone marrow transplants
Nonspecific	Chemical immunostimulants Biologic immunostimulants (such as BCG, *Corynebacterium parvum*) Cytokines (interferon, IL-2, tumor necrosis factor [TNF]) Chemotherapy	Lymphokine-activated killer cells (LAKC) Activated macrophages

From Phipps WJ, Long BC, and Woods NF: Medical-surgical nursing: concepts and clinical practice, ed 4, St Louis, 1990, Mosby–Year Book, Inc.

lists basic radiotherapy information and the principles of staff protection.

Cancer chemotherapy is based on the actions of certain drugs that create changes in the cell cycle phases as the cells replicate. They particularly affect rapidly dividing cells, both cancerous and noncancerous. Chemotherapy is used for both cure and palliation of symptoms. Drugs are frequently given in combination because this approach consistently demonstrates a therapeutic effect superior to single-agent treatment. Drugs are chosen on the basis of tumor size and rate of growth and may be administered orally, IV, arterially, intrathecally, and by regional perfusion. Table 2-2 lists the categories of chemotherapeutic drugs in common use and examples of each.

The role of the immune system in the development of cancer is being intensely studied. It is theorized that a natural immunity to cancer exists that normally destroys cancerous cells as fast as they develop. The development of clinical cancer may represent a failure of immune regulation, and immunotherapy attempts to stimulate the patient's own immune system to recognize cancer cells as "non-self" and destroy them. It includes approaches using nonspecific substances such as BCG and the antitumor effects of interferon or interleukin. Table 2-3 lists the three major types of immunotherapy being utilized.

NURSING MANAGEMENT OF THE PATIENT WITH CANCER

THE DIAGNOSTIC PERIOD

The diagnostic period is one of significant anxiety for patients and families. They are confronting the reality of the diagnosis, its impact on today and implications for the future, and concerns over the proposed plan of treatment and its effects.

Assessment

The following subjective factors should be assessed:
Knowledge of diagnosis—establish what physician has told patient
Response to diagnosis—anxiety, fear, anger
Coping skills of patient and family
Local/systemic effects of the tumor
General health state of patient
Family and social resources available to patient

Nursing Diagnoses

Pain related to local or systemic effects of tumor
Ineffective individual or family coping related to the diagnosis of cancer
Fear related to the diagnosis of cancer and the treatment protocol
Knowledge deficit related to the prognosis and treatment protocols

Expected Outcomes

Patient will experience decreased symptoms related to the local or systemic effects of tumor growth.
Patient and family will effectively cope with diagnosis.
Patient and family will be able to discuss advantages and disadvantages of various treatment options and participate actively in all treatment decisions.
Patient will feel supported during the period of uncertainty associated with diagnostic workup.
Patient will exhibit no overt signs of anxiety and will discuss areas of concern.

Nursing Interventions

Discuss patient and family's prior experiences with and attitudes toward the disease.
Explore with patient feelings and concerns about diagnostic tests and outcomes.
Avoid false reassurances and cliches that block honest communication.
Explain all tests and procedures thoroughly.
Include patient and family in all decisions about treatment options.
Refer patient and family to the American Cancer Society and other community agencies.
Provide symptomatic relief where feasible.

Evaluation

Patient and family understand diagnosis and treatment plan.

Patient and family experience no more than moderate anxiety.

Patient and family maintain effective coping patterns.

Patient expresses an increased level of comfort.

Patient receives psychosocial support from family, friends, and nursing staff.

CANCER SURGERY

The patient undergoing cancer surgery receives the same perioperative care provided to any surgical client. In addition, the nurse recognizes the radical and often mutilating nature of many cancer surgeries and the need for extensive psychosocial support.

Assessment

Assessment for cancer surgery should include the following:

Standard preoperative assessment, risk factors, patient's general health status

Patient's understanding of reason for surgery, nature of procedure, effects on body structure and function

Potential impact of surgery on patient's body image and role function

Nursing Diagnoses

There is a wide range of potential diagnoses depending on the specific procedure planned. Common diagnoses include the following:

Anticipatory grieving related to loss of body part or function

Body image disturbance related to effects of surgery

Spiritual distress related to dissemination of disease and prognosis

Knowledge deficit related to self-care protocols

Situational low self-esteem related to decreased self-care abilities

Expected Outcomes

Patient will be prepared for surgery physically and psychologically.

Patient will recover from surgery without physiologic complications.

Patient will appropriately grieve for physical loss.

Patient will successfully incorporate changes in body image and express feelings of self-worth.

Patient will express belief in meaning of life and begin to resolve feelings related to the prognosis.

Nursing Interventions

Provide standard postoperative nursing interventions to identify complications and promote healing.

Ensure adequate postoperative pain relief.

Provide teaching and reteaching as needed to keep patient informed about surgery and regimen of postsurgical care.

Teach patients skills and techniques needed to regain self-care ability.

Encourage patient to discuss feelings about surgical procedure and its effects on the body.

Assist patient and family to grieve over lost body part or function, or knowledge of widespread disease dissemination.

Refer patient to appropriate community support groups such as Reach to Recovery or Ostomy Club; describe the services of the American Cancer Society.

Evaluation

Patient recovers from surgery without complications and experiences only manageable pain.

Patient discusses surgical outcome and begins to display grief resolution.

Patient gradually resumes responsibility for self-care.

Patient faces the future with hope and optimism and speaks positively about self.

RADIOTHERAPY

Radiotherapy produces widespread symptoms that the nurse must be alert for. Interventions are based on the type of radiation used, the method of delivery (external or internal), and the tissue being treated.

Assessment

Factors to be assessed include:

General physical status of patient, especially area to be irradiated

Patient's understanding of nature and type of radiotherapy, its goals, and its expected side effects

Patient's prior experiences with, and misconceptions about, radiation therapy

Nursing Diagnoses

Common diagnoses for all forms of radiotherapy include the following:

Potential impaired skin integrity related to effects of radiation

Altered nutrition—less than body requirements, related to the anorexia, nausea, and vomiting of radiation syndrome

Activity intolerance related to the fatigue of radiation syndrome

Potential for infection related to immunosuppressive effects of radiation

Social isolation related to radiation precautions

Knowledge deficit related to radiation therapy and radiation precautions

Expected Outcomes

Patient will maintain an intact skin.

Patient will not develop infection or bleeding.

Patient in isolation will not experience social or sensory deprivation.

Patient will be knowledgeable about the effects of radiation and measures to deal with them.

Patient will ingest sufficient balanced nutrients to meet daily needs.

Patient will have sufficient energy to complete self-care activities.

Nursing Interventions: General

Teach patient about nature of radiotherapy and the general signs of early and late reactions.

Teach patient about how the treatment is given—the setting, equipment, and positioning used for therapy.

Encourage patient to space activities and take frequent rest periods.

Encourage patient to maintain usual self-care activities.

Nursing Interventions (external radiotherapy): Skin Care

Gently wash skin daily with tepid water and bland soap. *NURSING ALERT:* Do not remove markings.

Consult radiologist concerning skin care. Vaseline, A&D ointment, and corn starch are frequently employed. *NURSING ALERT:* Do not use cosmetics, lotions, or powders that may contain heavy metal base. Follow specific orders if skin reactions occur.

Teach patient to avoid tight or constricting clothing or friction.

Teach patient to avoid prolonged exposure to sun, wind, and extremes of temperature.

Nursing Interventions: Nutrition

Prepare patient for likelihood of anorexia and nausea.

Encourage small frequent meals throughout the day.

Explore use of high-protein, high-carbohydrate, low-fat meals. Sweet foods are frequently better tolerated.

Encourage patient to rest before and after meals.

Avoid use of "empty calorie" foods. Offer enriched supplements to meet nutritional needs.

Administer antiemetic medications as ordered prior to onset of nausea.

Assist patient to redistribute nutrients throughout the day to maximize nausea-free periods. Enrich breakfast nutrients if appropriate.

Encourage patient to avoid eating or drinking immediately before or after treatment.

Nursing Interventions: Infection and Injury

Monitor weekly blood tests.

Have patient avoid crowds and individuals with upper respiratory infections.

Monitor vital signs.

Observe bleeding precautions if patient is thrombocytopenic.

Encourage patient to follow scrupulous personal hygiene practices and increase the frequency of routine mouth care.

Interventions for Internal Radiotherapy (see box on p. 14 for methods of staff protection)

Teach patient about rationale for therapy, side effects, and reasons for required safety precautions.

Place patient in private room with signs that identify nature and extent of radiation hazard.

Restrict visitors to 15-minute visits per day.

Counter effects of isolation by frequent visits from doorway and encourage use of radio or television for stimulation.

Promote comfort measures.

Use Foley catheter and low-residue diet to protect against dislodgement of cervical implants.

Ensure that a lead container and long-handled forceps are present in the room at all times.

Reinforce the importance of maintaining bedrest and positioning restrictions as ordered.

Utilize the principles of distance, time, and shielding for all bedside care delivery.

Evaluation

Patient can state purpose of radiation therapy, nature of the treatment and side effects, and actions to be taken to manage side effects.

Patient has minimal discomfort from side effects—does not vomit; maintains normal bowel elimination.

Patient's skin remains intact without evidence of breakdown.

Patient remains afebrile and does not experience bleeding or injury.

Patient maintains a normal body weight and eats a diet that meets nutritional requirements.

Patient has sufficient energy to maintain self-care and participate in usual activities.

Patient maintains orientation to reality and experiences minimal depression from isolation.

CHEMOTHERAPY

The administration of chemotherapy usually produces a wide range of symptoms that may be quite severe. Specific responses depend upon the drugs used and the stage of treatment. Nurses who handle chemotherapeutic agents need to take appropriate precautions to protect themselves. They should observe the basic principles outlined in the box on p. 19.

Assessment

Factors to be assessed include the following:

Patient's understanding of the nature and goals of chemotherapy—drugs to be used, expected side effects and their management

PRECAUTIONS FOR HANDLING CHEMOTHERAPEUTIC AGENTS

1. Drugs should be prepared in strict laminar flow environments.
2. Surgical gloves and a long-sleeved, closed-front gown should be worn during preparation of drugs.
3. Wash skin areas thoroughly with soap and water in the event of skin contact with drugs.
4. Dispose of all needles and IV materials carefully in appropriately labeled containers.
5. Wash hands thoroughly before and after giving drugs.

General health and nutritional status of patient
Patency of patient's veins and IV lines

Nursing Diagnoses
Common diagnoses include the following:
Knowledge deficit related to chemotherapy and its effects
Pain related to stomatitis or vomiting
Altered nutrition—less than body requirements, related to anorexia, stomatitis, nausea, or vomiting
Potential impairment in skin integrity related to tissue sloughing
Body image disturbance related to alopecia
Potential for infection or injury related to immunosuppression
Alteration in oral mucous membranes related to cell destruction

Expected Outcomes
Patient will be knowledgeable about drugs to be used and the management of their expected side effects.
Patient will maintain intact mucous membranes.
Patient will maintain an adequate and nutritious oral intake.
Patient will maintain intact veins.
Patient will maintain social interactions and make positive references to self.
Patients will be free of infection and not develop bleeding.

Nursing Interventions: General
Teach patient names of drugs, expected side effects, and management of side effects.
Encourage patient to maintain self-care and usual activities, as tolerated.
Provide specific counseling about drug effects on fertility; include information on birth control and sperm banking as appropriate.
Remind patient of importance of close follow-up if treatment is given on an outpatient basis.

Nursing Interventions: Infection and Injury
Monitor daily or weekly blood counts. Be aware of expected nadir (low point).
Monitor vital signs and assess oral mucous membranes and lungs regularly for early signs of infection.
Teach patient signs of infection and thrombocytopenia.
Avoid use of Tylenol or aspirin products, which may mask the signs of infection.
Teach patient importance of scrupulous personal hygiene, for example, bathing and changing clothing regularly, performing mouth care and perineal care, and keeping fingernails short. Emphasize the importance of frequent careful handwashing.
Use creams and lotions to prevent drying and cracking of skin.
Instruct family and friends with colds or flu not to visit. Avoid all sources of infection.
Institute reverse isolation if prescribed. Follow scrupulous aseptic technique for all care.
Give no enemas or rectal medications; do not take rectal temperatures.
Institute bleeding precautions: give no intramuscular injections, inspect for bruises, test stool and urine for blood.
Administer packed red blood cells and platelets as ordered.

Nursing Interventions: Nutrition
Prepare patient for anorexia or nausea if expected with drugs.
Administer emetics as prescribed. *NURSING ALERT*: Administer drugs *before* anticipated nausea so oral forms may be used (usually 30 to 45 minutes before therapy).
Determine from patient best time for food and fluid intake in relation to treatment. Avoid food at time of treatment.
Avoid empty-calorie foods. Offer enriched supplements to meet nutritional needs if they can be tolerated.
Experiment with food groups useful during periods of nausea: dry bulky foods, sweet foods, clear liquids, soft bland foods. Avoid dairy products and red meats.
Keep environment clean and odor free.
Maintain fluid intake.
Teach relaxation and distraction techniques if appropriate.

Nursing Interventions: Mucous Membranes
Inspect mouth carefully for signs of irritation or ulceration at least twice daily.
Encourage frequent oral hygiene with soft toothbrush and mild mouth washes such as saline or dilute peroxide solutions. Use a water pick if platelets are low.
Stimulate the flow of saliva with gum and hard candies.

Assess frequently for *Candida* infection. Use nystatin tablets or suspension for prevention.

Use rinses and viscous lidocaine (Xylocaine) before meals for analgesia. Apply mineral oil or KY jelly to cracked lips.

Adjust diet toward bland, mechanically soft foods.

Nursing Interventions: Alopecia

Teach patient about hair loss—when it will occur and to what degree. NOTE: All body hair is affected. (Not all drugs cause hair loss.) *NURSING ALERT:* Reassure client that drug-induced hair loss is not permanent.

Plan with client in advance of hair loss for the acquisition and use of wigs, scarves, and cosmetics.

Avoid frequent shampooing and hair care.

Encourage patient to express feelings about hair loss.

Employ ice caps if prescribed and patient desires. NOTE: Ice caps are not employed for patients with leukemia or other blood-borne cancers because cancer cells are sequestered from effects of drugs.

Nursing Interventions: Vein Integrity

Monitor all infusions carefully. Ensure that IV is patent before beginning drug administration.

Know which drugs cause widespread tissue necrosis, for example, vincristine, nitrogen mustard, and doxorubicin. Monitor these infusions continuously.

If extravasation occurs, immediately discontinue infusion and apply ice to site.

Encourage patient to use and exercise arms between treatments if possible, but avoid injury.

Evaluation

Patient can state purpose of chemotherapy, drugs to be used, expected side effects and their management.

Patient has minimal discomfort from side effects—experiences minimal vomiting, maintains normal bowel elimination.

Patient's mucous membranes and veins are intact.

Patient is afebrile and does not experience bleeding, injury, or infection.

Patient maintains a stable body weight and eats sufficient nutrients to meet basic body needs.

Patient maintains normal social interactions and chooses satisfactory method to deal with alopecia.

PAIN

Pain is one of the most feared aspects of cancer. Contrary to popular belief, pain is rarely a problem in early stages of cancer but it is a significant challenge for one out of three persons with metastatic disease. Its presence requires vigorous management before it consumes the patient's entire life. (See Chapter 15 for additional discussion of pain management.)

Assessment

Factors to be assessed include the following:

Nature of pain experience—location, quantity, severity, duration, influencing factors

Patient's prior experience with pain and pain tolerance

Nursing Diagnosis

Pain or chronic pain related to local and systemic effects of cancer cell growth

Expected Outcomes

Patient will experience relief of pain.

Patient will achieve control of the pain experience and will continue to live as normal a life as possible.

Nursing Interventions

Administer narcotics and analgesics with a long duration of effect, promptly and as ordered.

Medications should be given routinely, in adequate doses around the clock.

Administer drugs orally if possible, or IV; avoid intramuscular route.

Start with larger doses to achieve initial control of the pain.

Psychological addiction is not a major concern.

Inadequate pain control increases anxiety and intensifies the pain experience.

Aspirin remains the most effective single medication for mild to moderate pain.

Explore use of oral morphine solutions, patient-controlled analgesia, or IV morphine drips for chronic severe pain.

Observe, record, and report the patient's responses to both the pain and the analgesia.

Augment analgesia with other measures, such as relaxation, distraction, and nursing comfort measures including massage, heat, or cold.

Prevent the side effects of high-dose narcotics, particularly constipation.

Tolerance, dependence, and respiratory depression are not major problems with oral delivery.

Evaluation

Patient experiences a decreased level of pain.

Patient is able to continue participating in activities of daily living.

SUPPORTIVE CARE FOR PATIENT AND FAMILY

The five-year survival rate for cancer is approximately 50%. Nursing intervention must shift its emphasis to assisting patients and families to live with the diagnosis of cancer. Cancer rehabilitation has become a major focus, emphasizing the highest level of physical and psychosocial well being.

Assessment

Factors to be assessed include the following:

Family interaction patterns

Support systems and resources available in the community

Family's and patient's knowledge about disease, its progression, and outcome

Nursing Diagnoses

Ineffective family coping related to diagnosis of cancer and potential of terminal illness

Alteration in family processes related to care for family member with cancer

Anticipatory or dysfunctional grieving related to death of family member in future

Expected Outcomes

Patient and family will be accurately informed about the progress and prognosis of patient's condition.

Patient and family will maintain supportive interaction.

Patient and family will resolve guilt feelings and begin disengagement when appropriate.

Patient and family will utilize resources and supports in community.

Nursing Interventions

Support and strengthen patient's and family's coping methods unless dysfunctional.

Involve patient and family in all decision making about care. Foster independence and support resilience.

Provide accurate information to patient concerning symptoms and prognosis. Cancer care is frequently chronic rather than terminal.

Encourage all efforts by patient to maintain independence in self-care.

Facilitate family participation in patient's care.

Encourage involvement with religious traditions if desired.

Encourage participation in programs designed to assist families to cope with cancer—refer to American Cancer Society.

Assist in planning alternatives to terminal hospitalization—hospice or home care—if family desires such help.

Provide and encourage time for patient and family to be alone together and talk about disease and impending death; encourage verbalization of feelings about death.

Assist family to establish appropriate goals and support hope.

Encourage patient to stay involved with the everyday routines of family life. Encourage enjoyment of the beauty of the moment.

Initiate contact with community agencies that may be of assistance to family.

Realize that patient and family will need extra support from nurses during periods when symptoms return or worsen.

Evaluation

Patient and family experience ongoing support from nursing staff.

Family has approached and is receiving support from community agencies.

Patient and family maintain normal activities and role relationships as long as symptoms permit.

Patient and family communicate openly about disease progress and incipient separation through death.

NURSING CARE PLAN

LARYNGECTOMY FOR CANCER OF THE LARYNX

Nursing Diagnoses	Expected Patient Outcomes	Nursing Interventions
Anxiety related to surgery and loss of ability to communicate	Patient does not exhibit signs of severe anxiety.	1. Maintain a calm, unhurried environment. 2. Assure patient that airway will be suctioned to facilitate breathing. 3. Provide simple explanations of activities and events. 4. Provide for some type of patient communication system. 5. Give family opportunities to share their concerns; provide them with information about patient's progress and how they can support patient. 6. Encourage self-care as soon as feasible. 7. Suggest visit by rehabilitated laryngectomee, if desirable. 8. Suggest patient and partner participate in special organization, such as Lost Chord Club, after hospital discharge.

Ineffective airway clearance related to copious postoperative secretions	Patient's airway is clear to auscultation.	1. Place patient in semi-Fowler's position.
		2. Monitor for noisy respirations, increased pulse and respiratory rate, and restlessness, indicating need for suctioning.
		3. Suction laryngectomy tube or stoma as needed (may be every 5 min initially).
		4. Provide tracheostomy care, if a tube is used.
		5. Provide air humidification.
		6. Encourage deep breathing and coughing.
		7. Minimize use of respiratory depressants (narcotics).
		8. Teach patient to protect stoma after discharge by:
		  a. Light covering (especially when shaving face)
		  b. Protection from water
		  c. Avoiding inhalation of powders, flour, or other substances in daily activities; avoiding smoky environments.

Pain related to tissue trauma and dry mouth	Patient experiences only manageable postoperative discomfort.	1. Provide mouth care while N/G tube is in place q 2–4 hr. 2. Give prescribed analgesics (aspirin, acetaminophen, or codeine preferred). 3. Teach patient to use hands to support the head and neck initially when changing positions. 4. Encourage ambulation when permitted.
Potential altered nutrition: less than body requirements, related to impaired swallowing after surgery	Patient maintains normal weight.	1. Give prescribed tube feedings during first week. 2. When N/G tube is removed, give fluids and stay with patient for initial meals until swallowing is tolerated. Assess for fistula development. 3. Encourage optimum food intake as tolerated. 4. Stop oral feedings if tracheal secretions show food particles. 5. Monitor weight two or three times/week. 6. Encourage frequent oral hygiene. Lack of oral stimulation dries the mouth.

NURSING CARE PLAN

LARYNGECTOMY FOR CANCER OF THE LARYNX—cont'd

Nursing Diagnoses	Expected Patient Outcomes	Nursing Interventions

Impaired verbal communications related to removal of larynx	Patient successfully communicates with others; patient begins speech rehabilitation.	1. Assist patient to communicate by hand signals or by writing during initial phase.
		2. Anticipate patient needs so requests are minimized. Answer call bell promptly.
		3. Support activities prescribed by speech therapist.
		4. For patient learning esophageal speech:
		  a. Encourage patient to practice burping
		  b. Monitor for gastric flatus or discomfort from swallowed air
		5. For patient with tracheal-esophageal prosthesis, teach patient:
		  a. How to remove, clean, and reinsert prosthesis
		  b. How to cover stoma when speaking
		  c. Avoidance of "sticky" foods that may clog prosthesis (such as cheese, pasta, beans)
		6. Discuss availability of mechanical devices for speech aid or for telephone use.

Knowledge deficit related to self-care needs	Patient understands self-care needs and can demonstrate appropriate stoma care.	1. Teach patient:
		  a. Nature of anatomical changes
		  b. Care of stoma, including self-suctioning
		  c. Methods to protect stoma from environment
		  d. Availability of community resources
		  e. Symptoms requiring medical follow-up
		  f. Activity or clothing adjustments needed for home care
		  g. Safety precautions associated with stoma.

BIBLIOGRAPHY

American Cancer Society: 1989 cancer facts and figures, New York, 1989, The Society.

Bender CM: Chemotherapy. In Ziegfeld CR, editor: Core curriculum for oncology nursing, Philadelphia, 1987, WB Saunders.

D'Agostino NS: Managing nutrition problems in advanced cancer, Am J Nurs **89**(1):50-56, 1989.

Derdiarian AK: Informational needs of newly diagnosed cancer patients, Nurs Res **35**:276-281, 1986.

Dudas S and Carlson CE: Cancer rehabilitation, Oncol Nurs Forum **15**:183-188, 1988.

Greenwald P and Sondik EJ: Cancer control objectives for the nation 1985-2000, Natl Cancer Inst Monogr No. 2:1, 1986.

Groenwald SL: Cancer nursing: principles and practices, Boston, 1987, Jones & Bartlett Publishers.

Gullo SM: Safe handling of antineoplastic drugs: translating the recommendations into practice, Oncol Nurs Forum **15**:596-602, 1988.

Hood LE: Interferon, Am J Nurs **87**:459-464, 1987.

Lewandowski W and Jones SL: The family with cancer: nursing interventions throughout the course of living with cancer, Cancer Nurs **11**:313-321, 1988.

Lewis F and Levita M: Understanding radiotherapy, Cancer Nurs **11**:174-185, 1988.

Sticklin LA: Interleukin-2 and killer T-cells, Am J Nurs **87**:468-469, 1987.

Strohl RA: The nursing role in radiation oncology: symptom management of acute and chronic reactions, Oncol Nurs Forum **15**:429-434, 1988.

Whipple B: Methods of pain control: review of research and literature, Image **19**:142-146, 1987.

CHAPTER 3

Disorders of the Musculoskeletal System

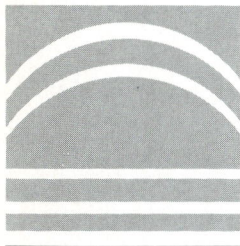

Disorders and injuries of the musculoskeletal system range from those that cause the client only minor discomfort and inconvenience to those that are life threatening. Included here are musculoskeletal disorders that commonly require hospitalization.

Regardless of the precipitating factors, patients with musculoskeletal disorders need to be assessed before care for them can be effectively planned. Areas to be assessed include the following:

Subjective factors
  Patient's current health status
  History of present illness or injury
  Pain assessment—nature, location, duration, and severity
  Impact of illness or injury on activities of daily living
  Presence and degree of weakness
  Diet and activity patterns
Objective factors
  Presence of obvious deformities
  Posture, gait, and balance
  Joint range of motion
  Muscle strength
  Peripheral pulses
  Use of assistive devices

Figure 3-1 shows the major anatomical structures of the musculoskeletal system. The following are common terms used in describing musculoskeletal function.

adduction Movement toward the midline of the body.
abduction Movement away from the midline of the body.
flexion Joint movement that decreases the angle between the two bones.
extension Joint movement that widens the angle between the two bones.
internal rotation Movement along the longitudinal axis in the direction of the midline of the body.
external rotation Movement along the longitudinal axis away from the midline of the body.

FRACTURES

Fractures represent one of the most common problems of the musculoskeletal system. A fracture is an injury to a bone, usually as a result of trauma, in which the continuity of the bone is interrupted. A number of classifications are used to describe fractures, and some of these are included in Table 3-1.

PATHOPHYSIOLOGY

Any force significant enough to cause a bone fracture may also injure the surrounding muscles, nerves, ligaments, tendons, blood vessels, and soft tissues. The immobilization necessary for bone healing may produce additional problems.

Bone healing occurs by a process known as callus, or new bone, formation. This is a multistage process that begins with hematoma formation at the fractured bone ends. Gradually this hematoma transforms into a fibrous network with calcium deposits, new bone formation, and destruction of dead bone. Optimal bone healing may be impeded by poor approximation of the fracture fragments, excessive edema at the site, infection, or necrosis of the bone.

Bone fractures may be complicated by fat emboli created by the release of fat molecules from the bone marrow or by the development of compartment syndrome as a result of the accumulation of blood and tissue fluid within the fascia compartments of the muscles of the extremities. Osteomyelitis may also occur if infection develops in the bone marrow spaces.

MEDICAL MANAGEMENT

The cornerstone of medical treatment of fractures is the realignment of the bony fragments of the fracture plus immobilization to allow healing to occur. Depending on

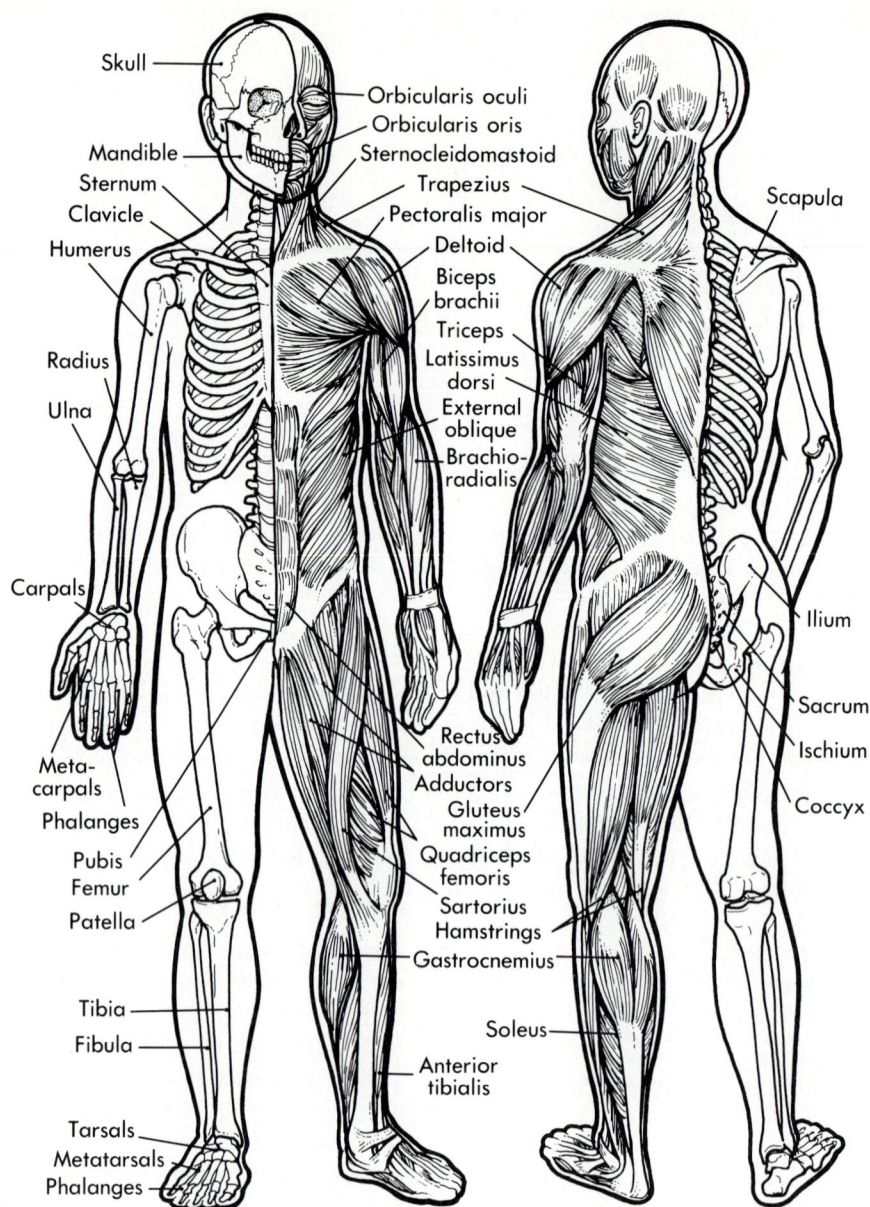

FIGURE 3-1 Musculoskeletal system.

the severity and the location of the fracture, medical management may involve reduction and realignment with either a cast or traction.

Reduction and fixation may be either external or internal. External fixation (closed reduction) involves manual realignment of the fractured bone parts, which is verified by x-ray. Internal fixation (open reduction) employs direct operative visualization and realignment of the bone parts. It frequently involves the use of pins, plates, screws, wires, or prostheses, as well as surgical debridement of the wound.

Traction involves the application of a continuous pull on a bone and surrounding tissue to reduce and immobilize the fracture, overcome muscle spasm, and correct deformities. There are numerous forms of traction. Most fit into one of the following categories:

skin traction Traction is applied to the skin through moleskin or adhesive, and the traction weight is applied indirectly to the bone through the skin (examples: Buck's, Russell, pelvic).

skeletal traction Traction is applied directly to the bone through the insertion of wires or pins usually positioned distally to the fracture site (examples: overhead arm, balanced suspension).

TABLE 3-1 Types of fractures

Type	Description
Complete	Bone is completely separated, producing two fragments.
Incomplete	There is a partial break in the bone without separation.
Simple or closed	Bone is broken; skin is intact.
Compound or open	Fracture parts extend through the skin.
Fracture without displacement	Bone is broken; bone fragments are in alignment in normal position.
Fracture with displacement	Bone fragments have separated at the point of fracture.
Comminuted	Bone has broken into several fragments.
Impacted (telescoped)	One bone fragment is forcibly driven into another.
Greenstick	Fracture is limited to splintering of one side of the bone (occurs most often in children with soft bones).
Transverse	Break is across the bone.
Oblique	Line of fracture is at an oblique angle to the bone shaft.
Spiral	Line of fracture encircles the bone.

From Long BC and Phipps WJ: Essentials of medical-surgical nursing: a nursing process approach, ed 2, St Louis, 1989, The CV Mosby Co.

running traction Direct pull is applied without support of the part (examples: Buck's, cervical).

balanced traction Direct pull on the part is applied with the extremity supported in a splint and held in place with balanced counterweights (examples: Thomas splint with Pearson attachment).

NURSING MANAGEMENT

Assessment

Subjective

History of trauma

Health history for conditions that may influence healing and treatment

Degree of pain, weakness

Usual diet and activity patterns

Objective

Loss of function, obvious deformity

Swelling and discoloration

Presence of bleeding or tissue damage

Baseline vital signs, neurocirculatory data

Crepitus (grating sound) with movement

Nursing Diagnoses

Nursing diagnoses are variable and are based on the location and extent of the injury as well as the type of treatment. Commonly encountered diagnoses include the following:

Pain related to bone displacement and muscle spasm

Impaired physical mobility related to presence of cast or traction

Actual or potential impairment of skin integrity related to trauma, cast irritation, skeletal traction, or immobility

Potential for infection related to bone or soft tissue injury or insertion of skeletal pins

Altered peripheral tissue perfusion related to edema and cast constriction

Constipation related to immobility

Altered nutrition: more than body requirements, related to immobility and decreased energy expenditure

Feeding, bathing/hygiene, dressing/grooming, or toileting self-care deficit related to presence of casts or traction

Knowledge deficit related to the correct use of ambulatory assistive devices

Expected Outcomes

Patient will experience minimal discomfort from fracture once reduction and realignment have been completed.

Patient will continue maximal activity level permitted by treatment.

Patient's skin will remain intact; tissue injuries will heal without infection or complications.

Patient will maintain adequate circulation and nerve conduction to areas distal to cast or traction setup.

Patient will pass soft stool daily or at usual frequency.

Patient will maintain desired body weight.

Patient will participate in self-care to the extent allowed by injury, cast, or traction.

Patient will learn the correct use of canes, crutches, walkers or other self-help devices.

Patient's fracture and other injuries will heal without the development of infection.

Nursing Interventions: Care of Casts

Cast materials include plaster of Paris, fiberglass, and plastic. All come in rolls and can be applied in a manner similar to the use of an Ace bandage.

Plaster casts are heavy, dry slowly, and will lose strength and integrity when wet. They are relatively inexpensive.

Fiberglass and plastic casts are light in weight, dry quickly, and can be immersed in water and redried.

They are more expensive and have the potential to macerate underlying skin.

Nursing Interventions: Immediate

Position patient on firm mattress with overbed trapeze.

Support fresh cast on pillows until dry. Place absorbent material beneath cast until dry.

Use flat of hand to move cast if necessary—do not embed fingers. Support at normal joint positions.

Allow free air circulation for drying; do not use heat lamps or hot hair dryers. Drying plaster casts generate heat.

Change patient's position frequently.

Institute neurocirculatory checks hourly—observe color, temperature, swelling, circulation, capillary refill, sensation, movement, pain. See Table 3-2 for detailed signs and symptoms of neurocirculatory impairment.

Medicate as prescribed. NOTE: Pain should decrease after realignment and resolution of tissue damage.

Assess bleeding through cast and monitor systemic signs.

TABLE 3-2 Signs and symptoms of neurocirculatory impairment

Observation	Interpretation
Tissue color white	Decreased arterial blood supply
Tissue color blue	Venous stasis and poorly oxygenated tissue
Color slow to return to nail bed after application of moderate pressure	Decreased arterial blood supply
Edema	Fluid accumulating in tissues; poor venous return
Tissue cold or cool to touch	Decreased arterial blood supply
Patient unable to move parts distal to cast or external fixation device	Pressure on nerves innervating parts distal to cast or underlying external fixation device
Patient complaint of heightened or decreased sensation or paresthesia in part underlying or distal to cast or external fixation device	Pressure on nerves innervating parts underlying or distal to cast or underlying external fixation device
Patient complaint of extreme pain unrelieved by elevation, analgesic, or repositioning	Pressure on nerves in parts underlying or distal to cast or external fixation device

Note: Compare uninvolved limb to determine extent of deviation from normal.
From Phipps WJ, Long BC, and Woods NF: Medical-surgical nursing: concepts and clinical practice, ed. 4, St Louis, 1990, Mosby–Year Book, Inc.

Apply ice pack to reduce swelling.
Pad or smooth all rough cast edges.

Nursing Interventions: Ongoing

Maintain neurocirculatory checks each shift.

Do not tightly cover cast with any substance (cloth, paint, varnish). Skin breathes through porous plaster.

Clean cast application debris from skin and petal cast margins with stockinette to prevent skin irritation.

Protect casts exposed to body excretions with waterproof material around perineal area. Remove soiling with scouring powder on a damp cloth.

Provide regular skin care to skin around cast and that affected by decreased mobility.

Note any odor that may indicate necrotic tissue or infection.

Nursing Interventions: Patient Teaching

Teach patient who will recover at home the signs and symptoms indicative of complications.

Teach patient to transfer safely and move comfortably in bed.

Teach patient to keep cast clean and dry, and not put foreign objects into the cast for scratching.

Teach patient to report any symptoms of burning beneath the cast.

Teach patient to adjust fluids and diet to prevent constipation, urinary calculi, and weight gain.

Teach patient to be as active as possible. Perform isometric muscle toning exercises on a regular basis, and follow exercise program established by physical therapy.

Teach patient how to ambulate safely using crutches or walker. A cast shoe permits weight bearing without damage to the cast. The box below describes the common crutch walking gaits.

COMMON CRUTCH WALKING GAITS

WEIGHT BEARING

Two-point gait—crutch on one side moves forward simultaneously with opposite leg; same motion is repeated on other side.

Four-point gait—two-point gait is broken down and performed more slowly. Crutch is placed and then followed by the opposite leg. Both motions are then repeated with the opposite side.

Swing-through gait—both crutches are moved forward together, then both legs are swung past the crutches by lifting both lower limbs.

NON-WEIGHT BEARING

Three-point gait—both crutches are moved forward together. Then the body swings forward to that position by lifting placed leg. Second limb is held off the ground at all times.

Nursing Interventions: Patient in Traction

Inspect apparatus regularly to ensure proper application.

Do not release or alter traction weights. Traction weights and pulley ropes must hang freely.

Teach patient how to move safely within the limits of the traction apparatus.

Prevent complications related to immobility:

Increase fluids.

Decrease calories and increase roughage in diet; offer stool softeners.

Provide regular, thorough skin care, and inspect all areas in contact with traction apparatus; use sheepskin or alternating pressure matress.

Provide patient with age-appropriate diversions.

Promote circulation by use of range of motion and isometric exercises as permissible.

Encourage movement and turning as permitted.

Teach patient to cough and deep breathe.

Monitor patient for incidence of fat emboli: dyspnea, pallor, alteration in mental status, petechiae in neck and shoulder region.

Provide pin care as ordered:

Inspect pin insertion sites carefully every shift per routines.

Cleanse sites with saline, peroxide, or Betadine solutions if ordered.

Use antibiotic ointments and dry sterile dressings if ordered.

Evaluation

Patient states that pain is minimal or absent.

Patient maintains maximal allowable activity and participates in self-care activities.

Patient's skin is intact; pin sites and soft tissue injuries heal without infection.

Patient maintains adequate circulation and nerve conduction to areas treated by cast or traction.

Patient maintains a normal elimination pattern.

Patient's weight remains stable.

Patient can demonstrate correct use of cane, crutches, walker, or other self-help device.

Patient can state exercise, diet, or activity restriction to be followed at home and has made plans for follow-up care.

FRACTURED HIP

Fractures of the hip are one of the most common fractures seen in the hospital. They generally fall into two categories. Intracapsular fractures occur within the hip joint and capsule. Extracapsular fractures occur outside the capsule to an area below the lesser trochanter. Fractured hips occur most frequently in older adults and are more common in women because of the osteoporotic and degenerative changes of the postmenopausal period.

PATHOPHYSIOLOGY

The clinical signs of a hip fracture include pain, loss of movement, shortening of the leg on the affected side, abduction, and external rotation. Displaced fractures may cause serious disruption to the blood supply of the femoral head and can result in avascular necrosis.

MEDICAL MANAGEMENT

The treatment of choice is surgical repair, which allows for early mobilization of the patient. Either pinning with screws, nails, and pins or prosthetic replacement of the femoral head and neck is the usual approach. The site of the fracture, condition of the bone, and adequacy of the blood supply to the hip will dictate the approach and device used. Patient management for both treatments is similar. Surgery may be delayed while the patient's overall health status is evaluated. Buck's traction is frequently employed to relieve pain and muscle spasm prior to surgery.

NURSING MANAGEMENT

Assessment

Preoperative

Circumstances of injury

Current general health and mental status

Degree of pain and muscle spasm

Patient's ability to urinate

Traction setup

Postoperative

Routine surgical assessment: vital signs, respiratory, circulatory, wound

Position of operative leg and condition of dressing

Family support available for rehabilitation period

Orientation and alertness

Nursing Diagnoses

Diagnoses are variable depending on the general health status of patients and their responses to surgery. Diagnoses that are common with and specific to the fractured hip procedure include the following:

Preoperative

Pain related to displaced fracture

Impaired physical mobility related to fracture and traction

Altered pattern of urinary elimination related to swelling in pelvic region.

Altered thought processes related to shock and pain of trauma

Knowledge deficit related to surgical repair and postoperative interventions

Postoperative

Impaired physical mobility related to non–weight-bearing orders

Self-care deficit related to positioning and immobility

Knowledge deficit related to correct use of walker or crutches

Impaired home maintenance management related to inadequate support systems and limitations of injury.

Expected Outcomes: Preoperative

Patient will have pain and spasm decrease to a tolerable level.

Patient will adhere to activity restrictions before surgery.

Patient will establish an adequate pattern of urinary elimination.

Patient will remain oriented to circumstances and surroundings.

Patient will be able to explain the nature of proposed surgery and the associated requirements for positioning and activity.

Expected Outcomes: Postoperative

Patient will be free of complications related to immobility.

Patient will successfully adapt self-care patterns to the limitations of the surgery.

Patient will demonstrate the correct use of a walker or crutches

Patient and family will make safe and mutually satisfactory plans for care after discharge.

Nursing Interventions: Preoperative

Maintain patient on bed rest in Buck's traction if ordered.

Administer analgesics as ordered.

Elevate the head of the bed no more than 45 degrees.

Turn slightly to unaffected side if tolerated.

Use fracture pan for voiding or insert Foley catheter if patient is unable to void.

Encourage hourly deep breathing and coughing; apply TED stockings to unaffected leg; assess for cardiac and respiratory complications.

Teach patient about the planned surgery and position restrictions in the postoperative period.

Nursing Interventions: Postoperative

Position

Maintain abduction of affected leg with splints or pillows at all times.

Use trochanter rolls to prevent external rotation.

Avoid hip flexion by keeping head of bed low.

Turn every two hours to unaffected side, supporting the operative leg in an abducted position.

Activity

Begin getting patient out of bed according to physician's order.

Teach non–weight-bearing or partial weight-bearing techniques.

Teach patient quadriceps and gluteal set exercises for strengthening the muscles of ambulation.

Work with physical therapy plan to teach safe ambulation, transfer techniques, and range of motion.

Use chairs with firm, nonreclining seats and arms.

Nursing Interventions: General

Aggressively employ standard interventions to combat effects of immobility. Observe patient for signs of atelectasis, wound infection, skin breakdown, thrombophlebitis, or pulmonary embolus.

Encourage patient to remain active in self-care.

Provide meaningful stimuli to keep patient oriented and hopeful about the future.

Assist patient and family to explore resources available in community for postdischarge care.

Assist patient and family to acquire equipment and supplies needed for safe self-care at home.

Evaluation: Preoperative

Patient has minimal pain.

Patient maintains bed rest with affected leg in abduction.

Patient exhibits no early complications of immobility.

Patient maintains an adequate urinary output.

Patient remains oriented to time, place, and person.

Patient can explain the proposed surgery and the postoperative care.

Evaluation: Postoperative

Patient is free of the complications of immobility.

Patient resumes responsibility for self-care and completes activities of daily living.

Patient demonstrates the correct use of crutches or walker.

Patient and family express satisfaction with the arrangements for the patient's postdischarge care.

Patient verbalizes understanding of ongoing positioning and weight-bearing restrictions.

ARTHRITIS

Rheumatic diseases include a wide range of clinical conditions. The term *arthritis* means inflammation of a joint. It is a condition that exists in a number of specific diseases, but the term is frequently used to describe any condition involving pain and stiffness of the musculoskeletal system. It is estimated that arthritis affects some 20 million people (one in every seven persons) in the United States at an annual economic cost of billions of dollars. The three most common forms of arthritis are rheumatoid arthritis, osteoarthritis, and gouty arthritis.

FRACTURED HIP AND PROSTHETIC IMPLANT

Nursing Diagnoses	Expected Patient Outcomes	Nursing Interventions
Pain related to surgical procedure	Patient is comfortable and able to participate in self-care activities.	1. Give prescribed analgesics at timely intervals during initial postoperative period. 2. Teach relaxation techniques, as appropriate. 3. Use other appropriate pain-relieving techniques. 4. As pain decreases, use milder analgesics.
Impaired physical mobility related to pain and weight-bearing restrictions	Patient is active within prescribed limitations and remains free of the complications of immobility.	1. Determine from physician the limits of movement and weight bearing permitted. 2. Encourage activity within the prescribed limits. 3. Encourage isometric exercises (gluteal and quadriceps). 4. Assist patient to ambulate, when permitted, using the appropriate ambulatory aid.

Potential for injury related to surgical procedure and decreased mobility	Patient does not experience neurocirculatory or respiratory complications.
	Hip remains in alignment.
		1. Perform neurocirculatory checks once an hour for first 24 to 48 hours.
		2. Notify physician of any changes from preoperative status.
		3. Encourage active range of motion exercises of unaffected limbs.
		4. Encourage deep breathing and coughing exercises.
		5. Avoid hip flexion and adduction:
		  a. Assist patient to turn by supporting leg in abduction.
		  b. Use pillows to maintain abduction when patient is lying in bed.
		  c. Patient should avoid sitting initially; when sitting is permitted, elevate sitting surface with pillows to keep angle of hip within prescribed limits.
		  d. Patient should avoid elevating leg when sitting.
		6. Avoid positioning patient on operative side.

Potential impairment of skin integrity related to immobility and surgical incisions	Patient's skin remains intact; infection does not occur.	1. Monitor back and sacrum for signs of pressure. 2. Apply deep foam mattresses or other devices as appropriate. 3. Use heel pads and other protective pads as necessary. 4. Use aseptic technique for any dressing changes.
Potential for constipation related to decreased mobility	Stools are soft and occur at usual frequency.	1. Encourage fluid intake of 2000 to 3000 ml/day. 2. Encourage activity within prescribed limits. 3. Encourage high-fiber foods in diet. 4. Monitor bowel elimination pattern. Give prescribed stool softeners, suppositories, or laxatives.

Knowledge deficit related to treatment regimen and restrictions	Patient understands treatment regimen and follows positioning and weight-bearing restrictions.	1. Teach patient:
		  a. Rationale for activity restrictions as prescribed by physician.
		  b. No flexion of affected hip beyond 60 degrees in first week. No flexion beyond 90 degrees until cleared by physician.
		  c. No adduction of affected leg beyond midline.
		  d. Maintenance of partial weight-bearing status until cleared by physician.
		  e. No elevation of leg when sitting.
		  f. Need for follow-up care until fracture is fully healed.

Rheumatoid arthritis is a chronic, systemic inflammatory disease characterized by recurrent inflammation in joints and related structures that can result in crippling deformities. It is more prevalent in women than men by a 2:1 to 3:1 ratio, and usually appears during the young adult years. Possibly autoimmune in nature, it follows a pattern of exacerbation and remission. Rheumatoid arthritis primarily affects proximal joints, although virtually any joint can become involved. Involvement is usually bilaterally symmetric. Lesions of the vasculature, lungs, and other major organs also occur.

Osteoarthritis is a slow, progressive, noninflammatory, chronic disease primarily affecting the weight-bearing joints. It is characterized by pain, stiffness, and limitation of motion. Most prevalent in the 50- to 70-year-old group, it is believed to be a degenerative process that accompanies aging but can occur secondary to trauma or excess strain. Table 3-3 compares major characteristics of rheumatoid arthritis and osteoarthritis.

Gouty arthritis is a metabolic disorder of purine metabolism in which excess uric acid leads to the formation of urate crystals in the synovial tissue, producing intense inflammation. It is an inherited disorder affecting men eight to nine times more often than women. The peak age of onset is the fifth decade, but it can occur at any age. The great toe is most commonly involved. Patients may develop tophi, deposits of monosodium urate, in the tissues.

PATHOPHYSIOLOGY

Rheumatoid Arthritis

The disease process of rheumatoid arthritis begins with synovial inflammation with edema, congestion, and fibrin exudate. Continued inflammation produces synovial thickening and formation of pannus where it joins the articular cartilage, interfering with the nutrition of the cartilage, which may become necrotic. Pannus also invades the subchondral bone and soft tissue structures and may destroy them. The destruction of cartilage and bone and the weakening of tendons and ligaments can lead to dislocation, subluxation, and ankylosis. Common problems include the following:

subluxation Partial dislocation of a joint.
valgus deformity The distal arm of the angle of the joint points away from the midline of the body (bow legged).
varus deformity The distal arm of the angle of the joint points toward the midline of the body (knock knees).
ulnar deviation Condition in which fingers deviate at the metacarpophalangeal joints toward the ulnar aspect of the hand.
swan neck deformity Combination deformity in which there is flexion contracture of the metacarpophalangeal joint, hyperextension of the proximal interphalangeal joint, and flexion of the distal interphalangeal joint.
boutonniere deformity Flexion of the proximal interphalangeal joint and hyperextension of the distal interphalangeal joint.
Z deformity of thumb Hyperextension of the interphalangeal joint of the thumb with flexion of the metacarpophalangeal joint.

Rheumatoid arthritis is accompanied by an elevated erythrocyte sedimentation rate, decreased red blood cell count, and mild elevation in white blood cell count; 50% to 90% of patients exhibit a positive rheumatoid factor. Painless subcutaneous nodules may develop near joints and along extensor surfaces of the bones.

Osteoarthritis

In osteoarthritis the articular cartilage becomes yellow and opaque. It softens and the surfaces become roughened, frayed, or cracked. Cartilage may be destroyed and underlying bone altered. New bone (Heberden's nodes and Bouchard's nodes) appears at joint margins and may even break off in the joint. Serologic and synovial fluid examinations have essentially normal outcomes.

TABLE 3-3 Differential characteristics between rheumatoid arthritis and osteoarthritis

Rheumatoid Arthritis	Osteoarthritis
Systemic disease; people are sick with malaise, fever, fatigue	Local joint disease; people have no systemic symptoms
Signs of inflammation present both locally in joints and systemically as pain, fever, soreness, malaise	Inflammatory signs are less prominent and are local (not systemic) when present
Fingers and proximal interphalangeal joints are involved more commonly	Distal interphalangeal joints are involved more commonly
Subcutaneous, extraarticular (rheumatoid) nodules are present in tissues around (not in) the joints in 20% of clients	No periarticular or subcutaneous nodes are present; Heberden's nodes are bony enlargements within the joints
Bony ankylosis and osteoporosis are common	Ankylosis and osteoporosis are uncommon
Elevated sedimentation rate; elevated serum rheumatoid factors	Normal sedimentation rate and blood chemistries
Young adults to older adults are affected (25-50 years of age)	Adults are affected during later years (from 45 years of age)

From Mourad L: Nursing care of adults with orthopedic conditions, ed 2, New York, 1988, John Wiley & Sons, Inc.

NURSING CARE PLAN

RHEUMATOID ARTHRITIS

Nursing Diagnoses	Expected Patient Outcomes	Nursing Interventions
Pain related to joint inflammation and stiffness	Patient experiences decreased pain and stiffness.	1. Assess pain characteristics. 2. Provide prescribed medications on time. 3. Apply heat or cold, as appropriate, especially prior to exercise or at bedtime. 4. Encourage patient to change position frequently. 5. Provide rest periods. 6. Encourage use of resting splints during acute periods.
Impaired physical mobility related to joint destruction and decreased muscle strength	Patient demonstrates improved active range of motion and muscle strength.	1. Encourage regular active range of motion exercises of joints to greatest degree possible. 2. Encourage patient to assist with ADL to greatest degree possible. 3. Give analgesic or heat/cold treatments prior to exercise. 4. Provide support and assistance to patient during exercise prescribed by physician or physical therapist. 5. Avoid active exercises if joint is acutely inflamed.
Potential for injury related to impaired mobility and weakness	Patient uses assistive devices effectively to avoid injury. Patient does not experience joint deformity.	1. Position joints to support joint function; avoid positions of flexion. 2. Encourage active range of motion exercises. 3. Encourage other prescribed exercises and ambulation alternated with rest periods. 4. Encourage isometric exercises when joints are acutely inflamed. 5. Provide appropriate ambulatory devices (walker, cane). 6. Encourage use of shoes rather than slippers when ambulating. 7. Teach joint protective techniques. 8. Teach use of safety devices as appropriate (such as safety arms on toilets or grab bars on tubs or showers).
Self-care deficit in personal hygiene and feeding related to pain and limitation of movement	Patient demonstrates ability to perform self-care activities.	1. Encourage patient to participate in ADL to greatest degree possible. 2. Give patient sufficient time for ADL. 3. Use comfort measures as needed before required activities. 4. Encourage patient to acquire and use assistive devices for dressing, feeding, and activities of daily living, as appropriate.
Body image disturbance related to deformed joints and impaired mobility	Patient has a more positive self-concept.	1. Provide patient with opportunities to discuss feelings about body changes and increased dependence on others. 2. Help patient identify personal strengths. 3. Allow patient maximum independence possible within physical limitations. 4. Anticipate patient needs for assistance and provide help as necessary. 5. Assist family to participate in patient's care so they can see what patient can do and thus provide positive encouragement and help patient maintain optimal independence.

Continued.

NURSING CARE PLAN

RHEUMATOID ARTHRITIS—cont'd

Nursing Diagnoses	Expected Patient Outcomes	Nursing Interventions
Knowledge deficit related to the control and management of arthritis and its complications	Patient describes disease process and therapeutic regimen.	1. Teach patient: a. Nature of disorder. b. Medication program. c. Exercise program; use of splints if appropriate. d. Balance of activity with rest. e. Correct use of heat/cold packs and assistive devices. f. Measures to prevent injury and protect joints. g. Basics of good nutrition and importance of avoiding overweight. h. Community resources.

Gouty Arthritis

In gouty arthritis uric acid deposits trigger intense inflammation and pain in the joint and surrounding tissue. Deposits and tophi cause gradual destruction of joints and bone. If unchecked, the disease can also produce renal damage. It is accompanied by elevated serum uric acid levels and by urate crystals in the synovial fluid.

MEDICAL MANAGEMENT

Rheumatoid Arthritis and Osteoarthritis

Treatment for arthritis involves a balanced program of exercise and rest, patient education, joint protection, and control of inflammation through the use of salicylates and nonsteroidal antiinflammatory drugs. Medica-

tions are progressively added on the basis of the patients response to therapy. Adjunctive therapy may include analgesics, intraarticular steroids, antidepressants, and surgery. Table 3-4 summarizes arthritis drug therapy, and Table 3-5 describes commonly used surgical procedures.

Gouty Arthritis

Acute gouty arthritis attacks can be controlled and recurrent attacks can be prevented through administration of antiinflammatory drugs and reduction of the body pool of urates and uric acid. Colchicine is the drug of choice for treatment of acute attacks. Allopurinol (Zyloprim), probenicid (Benemid), and sulfinpyrazone (Anturane) are used to decrease uric acid levels. Dietary re-

---

TABLE 3-4 Medications prescribed in the treatment of rheumatoid arthritis

Medication	Action	Side Effects/Toxic Effects	Precautions
Salicylates			
Examples: acetylsalicyclic acid, choline salicylates	Analgesic, antipyretic, antiinflammatory	Gastric irritation; dose-related salicylism; skin rash; hypersensitivity; decreased platelet aggregation	Take with food, milk, or antacid; space every 4 to 6 hr to maintain antiinflammatory effect; report incidence of bleeding or hearing changes
Nonsteroidal Antiinflammatory Agents			
Indomethacin (Indocin)	Analgesic, antiinflammatory	Headache; dizziness; insomnia; confusion; gastrointestinal irritation	Take with food, milk, or antacid; discontinue if CNS symptoms develop and notify physician
Ibuprofen (Motrin)	Same as indomethacin	Same as indomethacin but believed less irritating to gastrointestinal tract	Delayed absorption if taken with food
Tolmetin sodium (Tolectin)	Same as ibuprofen	Same as ibuprofen	Take with food or milk
Naproxen (Naprosyn)	Same as ibuprofen	Same as indomethacin; also drowsiness	Take with food, milk, or antacid; avoid driving until dosage effect is established
Fenoprofen calcium (Nalfon)	Same as ibuprofen	Same as naproxen	Delayed absorption if taken with food; avoid driving until dosage effect is established
Sulindac (Clinoril)	Same as ibuprofen	Same as ibuprofen; plus skin rash	Take with food, milk, or antacid; do not use with acetylsalicylic acid
Diflunisal (Dolobid)	Analgesic, antiinflammatory	Gastric irritation; headache; dizziness; skin rash; tinnitus; fluid retention	Take with food or milk; do not use with salicylates or other antiinflammatory medications
Piroxicam (Feldene)	Analgesic, antiinflammatory	Gastric irritation; anemia; skin rash; fluid retention; dizziness; headache	Take with food or antacid
Diclofenac sodium (Volteran)	Analgesic, antiinflammatory	Possible intestinal irritation; headache; drowsiness; fatigue	Enteric coated; may be taken with food or milk

Continued.

TABLE 3-4 Medications prescribed in the treatment of rheumatoid arthritis—cont'd

Medication	Action	Side Effects/Toxic Effects	Precautions
Slow Acting Antiinflammatory Agents			
Antimalarials			
Hydroxychloroquine (Plaquenil)	Antiinflammatory (mechanism unknown); effect not expected to be noted for 6-12 mo after beginning therapy	Gastrointestinal disturbances; retinal edema that may result in blindness	Eye examination before beginning therapy and every 6 mo thereafter
Chloroquine (Aralen)	Same as hydroxychloroquine	Same as hydroxychloroquine	Same as hydroxychloroquine
Quinacrine (Atabrine)	Same as hydroxychloroquine	Same as hydroxychloroquine but may be better tolerated; yellow discoloration of the skin	May be stopped periodically to prevent deepening of skin discoloration
Gold salts—IM Gold Sodium Thiomalate (Myochrysine), Gold Thioglucose (Solganol) Gold—oral Auranofin (Ridaura)	Antiinflammatory; effect not noted for 3-6 months after beginning therapy	Renal and hepatic damage; corneal deposits; dermatitis; ulcerations in mouth; hematologic changes	Urinalysis and CBC before each injection; report dermatitis, metallic taste in mouth, or lesions in mouth to physician. Oral gold may produce fewer side effects, than injectable, but periodic laboratory tests are required
Penicillamine (Cuprimine)	Antiinflammatory (mechanism unclear); effect not expected to be noted until several months after beginning treatment	Fever; rash; nephrotic syndrome; hematologic changes; gastrointestinal irritation; lupuslike syndromes; allergic reactions (33% probability if allergic to penicillin); retarded wound healing	Urinalysis, CBC, differential, hemoglobin and platelet count at least weekly for 3 mo, then monthly; report skin rash, fever to physician; food interferes with absorption—take on empty stomach between meals
Potent Antiinflammatory Agents			
Adrenocorticosteroids (e.g., prednisone)	Interfere with body's normal inflammatory response	Fluid retention; sodium retention; potassium depletion; hypertension; decreased healing potential; increased susceptibility to infection; gastrointestinal irritation; hirsutism, osteoporosis, fat deposits; diabetes mellitus; myopathy; adrenal insufficiency or adrenal crisis if abruptly withdrawn	Take with food, milk, or antacid; dosage not to be increased or decreased without physician's supervision; take in morning if taken on once-a-day basis
Phenylbutazone (Butazolidin)	Antiinflammatory; analgesic at subcortical site in brain	Gastrointestinal irritation; hematologic toxicity; hypertension, impaired renal function	Used for a short term (7-10 days); take with food or milk

From Phipps WJ, Long BC, and Woods NF: Medical-surgical nursing: concepts and clinical practice, ed 4, St Louis, 1990, Mosby–Year Book, Inc.

NOTE: It should also be noted that the immunosuppressive agents azathioprine (Imuran), cyclophosphamide (Cytoxan), and chlorambucil (Leukeran) have been used on an investigational basis in patients with severe disease that has not responded to the conventional medications. These agents are used with great care because of their severe side effects and the attendant risks of the development of neoplasms. The drug methotrexate has recently received FDA approval for use in rheumatoid arthritis.

TABLE 3-5 Surgical interventions for arthritis

Procedure	Description	Expected Outcome
Synovectomy	Removal of synovial tissue to arrest the arthritic process in a particular joint	Maintains joint function Prevents recurrent inflammation
Arthrotomy	Exploration of a joint	Drains Removes damaged tissue
Arthroplasty	Joint reconstruction by reshaping bones, replacement of all or part of a joint with prosthetic parts	Restores motion and function Relieves pain Corrects deformity
Arthrodesis	Surgical fusion of joint performed to eliminate pain and provide stability	Relieves pain Improves stability Restores function

striction of purine intake (found in red meats and legumes) may also be recommended. Increasing fluid intake helps to prevent crystal formation in the urine.

NURSING MANAGEMENT

Assessment

Both subjective and objective factors should be assessed in patients with rheumatoid arthritis and osteoarthritis.

Subjective
Current health status
History and management of disorder
Diet and medication history
Pain pattern and severity
Patient and family coping patterns
Complaints of fatigue, weakness, and stiffness, especially early morning and following periods of inactivity
Effects of disease on usual patterns of activities—work and recreation

Objective
Joint range of motion, muscle strength/atrophy, swelling
Presence of obvious joint deformities
Functional abilities for self-care—gait and ambulation, bathing, feeding, toileting activities
Presence of bony protuberance, such as Heberden's or Bouchard's nodes (osteoarthritis only)
Systemic symptoms of fever, tachycardia, weight loss, subcutaneous nodules, anemia (rheumatoid arthritis only)

Nursing Diagnoses

Diagnoses are variable according to extent and severity of the disease process. Common diagnoses encountered with rheumatoid and osteoarthritis include the following:

Pain in joints related to inflammation or degeneration
Activity intolerance related to weakened muscles, pain, or anemia

Potential for injury related to decreased muscle strength, balance, and coordination
Impaired physical mobility related to joint destruction and decreased muscle strength
Self-care deficit in feeding, bathing/hygiene, dressing/grooming or toileting related to pain and limitation of movement
Body image disturbance related to deformed joints and impaired mobility
Knowledge deficit related to disease management, joint protection strategies, and use of assistive devices

Expected Outcomes

Patient will experience a decrease in pain and stiffness.
Patient will demonstrate increased energy through involvement in self-care activities.
Patient will not fall or experience injury.
Patient will have increased joint mobility and muscle strength.
Patient will incorporate altered body image into a positive self-concept.
Patient will understand disease process and the management of symptoms.
Patient will incorporate joint protection strategies into daily activity routines.

Nursing Interventions: Pain

Teach patient to balance rest and activity.
Teach patient about medications and their side effects.
Caution about gastrointestinal effects of drugs and importance of buffering with food or antacid.
Tell patient to maintain adequate blood levels of antiinflammatories and avoid PRN use.
Apply heat or cold to joints for comfort and muscle relaxation.
During acute attack, rheumatoid arthritis patient should be on bed rest with joints held in position of function.

JOINT PROTECTION

Use the largest or strongest joint possible for all activities.
Use shoulder or arm instead of hand or fingers.
Lift heavy objects with knees not the back.
Avoid positions of possible joint deformity.
Avoid twisting motions with small joints.
Do not maintain positions of flexion for long periods of time.
Use joints in their best and most stable positions.
Maintain good posture.
Avoid unnecessary twisting, bending, or stretching.
Avoid maintaining joints in one position for a long time.
Change positions frequently.
Incorporate full joint movement into all activities.
Conserve energy.
Organize work and eliminate unnecessary tasks.
Take frequent planned breaks during work.

Nursing Interventions: Mobility

Encourage patient to perform prescribed exercises. Use heat to reduce stiffness prior to exercise.

Patient should avoid AM exercise when stiffness is acute.

Teach patient to exercise only to the point of pain.

Assist patient with range of motion exercises as needed.

Focus on exercise directed at increasing functional capacities.

Avoid positioning in a way to encourage contracture.

Explore use of splints, braces, and assistive devices with physical therapy.

Assist patient to utilize joint protection principles in planning daily activities. (See box above.)

Nursing Interventions: Adjustment

Encourage use of basic nutritious diet to foster optimal general health.

Encourage weight loss if indicated.

Encourage patient to express fears and frustration about chronic progressive nature of the disease.

Teach environmental modifications for safety and comfort such as supportive shoes, hand rails in bathtub, and raised toilet seats.

Explore use of self-help devices to foster independence in activities of daily living.

Teach patient and family to maintain regular medical supervision and avoid quack therapies.

Evaluation

Patient reports a decrease in pain and stiffness.

Patient has sufficient energy to participate in self-care and social activities of daily living.

Patient reports increased range of motion and muscle strength.

Patient states improved feelings about self.

Patient can describe purpose and side effects of medica-

tions, select appropriate foods for healthy diet, and demonstrate prescribed exercise program.

Patient and family modify environment to improve safety and incorporate joint protection principles into daily routines.

TOTAL JOINT REPLACEMENT

Total joint replacement is increasingly being used to correct deformities and maintain functional capacities in patients with arthritis. Table 3-6 discusses the pre- and postoperative care involved in the two most common procedures, total hip replacement and total knee replacement. Preventing infection and understanding mobility restrictions are the most important aspects of care.

Table 3-7 presents characteristics of some common nonarticular rheumatic diseases. They include rheumatic diseases involving supportive structures near the joints but not the joints themselves.

COLLAGEN DISEASE

Collagen disorders are a group of diseases involving the connective tissue of the body. These diseases share some pathological features. The cause of these diseases is unknown and they are grouped together largely on the basis of signs and symptoms. Management is largely treating symptoms and providing support. The category includes systemic lupus erythematosus (SLE), polymyositis, progressive systemic sclerosis (scleroderma), necrotizing arteritis, and Sjögren's syndrome. See Table 3-8 for the major characteristics of SLE and the other disorders.

SYSTEMIC LUPUS ERYTHEMATOSUS

SLE is a chronic inflammatory disease of unknown etiology that affects women, particularly adolescents and young adults, 8 to 10 times more often than men. It was named for the characteristic rash that accompanies it.

PATHOPHYSIOLOGY

Common pathologic manifestations include the following:
Severe vasculitis with necrosis of small arterial walls
Thickening of glomerular basement membrane and necrosis of glomerular capillaries
Lymph node necrosis
Fibrous villous synovitis

It is suspected that a disorder of immunity may cause immune complexes to be deposited in the tissue. A second possibility is the presence of a viral infection resulting from an immunologic abnormality. Depending on the organ involved, the patient may have findings of

TABLE 3-6 Nursing interventions for the patient with a total hip or total knee replacement

Procedure	Preoperative Interventions	Postoperative Interventions	General Surgical Interventions
Total hip replacement	Scrupulously clean skin and prepare patient per surgeon's routine. Administer prophylactic antibiotics as prescribed. Teach patient and family about surgical procedure and postoperative restrictions concerning movement and positioning.	Position according to surgeon's practice and preference: usually hip is kept in wide abduction with slings or pillows. Avoid external rotation by using sandbags or trochanter rolls. Keep head of bed elevated less than 45 degrees except for meals. Turn to unaffected side with operative leg maintained in abduction. Encourage patient to do bed exercises (quadriceps and gluteal sets exercises) to strengthen muscles for ambulation and prevent venous stasis. Assist with ambulation and progressive weight bearing as ordered—may be as early as postoperative day 1. Patient will probably use crutches or a walker. Increase amount of ambulation daily. Teach patient in preparation for discharge to avoid hip flexion greater than 90 degrees, use raised toilet seat for at least 2 months, observe activity and weight-bearing restrictions, use self-help devices to avoid bending and stooping. Warn against adduction beyond the midline. Reinforce importance of prophylactic prevention of systemic infection. Inform all dentists and doctors of presence of prosthesis.	Maintain drainage system; note type and amount of drainage. Keep operative area free from contamination: Assess site regularly. Change dressing as needed. Administer antibiotics as ordered. Administer anticoagulant if prescribed for risk of thrombus. Administer narcotics as needed for pain control
Total knee replacement	Scrupulously clean skin and prepare patient per surgeon's routine. Teach patient and family about surgical procedure and exercises to be employed in postoperative period (quadriceps sets and straight leg lifts).	Provide sufficient analgesia to allow patient to perform exercises. Begin active flexion exercises after dressing removal. Continuous passive motion machines may be employed. Assist with ambulation (partial weight bearing) once patient demonstrates quadriceps muscle control. Use of resting knee immobilizer is common.	Maintain drainage system; note type and amount of drainage. Keep operative area free from contamination: Assess site regularly. Change dressing as needed. Administer antibiotics as ordered.

TABLE 3-7 Nonarticular rheumatic diseases

Disorder	Description	Signs and Symptoms	Medical Management
Bursitis	Inflammation of the bursa, acute or chronic, is caused by trauma, strain or over-use of the joint. Shoulder bursa is most commonly affected.	Severe pain; limitations in joint movement	Rest for involved area Antiinflammatory analgesic agents Application of cold during acute period
Carpal tunnel syndrome	Pressure is exerted by the flexion tendon sheaths on the median nerve at the wrist. Condition usually localized.	Disorders in sensation (burning, tingling) in the thumb, index, and middle fingers—especially during prolonged flexion Referred pain to upper extremity	Rest Splinting of wrist Surgical release of transverse carpal ligament
Dupuytren's contracture	Palmar fascia on ulnar side of one or both hands becomes thickened and shortened, pulling the fingers into fixed flexion.	Progressive inability to extend fourth and fifth fingers; painless Palmar skin is tense with puckers and nodules	As condition worsens, surgical intervention to remove involved palmar fascia and release contracture
Fibrositis and fibromyositis	Commonly occurring self-limiting symptom complex	Pain and stiffness in neck, shoulder girdle, and extremities Pain worsens with activity and subsides with rest	Management directed at specific symptoms Rest, analgesics, and physical therapy

glomerulonephritis, pleuritis, pericarditis, peritonitis, neuritis, or anemia.

MEDICAL MANAGEMENT

The use of adrenocorticosteroids is the cornerstone of medical intervention and frequently is successful in controlling the course of the disease. Joint pain may be treated by salicylates. Other care is aimed at dealing with the specific symptoms confronting a patient. Lesions affecting major organ systems can be fatal.

NURSING MANAGEMENT

Assessment

Factors to be assessed include the following:
   History, symptoms, and course of the disease
   Patient's medication regimen and compliance
   Side effects of high-dose steroids
   Patient response to chronic progressive disorder
   Presence of arthritislike symptoms or skin rashes (butterfly pattern of erythema over cheeks and bridge of nose)
   Other specific system assessments as suggested by symptoms

Nursing Diagnoses

Diagnoses will be variable based on the patient's disease course and current symptoms. Common diagnoses include the following:

Pain related to joint inflammation
Activity intolerance related to fatigue and weakness
Body image disturbance related to skin rashes and side effects of adrenocorticosteroids
Knowledge deficit related to disease management, use of adrenocorticosteroids, and the management of side effects

Expected Outcomes

Patient will experience less pain, increased comfort.
Patient will have sufficient energy to complete self-care and normal social activities.
Patient will incorporate body changes into a satisfactory body image.
Patient will be knowledgeable about prescribed medications, side effects, and their management.

Nursing Interventions

Administer prescribed medications.
Discuss the management of side effects through diet modification and fluid balance.
Plan with patient a balanced program of rest and exercise.
Teach patient to avoid excessive sun exposure by covering body surfaces, wearing a wide brimmed hat, and using a sunscreen when exposed to direct sunlight.
Provide symptomatic and supportive care as indicated by patient symptoms.

TABLE 3-8 Collagen disorders: pathophysiology, signs and symptoms, and medical management

Disorder	Pathophysiology	Signs and Symptoms	Medical Management
Systemic lupus erythematosus (SLE) (chronic inflammatory disease)	Severe vasculitis with necrosis of walls of small arteries Thickening of glomerular basement membrane Lymph node necrosis Fibrous villous synovitis Lesions in nervous system	Arthritis symptoms Weakness, fatigue Sun sensitivity—rash reaction Erythema in butterfly pattern over nose and cheeks Specific organ symptoms Positive LE cell reaction	High-dose glucocorticosteroids Salicylates General supportive care
Polymyositis (dermatomyositis) (inflammatory disease involving striated, voluntary muscle)	Primary degeneration of muscle fibers Necrosis of parts or entire groups of muscle fibers Interstitial fibrosis	Muscle weakness and fatigue, especially in pelvic and shoulder muscles Muscle pain or tenderness Eventual contractures and atrophy if weakness persists Dusky red skin rash if dermatomyositis form EMG, muscle biopsy results Elevated serum enzymes	High-dose glucocorticosteroids to effect remission Physical therapy and occupational therapy for exercise regimen; rest
Progressive systemic sclerosis (PSS, scleroderma) (sclerosis involving connective tissue throughout the body)	Involved tissue becomes fibrotic Changes may be accompanied by vascular lesions	Gradual thickening and tightening of the skin on face and body Telangiectasis on lips, tongue, face Pain and stiffness; muscle weakness Local effects produced by fibrosis of vital organs	Glucocorticosteroids for those with myositis symptoms Salicylates Range of motion exercise
Necrotizing arteritis (inflammation of the blood vessels)	Inflammation and necrosis of arterial wall Fibrosis and intimal proliferation result from body's attempts to clear necrosis Partial or complete vessel occlusion, infarction, or aneurysm	Involvement of vessels anywhere in body—angina, myocardial infarction, hypertension, peripheral neuropathy, intractable headaches Elevated white blood count (WBC) and erythrocyte sedimentation rate (ESR). Angiography results show vessel destruction	High-dose glucocorticosteroids to effect remission Rest
Sjögren's syndrome (chronic inflammation of lacrimal and parotid glands)	Infiltration of lacrimal and parotid glands by lymphocytes and plasma cells Decrease in flow of tears and saliva	Dry gritty sensation in eyes—redness and itching Difficulty in chewing or swallowing or with speech Corneal, tongue, and lip ulceration	Symptomatic care with eye drops, increased fluids, and hard candy to stimulate saliva

Encourage patient to verbalize feelings about chronic progressive disease.

Evaluation

Patient reports increased comfort and is able to participate in self-care activities.

Patient reports an increased energy level and resumes normal patterns of work and social activities.

Patient remains involved socially and makes positive references to self.

Patient and family can discuss prescribed medications and activities to control and manage their side effects.

HERNIATED NUCLEUS PULPOSUS

Herniated nucleus pulposus is a condition in which the gelatinous intravertebral disk protrudes through the surrounding cartilage, causing pressure on the spinal nerve roots. Degeneration of the disk cartilage results in a loss of elasticity.

PATHOPHYSIOLOGY

Herniation may be triggered by a sudden strain or trauma in spinal region. The condition may also be predisposed by damage resulting from rheumatoid arthritis or osteoarthritis. Nerve compression produces low back pain radiating down path of the sciatic nerve in the posterior thigh. There will frequently be paresthesias in the leg and foot, muscle weakness, and muscle spasm. The most common sites of herniation are at L3-4, L4-5, and L5-S1. A myelogram may be used to confirm the diagnosis.

MEDICAL MANAGEMENT

Conservative medical management includes bed rest with a firm mattress, muscle relaxants and analgesics, physical therapy for deep heat and massage, and pelvic traction to relieve spasms.

Surgical interventions are designed to relieve pressure on the nerve root and stabilize the spine and may include diskectomy, laminectomy, or spinal fusions if multiple vertebrae are involved or the spine is unstable.

NURSING MANAGEMENT

Assessment

Factors to be assessed include the following:
Pain pattern and extent, duration, and severity
Presence of paresthesias or muscle weakness
History of trauma or degenerative disease
Actions that relieve or improve pain
Patient's normal daily living, occupational, and leisure activities
Patient's knowledge of surgery or therapy prescribed

Nursing Diagnoses

Diagnoses will vary slightly depending on patient's symptoms, treatment, and general health status. Common diagnoses include the following:
Pain related to spinal nerve compression
Activity intolerance related to pain and muscle spasm
Impaired physical mobility related to pain and weakness
Knowledge deficit related to therapy, surgery, postoperative positioning, normal body mechanics, or back-strengthening exercises.

Expected Outcomes

Patient will experience decreased pain and muscle spasm.
Patient will be able to resume normal activity patterns.
Patient will demonstrate understanding of therapy, surgical procedure, body mechanics, and exercises to strengthen back.

Nursing Interventions: Conservative

Encourage patient to maintain bed rest with head of bed low and knees slightly flexed.
Establish and maintain pelvic traction if ordered.
Administer analgesics and muscle relaxants as ordered.
Use nursing measures to augment pain relief, such as diversion, application of heat, and back rubs.
Monitor for and prevent complications of immobility by increasing roughage and fluids, giving frequent skin care and position changes, encouraging deep breathing and range of motion exercises, and observing for Homans' sign (calf tenderness).

Nursing Interventions: Surgical

Teach patient about procedure and restrictions for postoperative positioning.
Teach patient about log rolling, coughing, and deep breathing.
Obtain baseline preoperative neurologic assessment.
Check movement and sensation in lower extremities frequently in postoperative period.
Encourage ambulation—patient should avoid sitting.
Administer stool softeners to prevent straining.
Teach patient principles of good body mechanics. Patient should:
Maintain broad base of support.
Use large groups of muscles.
Maintain good posture.
Squat, not bend.
Pull objects rather than pushing.
Teach patient back-strengthening exercises.
NOTE: If patient undergoes spinal fusion, a period of bedrest may be required. A brace or corset may be utilized, and care will include a second surgical incision from the bone graft. Meticulous attention to monitoring and preventing complications related to immobility is essential.

Evaluation

Patient is free of pain and muscle spasm.
Patient gradually resumes normal activity pattern and experiences no residual weakness.
Patient demonstrates good posture and the principles of body mechanics in moving. Patient incorporates back-strengthening exercises into daily activities.

AMPUTATION

Amputation is the surgical removal of a limb as a result of trauma or disease. The lower extremities are the limbs amputated most commonly, and approximately 80% of amputations involve peripheral vascular disease, usually as a result of diabetes.

PATHOPHYSIOLOGY

Although trauma or tumor may result in amputation, chronic limb ischemia is the most common pathology. When the development of collateral blood flow cannot compensate for the decrease in arterial flow, the chronic tissue ischemia can gradually lead to necrosis, ulceration, and eventually gangrene.

MEDICAL MANAGEMENT

The operative procedure and level of the amputation are determined by the extent of damaged tissue and the adequacy of the arterial blood supply. The level must ensure that adequate nutrition and blood supply are available for healing. The limb stump may be treated with pressure dressings or the immediate application of a cast with a temporary prefitted prosthesis according to surgeon preference.

NURSING MANAGEMENT

Assessment
Preoperative
History of disease and treatment
General health status
Condition of affected limb
Knowledge of planned surgical procedure and outcomes
Psychological response to need for surgery
Postoperative
Routine surgical assessment: vital signs, respiratory, wound status
Position of stump and condition of dressings
Pain—amount and location
Psychological response—grieving state
Social supports available for rehabilitation period

Nursing Diagnoses
Diagnoses are variable depending on the general health status of the patients and their responses to surgery. Common diagnoses include the following:
Pain related to swelling, tissue injury, and phantom sensation
Impaired physical mobility related to pain, decreased muscle strength, or decreased range of motion
Knowledge deficit related to ongoing care of stump and prosthesis
Body image disturbance related to effects of limb loss
Potential for dysfunctional grieving related to unresolved feelings of loss

Expected Outcomes
Patient will experience a decreased level of pain.
Patient will utilize assistive devices as needed to manage activities of daily living.
Patient will maintain full range of motion to affected limb.
Patient will demonstrate appropriate care for stump and apply wrappings correctly.
Patient will successfully incorporate amputation into a revised body image.
Patient will successfully resolve grief associated with the loss of a limb.

Nursing Interventions
Elevate stump for first 24 hours to reduce swelling.
Assess frequently for excessive bleeding.
Administer analgesics as needed.
Begin active range of motion exercise and encourage isometric exercise to gluteals, quadriceps, and triceps muscles for crutch walking.
Encourage patient to lie prone three or four times daily to prevent flexion contractures.
Reinforce crutch walking regimen developed by physical therapy. Assist patient to compensate for altered balance and center of gravity.
Instruct patient in proper technique for stump wrapping. Maintain appropriate wrapping at all times except for skin care.
Monitor stump carefully for signs of infection or irritation.
Teach patient to provide skin care daily using a mild soap. Avoid use of creams or ointments that may excessively soften skin.
Discuss concept of phantom limb sensation and reinforce that it is a normal occurrence.
Encourage patient to discuss concerns over losses. Reinforce importance of normal grieving for missing part.

Evaluation
Patient is able to deal with occurrence of phantom limb sensation.
Patient resumes normal activities and uses crutches effectively.
Patient demonstrates appropriate skin care for stump and applies wrappings correctly.
Patient successfully incorporates amputation into revised body image.
Patient resolves feelings of loss and grief concerning loss of limb.

BIBLIOGRAPHY

Clay KL and Stirn ML: Documentation of discharge teaching of patients who have had hip surgery, Orthop Nurs **5**(6):22, 1986.
Gamron R: Taking the pressure out of compartment syndrome, Am J Nurs **88**:1076-1080, 1988.
Hansell M: Fractures and the healing process, Orthop Nurs **7**(1):43, 1988.

Henning LM and Burrows SK: Keeping up on arthritis meds., RN 32, February 1986.

Hines NA, and Bates MS: Discharging the patient in skeletal traction, Orthop Nurs **6**(4):21, 1987.

Ignatavicius DD: Meeting the psychosocial needs of patients with rheumatoid arthritis, Orthop Nurs **6**(3):16-21, 1987.

Joseph N: Arthritis medications from A to Z, Caring **8**(1):14-16, 1989.

Lambert VA, and others: Coping with rheumatoid arthritis, Nurs Clin North Am **22:**555-558, 1987.

Maher AB: Early assessment and management of musculoskeletal injuries, Nurs Clin North Am **21:**717-727, 1986.

Morris L: Nursing the patient in traction, RN 26, January 1988.

Osterman H and Pinzur M: Amputation: last resort or new beginning, Geriatr Nurs **8**(5):246, 1987.

Schoen D: Assessment for arthritis, Orthop Nurs **7**(20):31, 1988.

Wise LB: A comparison of orthopedic casts: breaking the mold, Maternal Child Nurs J **11:**174, 1986.

CHAPTER 4

Neurologic Disorders

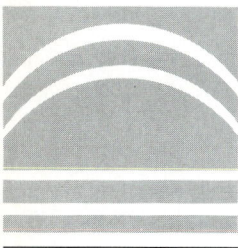

The nervous system functions as the coordinator and regulator of all body activity, collecting and processing sensory data and transmitting impulses along motor pathways to effector muscles and glands for action. Neurologic problems may be related to trauma, infection, neoplasm, vascular impairment, or degenerative processes. The effects of neurologic disorders range from decreased or absent function to excessive uncontrolled function. Nursing care for common neurologic disorders is described in this chapter. Figure 4-1 illustrates the basic anatomic structure of the nervous system.

CHRONIC/DEGENERATIVE NEUROLOGIC DISORDERS

Neurologic disorders often require individuals to make multiple adjustments in their life-style. Diseases that are chronic or degenerative add additional stress and create the need for comprehensive and creative nursing management.

CONVULSIVE DISORDERS (EPILEPSY)

Seizures may be defined as transitory disturbances in motor, sensory, or autonomic functions with or without loss of consciousness, resulting from uncontrolled electrical discharges in the brain. Seizures may be triggered by a wide variety of causes including the following:

Cerebral anoxia
Hypoglycemia
Infections accompanied by high temperature
Neoplasms
Trauma and scar tissue
Metabolic disturbances
Electrolyte imbalances
Drugs and poisons
Inflammation and abscess
Increased intracranial pressure

In idiopathic epilepsy the actual cause of the seizures may remain unknown; the role of heredity remains unclear. There are several types of seizures, the most common of which are described in Table 4-1.

PATHOPHYSIOLOGY

Seizures represent sudden, excessive, disorderly discharges of the neurons of the brain. The process may last from a few seconds to as long as 5 minutes. Fatigue of the precipitating neurons is believed to help end the seizure, which is generally followed by a period of inhibition of cerebral function, usually incomplete. The seizure may involve only a minute focal spot in the brain or virtually all of it at once.

MEDICAL MANAGEMENT

If no correctable cause can be uncovered, medical management focuses on the control of seizures through anticonvulsant medication. Dosages of anticonvulsant medications are difficult to establish and regulate because of the high incidence of side effects and the toxicity of the drugs. Table 4-2 presents some of the common medications used to control seizures. Electroencephalograms (EEGs) are used extensively to diagnose and localize seizures.

NURSING MANAGEMENT

Assessment
Subjective
History of seizure disorder and manifestations
Patient's knowledge of seizure disorder
Patient's knowledge of prescribed medications, side effects; degree of compliance
Patient's description of aura experience, if any, and postictal feelings
Patient's social adjustment to seizure disorder

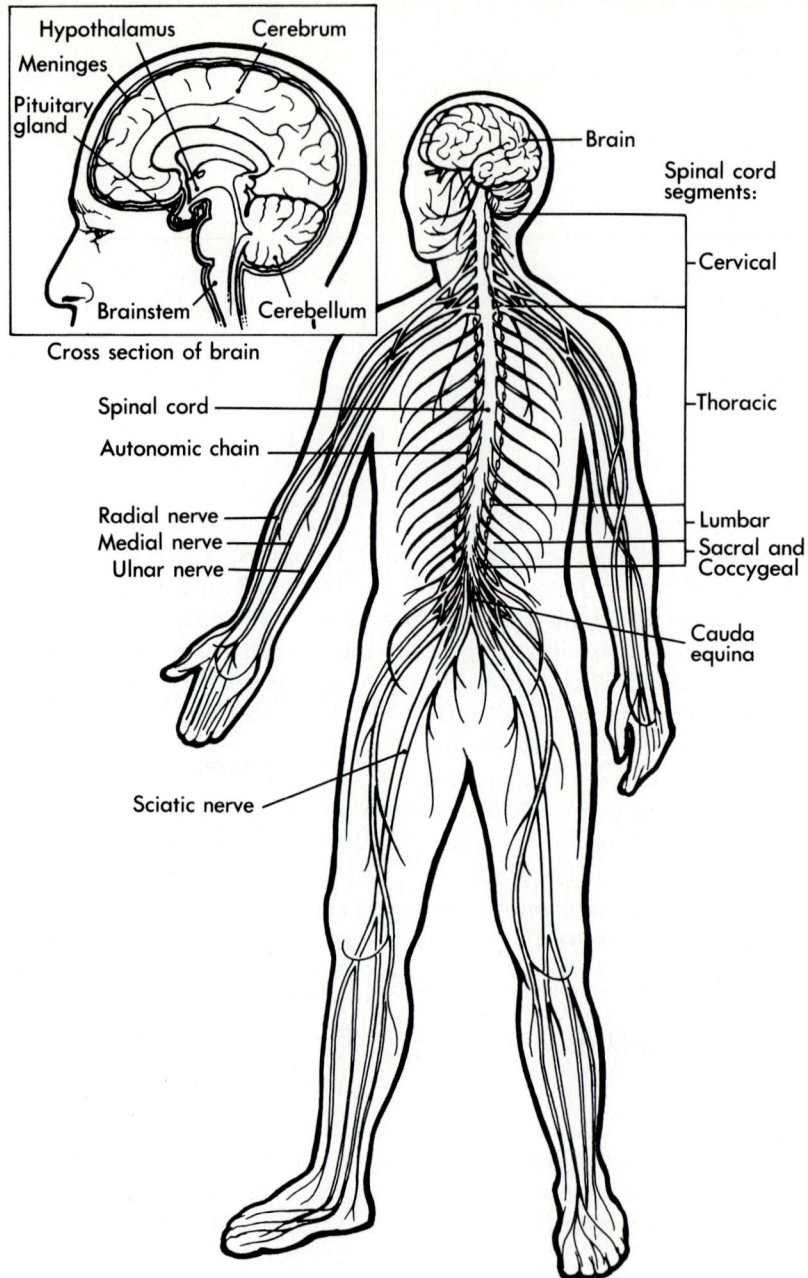

FIGURE 4-1 Nervous system.

Objective
Nature and duration of seizure if observed (Table 4-3)
Observed behavior before seizure—signs of stress or fatigue
Side effects of medications

Nursing Diagnoses
Common diagnoses include the following:
Potential for injury related to loss of consciousness and tonic clonic muscle movements

Knowledge deficit related to seizure management and control of drug side effects
Self-esteem disturbance related to socially stigmatizing aspects of seizures
Ineffective individual coping related to the diagnosis of epilepsy and its treatment restrictions
Potential for aspiration related to the glottal obstruction and loss of consciousness occurring during grand mal seizure

TABLE 4-1 Common types of seizures

Type	Characteristics
I. Generalized	Bilaterally symmetrical, with no local onset

A. Grand mal	Most common and dramatic type of seizure
	Progression:
	  1. Aura—change in sensation or affect that precedes seizure and occurs in about 50% of all patients; may include numbness, odors, lights, dizziness
	  2. Cry—caused by spasms of thorax expelling air through glottis or abrupt inspiratory effort
	  3. Loss of consciousness—sudden and profound, and variable in duration (usually several minutes)
	  4. Fixed dilated pupils
	  5. Tonic clonic contractions—immediate bilateral tonic contraction with cessation of respiration and cyanosis, followed by clonic rhythmic contractions of increasing strength and return of shallow respiration; urinary and fecal incontinence may occur
	  6. Postictal condition—patient experiences partial return of consciousness to a groggy confused state; headache, muscle pain, and need for deep sleep frequently follow, and general fatigue may persist for 1 to 2 days

B. Petit mal	Most common during childhood
	Progression:
	  1. Sudden impairment of or loss of consciousness with little or no motor movement.
	  2. Sudden vacant facial expression with eyes focused straight ahead
	  3. Duration is usually not more than 10 to 20 seconds, but may occur many times in a day

C. Status epilepticus	When recurrent generalized seizure activity occurs at such frequency that full consciousness is not regained between episodes:
	  1. It can lead to death from brain damage secondary to hypoxia and requires intensive care
	  2. The patient is usually in a coma for 12 to 24 hr or more

II. Partial seizures	Have a localized onset

A. Psychomotor—
    Temporal lobe
    Complex partial
	Complex seizures may occur at any age
	  1. Sudden change in awareness or consciousness—patient may have complex hallucination aura.
	  2. Patient may behave as if partially conscious or intoxicated and engage in antisocial behavior such as exposing self or perform repetitive meaningless acts such as buttoning and unbuttoning.
	  3. Patient may have autonomic complaints—chest pain, dyspnea, etc.
	  4. End of seizure—patient may be confused, amnesiac, and groggy.
	  5. Duration of seizure is much longer than petit mal

B. Focal seizures
    Jacksonian
	Arise in any localized motor or sensory portion of cortex
	  1. Symptoms depend on site of occurrence; limited almost exclusively to patients with structural brain disease
	  2. Progressive involvement of adjacent motor or sensory areas may occur
	  3. Consciousness is usually maintained unless seizure progresses to full grand mal seizure

TABLE 4-2 Drugs used to prevent seizures

Drug	Seizure Type	Toxic Effects
Phenytoin sodium (Dilantin)	Grand mal, focal, psychomotor	Ataxia, vomiting, nystagmus, drowsiness, rash, fever, gum hypertrophy, lymphadenopathy
Phenobarbital (Luminal)	Grand mal, focal, psychomotor	Drowsiness, rash
Primidone (Mysoline)	Grand mal, focal, psychomotor	Drowsiness, ataxia
Mephenytoin (Mesantoin)	Grand mal, focal, psychomotor	Ataxia, nystagmus, pancytopenia, rash
Ethosuximide (Zarontin)	Petit mal, psychomotor, myoclonic, akinetic	Drowsiness, nausea, agranulocytosis
Trimethadione (Tridione)	Petit mal	Rash, photophobia, agranulocytosis, nephrosis
Diazepam (Valium)	Status epilepticus, mixed	Drowsiness, ataxia
Carbamazepine (Tegretol)	Grand mal, psychomotor	Rash, drowsiness, ataxia
Valproic acid (Depakene)	Petit mal	Nausea, vomiting, indigestion, sedation, emotional disturbance, weakness, altered blood coagulation
Clonazepam (Clonopin)	Petit mal	Drowsiness, ataxia, hypotension, respiratory depression

Modified from Phipps WJ, Long BC, and Woods NF: Medical-surgical nursing: concepts and clinical practice, ed 4, St Louis, 1990, Mosby–Year Book, Inc.

Expected Outcomes

Patient will not experience injury during seizures.

Patient will be knowledgeable about medications and life-style adaptations related to seizure management.

Patient will maintain self-esteem and fulfill developmental tasks appropriate to age group.

Patient will successfully incorporate treatment limitations into preferred life-style.

Patient will maintain a patent airway and adequate oxygenation during seizure.

Nursing Interventions

Employ seizure precautions for any patient with seizure history:

Keep padded tongue blade or oral airway at bedside.

Use padded side rails. Avoid use of soft pillows because of risk of suffocation.

Supervise ambulation.

Ensure prompt access to oxygen, suction, and anticonvulsant medications.

Protect patient from injury. The box on this page outlines specific nursing interventions during a seizure.

Record nature and progression of seizure (see Table 4-3).

Encourage patient to verbalize feelings about diagnosis and problems encountered in social settings.

TABLE 4-3 Observations to be made about a person having a seizure

Aura	Presence or absence; nature if present; ability of patient to describe it (somatic, visceral, psychic)
Cry	Presence or absence
Onset	Site of initial body movements; deviation of head and eyes; chewing and salivation; posture of body; sensory changes
Tonic and clonic phases	Movements of body as to progression; skin color and airway; pupillary changes; incontinence; duration of each phase
Relaxation (sleep)	Duration and behavior
Postictal phase	Duration; general behavior; ability to remember anything about the seizure; orientation; pupillary changes; headache; injuries present
Duration of entire seizure	Measure by clock
Level of consciousness	Length of unconsciousness if present

From Phipps WJ, Long BC, and Woods NF: Medical-surgical nursing: concepts and clinical practice, ed 4, St Louis, 1990, Mosby–Year Book, Inc.

NURSING CARE DURING A SEIZURE

Never leave patient alone during seizure.

If patient is upright, lower to bed or floor and clear immediate environment to prevent injury.

Loosen constrictive clothing, especially around the neck.

Position patient: turn head to side if feasible to help keep airway open.

Cushion head.

Provide privacy.

No effort should be made to restrain the individual during the seizure.

A padded tongue blade or oral airway may be inserted between the back teeth to protect tongue and mouth if jaws are not already clenched. *Never attempt to pry open the mouth once jaws are clenched.*

Record sequence and progression of seizure accurately.

Gently reorient patient at end of seizure, and provide for postictal rest and sleep.

Teach patient about prescribed medications and expected side effects.

Encourage good mouth care, particularly if patient is receiving Dilantin.

Encourage patient to follow guidelines for a healthy life-style:

Nutritious diet

Balance of rest and activity

Avoidance of alcohol and acute stress, which frequently trigger seizures

Discuss restrictions on employment, driving, and leisure mandated by seizure activity.

Drivers license may usually be obtained after one seizure-free year.

Stress the importance of ongoing adherence to the medication regimen.

Encourage the patient to live as normal a life-style as possible.

Encourage patient and family to make contact with local epilepsy society for support.

Evaluation

Patient is free of physical injury related to seizures.

Patient maintains a patent airway and adequate oxygenation during seizures.

Patient and family can discuss prescribed medications, side effects, and life-style modifications that will enhance seizure control.

Patient maintains a life-style appropriate for age and speaks positively of self.

Patient expresses commitment to the treatment regimen and desire to gain control of seizures.

Patient successfully copes with social problems related to seizures and treatment regimen.

PARKINSON'S DISEASE

Parkinson's disease is one of the more common diseases of the nervous system and typically affects individuals in the late middle years (50 to 60 years of age). It involves a classic cluster of symptoms whose cause is usually unknown, but it can be induced by certain drugs, arteriosclerosis, and viral diseases. There is no known cure.

PATHOPHYSIOLOGY

The pathophysiologic process involves depigmentation of the substantia nigra of the basal ganglia with substantial loss of neurons. Selective depletion of dopamine occurs that can be correlated with striatal degeneration. Without dopamine (a neurotransmitter essential for proper muscle movement) there is a loss of inhibiting influence and excitatory mechanisms are unopposed. The result is impairment in the centers of coordination, in control of muscle tone, and in the control of the initiation and inhibition of movements.

MEDICAL MANAGEMENT

Care of parkinsonism is basically palliative and involves treating symptoms and providing support. Drug therapy is the cornerstone of medical care and includes the following:

Dopamine precursor drugs (levodopa) to restore striatal dopamine

Anticholinergic drugs (Artane, Cogenten, and Akineton) to lessen muscle rigidity

Antiviral agents that have antiparkinsonian activity (Symmetrol) by allowing the accumulation of dopamine at synaptic sites

Combination of levodopa and carbidopa, a drug limiting the peripheral metabolism of levodopa (Sinemet)

Drug therapy is supplemented by appropriate diet and exercise prescriptions. In certain cases medical management may be supplemented by stereotactic surgery that involves local destruction of portions of the globus pallidus or thalamus to relieve rigidity. Experimental adrenal medullary transplant is also performed in the hope of restoring dopamine balance.

NURSING MANAGEMENT

Assessment

Subjective

History and course of the disease

Patient's knowledge of disease process, medication and side effects

Patient's awareness that symptoms worsen with stress or fatigue

Patient's complaints of fatigue, incoordination

Defects in judgment and emotional instability

Objective

Presence of "classic triad" of symptoms:

Tremor (pill-rolling type—more prominent at rest)

Rigidity (jerky movements)

Muscle weakness with bradykinesia (slow or retarded movements)

Loss of postural reflexes

Absence of automatic associated body movements—stooped posture, deadpan expression, shuffling gait (may be propulsive), difficulty initiating movement, drooling saliva

Signs of complications—dysphagia, constipation, movement "freezing," incontinence, general debilitation, depression

General nutritional status

Elimination patterns and control

Nursing Diagnoses

Diagnoses associated with parkinsonism will vary depending on the stage of disease and severity of symptoms. Common diagnoses include the following:

Constipation related to decreased mobility and reduced food and fluid intake

Pain and soreness related to chronic muscle flexion and rigidity

Impaired physical mobility related to muscle rigidity and bradykinesia

Self-care deficit in feeding, bathing/hygiene, dressing/grooming, and toileting related to muscle rigidity and bradykinesia

Altered nutrition: less than body requirements related to dysphagia

Knowledge deficit related to medications and activities that will promote muscle function and control symptoms

Impaired verbal communication related to rigid facial muscles and decreased voice volume

Potential for injury related to posture defects, muscle rigidity, and propulsive gait

Potential for social isolation related to impaired mobility, communication disorders, and lack of affect

Expected Outcomes

Patient will maintain sufficient muscle strength and flexibility to remain independent in activities of daily living.

Patient will maintain a regular pattern of bowel elimination.

Patient will experience minimal discomfort from sore muscles.

Patient will eat a diet that maintains appropriate weight and meets body's baseline nutritional needs.

Patient and family will be knowledgeable about prescribed medications and their side effects as well as exercises and activities to decrease symptoms.

Patient will be able to communicate verbally and maintain active social interaction.

Patient will not experience injury related to disease symptoms.

Nursing Interventions: Rigidity

Administer medications as prescribed; teach about side effects (nausea, hypotension, palpitations, arrhythmias, confusion, and hallucinations are all common effects of dopaminergic drugs).

Promote regular exercise and ambulation, particularly muscle stretching. Consult physical therapist for exercise prescription and gait training.

Explore use of hot packs and massage to relieve stiffness.

Encourage active or passive range of motion every 4 hours.

Encourage patient to hold hands behind back to improve gait and posture.

Encourage patient to rest on firm mattress and lie prone at intervals to support full extension of all joints.

Nursing Interventions: Bradykinesia

Teach patient to use upright straight chair—raising back chair legs on blocks makes it easier to get up.

Remove scatter rugs and clutter furniture—encourage family to install hand rails and other safety devices.

Suggest that patient modify clothing with wide zippers or Velcro closures as needed to remain independent.

Encourage family to allow sufficient time for all activities so patient can remain independent and not feel rushed.

Encourage patient to change positions frequently and remain active to avoid freeze ups and prevent immobility-related complications.

Nursing Interventions: Nutrition

Plan nutritious meals high in roughage, easily chewed.
Cut all food into safe sizes.
Keep fluid intake high.

Provide smaller, more frequent meals to prevent exhaustion.

Allow sufficient time for eating. Do not attempt to hurry patient.

Monitor weight.

Nursing Interventions: Communication

Allow enough time and be patient.

Listen carefully. Encourage patient to speak aloud.

Encourage patient to do breathing and vocal exercises to exercise diaphragm and increase voice volume and strength.

Evaluation

Patient engages in regular planned exercise and has sufficient strength and flexibility to remain independent in activities of daily living.

Patient maintains regular bowel elimination.

Patient expresses absence of pain.

Patient maintains desired weight.

Patient and family are knowledgeable about disease, complications, medications and side effects, and plan of treatment.

Patient communicates verbally and maintains social contacts and interactions.

Patient and family plan together for home modifications to increase safety.

MULTIPLE SCLEROSIS

Multiple sclerosis is a degenerative disease that occurs primarily in northern temperate climates and typically affects young adults between the ages of 20 and 40. The disease usually follows a downhill course toward progressive disability over a period of about 20 years. Some evidence of a familial pattern exists.

PATHOPHYSIOLOGY

Despite significant research, the cause of multiple sclerosis remains unknown, although viruses and autoimmunity are believed to play a significant role. Multiple sclerosis produces random patches of demyelination of the white matter of the spinal cord and brain, which causes interruption or distortion of impulses so that they are slowed or blocked. Partial healing appears to take place early in the disease, which partially accounts for the early transitory symptoms. In late stages the degeneration extends into the gray matter and is irreversible. It follows a pattern of exacerbation and remission and, because of the widespread distribution of degeneration, produces a wider range of symptoms than any other neurological disease.

MEDICAL MANAGEMENT

There is no definitive diagnosis or treatment for multiple sclerosis. Diagnosis is often a matter of clinical judgment. Treatment is directed at symptom management, and although adrenocorticotropic hormone (ACTH) and high-dose steroids are widely used, their effectiveness remains controversial. Physical therapy is used to strengthen muscles, and patient education and support are directed at the maintenance of optimal health.

NURSING MANAGEMENT

Assessment
Subjective
History and course of the disease (early symptoms are usually transitory)

Patient's knowledge of disease process, treatment, and medication

Patient's complaints of weakness, numbness, fatigue, double vision, spots before eyes

Patient's response to chronic progressive nature of the disease

Objective

Bowel or bladder problems—frequency, urgency, incontinence

Presence of tremor, muscle spasm, spastic ataxia, loss of coordination

Nystagmus (rapid oscillation of eyeballs), speech disorders (scanning speech)

Behavior patterns, including euphoria or depression and crying spells

Nursing Diagnosis

Diagnoses associated with multiple sclerosis are highly variable depending on the individual patient's symptoms and stage of the disease. Common diagnoses include the following:

Activity intolerance related to generalized weakness

Constipation or incontinence related to interruption of motor impulses

Altered patterns of urinary elimination or stress incontinence related to irregular nervous stimulation

Impaired physical mobility related to tremor, muscle spasticity, and incoordination

Feeding, bathing/hygiene, dressing/grooming, and toileting self-care deficit related to muscle weakness, spasticity, and incoordination

Sensory perceptual alteration (visual) related to interruption of optic nerve pathways

Self-esteem disturbance related to impaired mobility and loss of control over self-care

Ineffective individual or family coping related to the chronic progressive nature of the disease

Expected Outcomes

Patient will remain involved in usual occupational, family, and recreational activities.

Patient will maintain control over bowel and bladder function.

Patient will maintain sufficient muscular function and control to remain independent in the activities of daily living.

Patient will not be injured during periods of disordered vision.

Patient will maintain a positive sense of self through continued involvement in family and occupational activities.

Patient and family will work together to cope effectively with condition and plan for the future.

Nursing Interventions

Administer prescribed medications; teach patient and family about drugs and side effects.

Mobility

Stretching and range of motion exercises every shift; provide gait training.

Encourage ambulation; teach use of assistive devices as indicated. Suggest use of eye patch if diplopia exists.

Encourage activity but avoid overfatigue.

Teach patient and family the importance of frequent position changes, use of foam mattresses, and other general measures to prevent immobility-related complications.

Good general health. Good general health is thought to decrease the likelihood of exacerbations

Teach patient to eat nutritious high-protein diet and take supplemental vitamins.

Encourage patient to balance rest and activity and avoid fatigue.

Encourage patient to avoid hot baths and extremes of heat and cold, which increase weakness.

Teach patient to avoid exposure to infection and treat all infection immediately.

Elimination

Teach patient the symptoms of urinary tract infection.

Teach patient to acidify the urine and keep the daily fluid intake high.

Explore the use of antispasmodics if urinary urgency occurs.

Follow intermittent catheterization program or bladder retraining program if incontinent.

Protect patient against soiling, leaking, and skin breakdown.

Initiate bowel program with stool softeners and suppositories.

Adjustment

Encourage patient to verbalize feelings and concerns.

Calmly assist patient and family to control and deal with mood swings.

Refer patient to support groups in community and services of the National Multiple Sclerosis Society.

Teach patient to follow a health-promoting life style that helps to limit the frequency of disease exacerbations.

Evaluation

Patient will follow a bowel and bladder program that supports regular elimination and a minimum number of accidents.

Patient maintains self-care independence, engages in

TABLE 4-4 Other degenerative disorders of the nervous system

Disorder	Description	Signs and Symptoms	Management
Myasthenia gravis	Disease affecting young adults in which nerve impulses fail to pass the myoneural junction to the muscle from: Inadequate secretion of acetylcholine Excessive amounts of cholinesterase Nonresponse of muscle fibers	Muscle weakness, generalized severe fatigue of rapid onset that disappears with rest. Primarily affects head, neck, and upper body: Weakness in arm and hand Drooping facial muscles, ptosis, diplopia Difficulty in chewing or swallowing Weakness or failure of muscles of respiration	Administration of anticholinesterase drugs—neostigmine (Prostigmin), pyridostigmine (Mestinon)—in rigid, carefully spaced schedules to block destruction of acetylcholine Life-style with a balance of rest and activity—spacing activities and maintenance of optimal health
Amyotrophic lateral sclerosis (ALS, or Lou Gehrig's disease)	Motor neuron disease in which myelin sheaths are replaced by scar tissue; affects nerves in brain, spinal cord, or both, distorting or blocking impulses	Early signs are fatigue, awkwardness, and dysphagia. Progresses to muscle weakness, atrophy, tremor, and spasticity of flexor muscles. No sensory loss occurs. Death is frequently from respiratory failure, usually within 5 years. Patient remains alert.	Treatment is aimed at relieving symptoms: Assistance with daily activities Prosthesis or assistive devices for weakened muscles Feeding tubes to maintain nutrition Emotional support
Alzheimer's disease	Cells of brain show plaque deposits and disruption of neurofibrils, which causes impairment of intellectual functioning	Stage 1—mild mental impairment, forgetfulness, impairment of judgment Stage 2—confusion, irritation, restlessness, fecal and urinary incontinence Stage 3—complete incapacity with inability to care for self	No available treatment Nursing measures aimed at maintaining good general health, environmental safety, and continence Supportive help for family

regular range of motion exercise, and ambulates effectively with assistive devices.

Patient modifies environment and visual stimuli appropriately to maintain safe, independent ambulation.

Patient maintains stable weight, plans and eats nutritious meals, and is free of frequent infection.

Patient and family verbalize their fears and concerns about the future and work together for realistic planning.

Table 4-4 presents basic information about less common degenerative neurologic disorders for which the care largely involves treating symptoms and providing support.

CEREBROVASCULAR ACCIDENT

Cerebrovascular accident (CVA) is the most common problem of the nervous system and is the third leading cause of death in the United States. The general term refers to disturbances in the cerebral circulation resulting from a thrombus/embolus (92%) or hemorrhage (8%). Clinically CVA refers to the sudden interruption of the blood supply to the brain that produces the dramatic development of focal neurologic deficits. Hemiplegia is the classic symptom. Some of the multiple specific causes of CVA are listed in the box on the next page.

PATHOPHYSIOLOGY

The brain has no reserve oxygen supply. Therefore any condition that alters perfusion can lead to cerebral hypoxia and rapid cell death. The effects seen are dependent on which cerebral vessels are involved, which areas of the brain are affected, and the adequacy of the collateral circulation to the area. Symptoms vary widely. The two vessels most frequently affected are the middle cerebral and internal carotid arteries. Cerebral edema often accompanies the hypoxia and worsens the initial defects.

Transient ischemic attacks (TIAs) occur when transient cerebral ischemia produces temporary episodes of neurologic dysfunction. They are a frequent precursor of thrombotic CVAs and are a warning of an underlying

CONDITIONS CAUSING CVA

THROMBUS

Atherosclerosis in intracranial and extracranial arteries
Adjacency to intracerebral hemorrhage
Arteritis caused by collagen (autoimmune) disease or bacterial arteritis
Hypercoagulability such as in polycythemia
Cerebral venous thromboses

EMBOLI

Valves damaged by rheumatic heart disease
Myocardial infarction
Atrial fibrillation (this arrhythmia causes variable emptying of left ventricle. Blood pools and small clots form, and then at times the ventricle will be emptied completely with release of small emboli)
Bacterial endocarditis and nonbacterial endocarditis causing clots to form on endocardium

HEMORRHAGE

Hypertensive intracerebral hemorrhage
Subarachnoid hemorrhage
Rupture of aneurysm
Arteriovenous malformation
Hypocoagulation (as in patients with blood dyscrasias)

GENERALIZED HYPOXIA

Severe hypotension, cardiopulmonary arrest, or severe depression in cardiac output caused by arrhythmias

LOCALIZED HYPOXIA

Cerebral artery spasms associated with subarachnoid hemorrhage
Cerebral artery vasoconstriction associated with migraine headaches

From Phipps WJ, Long BC, and Woods NF: Medical-surgical nursing: concepts and clinical practice, ed. 4, St Louis, 1990, Mosby–Year Book, Inc.

pathologic condition. Information about TIAs is presented in the box on this page.

MEDICAL MANAGEMENT

Patients with thrombotic strokes may be given anticoagulants or vasodilators to prevent further damage. Surgical intervention through carotid endarterectomy may be indicated in selected patients. Research protocols are testing reperfusion techniques using tissue plasminogen activator in a few settings. After a brief initial period of bedrest and stabilization the patient moves to active rehabilitation.

Patients with hemorrhagic strokes are initially placed on absolute bed rest to prevent additional bleeding. Meticulous monitoring of vital functions is necessary until their condition stabilizes. Surgery may be attempted if an aneurysm is the cause of the bleeding. Patients will gradually begin active rehabilitation.

TRANSIENT ISCHEMIC ATTACKS (TIAS)

DEFINITION

Transient episodes of reversible cerebral ischemia accompanied by temporary occurrences of neurologic dysfunction

CAUSE

May be produced by any of the conditions that cause CVA. Most commonly they precede a thrombotic stroke and may result from vessel spasm. Attacks may occur many times over the course of weeks or months or years. They warn of an underlying pathologic condition.

SYMPTOMS

Focal deficits are quite varied depending on the site of ischemia. The more common deficits include the following:
One-sided weakness of the lower face, hands and fingers, arm, or leg
Transient dysphasia
Some sensory impairment
Moment of clumsiness or incoordination

TREATMENT

Resolve associated risk factors and health conditions.
Vasodilators, anticoagulants, and aspirin may be used to decrease platelet aggregation and prevent clotting.
Surgical correction may be needed if cause is an isolated extracranial lesion.

NURSING MANAGEMENT

Assessment
Subjective
Onset and sequence of symptoms
Coexisting health problems
History of TIAs
Patient's complaints of headaches and sensory disturbances: visual, touch, hearing
Emotional response of patient and family
Patient's and family's understanding of symptoms and diagnosis
Objective
Level of consciousness—general thinking ability
Vital signs
Presence of motor deficits—hemiparesis or hemiplegia
Presence of expressive or receptive aphasia or dysarthria
Bowel and bladder function
Signs of increased intracranial pressure (see box on page 60)
Seizure activity

Nursing Diagnoses
Diagnoses will be variable dependent on the precipitating cause and degree of severity of the CVA. Common

NURSING CARE PLAN

CEREBROVASCULAR ACCIDENT

Nursing Diagnoses	Expected Patient Outcomes	Nursing Interventions
Altered tissue perfusion (cerebral) related to vascular thromboses or hemorrhage	Patient will experience increased blood flow to the brain and will not develop further damage.	1. Assess vital signs and level of consciousness at frequent intervals during first 2 days; be alert to signs of rising intracranial pressure. 2. Position patient to maintain patent airway and administer prescribed oxygen. 3. Maintain fluid intake at prescribed level; avoid overhydration which may lead to cerebral edema. 4. Give prescribed medications to prevent further cerebral thrombosis, hemorrhage or edema or to prevent seizures. 5. Provide rest and a quiet environment initially.
Potential for injury related to diminished or absent protective reflexes	Patient's eyes remain moist and unscratched. Patient's lung fields are clear to auscultation. Patient's swallowing ability is intact.	1. Assess for intactness of blink reflex and adequacy of lid closure. If needed, keep eyes moist with artificial tears and covered with eye patch. Inspect eyes for infection or irritation every 2 to 4 hours. 2. Assess intactness of swallowing and gag reflexes. 3. Avoid oral food or fluid if not intact. Position to support drainage of saliva. Keep suction apparatus at bedside.
Potential impairment of skin integrity related to decreased mobility	Patient's skin remains intact.	1. Monitor skin for signs of breakdown. 2. Use turning sheet when changing patient's position every 2 hours to prevent shearing effect on skin. 3. Encourage patient to assist in turning self as able. 4. Use foam mattresses, heel protectors, or other devices to prevent pressure sores. 5. Keep perineal skin clean and dry. 6. If patient is incontinent, monitor frequently and keep bed pads clean and dry at all times; wash and dry perineal area as needed.
Altered nutrition: less than body requirements related to decreased swallowing and self-care abilities	Patient takes in required nutrients and maintains stable weight.	1. Provide intravenous fluids and tube feedings as prescribed during initial period. 2. Assess ability to swallow before initiating oral feedings. 3. Position patient with head elevated and turned to unaffected side when feeding patient. 4. Provide foods initially that are easier to swallow (soft or pureed foods, except for mashed potatoes). Avoid clear liquids. 5. Place food in unaffected side of mouth. 6. Cleanse mouth after eating to remove retained food particles. Teach patient to use tongue to clear food from paralyzed side of mouth. 7. Be patient when feeding patient and provide directions for swallowing, as needed. 8. Encourage patient to chew food thoroughly. Remind patient to tilt head forward to facilitate swallowing. 9. Ensure adequate hydration if patient is having swallowing difficulties.

NURSING CARE PLAN

CEREBROVASCULAR ACCIDENT—cont'd

Nursing Diagnoses	Expected Patient Outcomes	Nursing Interventions
Altered nutrition—cont'd		5. Place food in unaffected side of mouth. 6. Cleanse mouth after eating to remove retained food particles. Teach patient to use tongue to clear food from paralyzed side of mouth. 7. Be patient when feeding patient and provide directions for swallowing, as needed. 8. Encourage patient to chew food thoroughly. Remind patient to tilt head forward to facilitate swallowing. 9. Ensure adequate hydration if patient is having swallowing difficulties. 10. Encourage patient to feed self as soon as able; provide self-help devices as necessary. 11. Assess food/fluid intake and offer supplementary feedings as needed.
Impaired physical mobility related to muscle weakness or paralysis	Patient maintains adequate muscle tone and achieves maximal independence in ambulation.	1. Emphasize full extension of joints in positioning. 2. Change positions at least every 2 hours. 3. Teach patient how to sit up on side of bed and to transfer to chair when permitted. 4. Support activities initiated by physical therapy. 5. Consider use of sling to prevent shoulder subluxation when ambulating. 6. Provide good shoe support for transfer and ambulation.
Self-care deficit in hygiene, dressing, and grooming related to muscle weakness and paralysis	Patient achieves independence in the activities of daily living.	1. Provide basic needs for activities of daily living as necessary during initial period, but encourage patient to begin to participate at ability level. 2. Transfer all self-care activities to unaffected side. 3. Provide sufficient time for activities of daily living. 4. Meet with physical therapist and occupational therapist to optimize patient's learning needs. 5. Facilitate use of self-help devices, as needed.
Functional incontinence related to disruption of normal voluntary control	Patient will achieve urinary continence.	1. Monitor urinary output and signs of retention or incontinence. 2. Reassure patient that reestablishing continence is a reasonable goal. 3. Provide catheter care if Foley catheter is used. 4. Offer bedpan or urinal after meals and at regular intervals. 5. Provide fluids to maximum amount prescribed; provide greater amounts before 4:00 PM. 6. Use disposable pads or external urinary system as indicated. 7. Teach patient symptoms of UTI and the importance of adequate fluids and acidifying the urine.

Continued.

Clinical Manual of Medical-Surgical Nursing

NURSING CARE PLAN

CEREBROVASCULAR ACCIDENT—cont'd

Nursing Diagnoses	Expected Patient Outcomes	Nursing Interventions
Impaired verbal communication related to expressive or receptive aphasia	Patient will successfully communicate with staff and family.	1. Speak slowly and distinctly. 2. Phrase questions that can be answered by yes or no (or by appropriate signals). 3. Try to anticipate patient needs. 4. Provide call signal within reach of unaffected hand. 5. Begin speech therapy as soon as possible. 6. Encourage patient to verbalize and practice speech. 7. Allow sufficient time for patient to respond. 8. Teach family about disorder and the importance of not "speaking for" the patient.
Sensory perceptual alteration (visual, kinesthetic) related to cerebral hypoxia	Patient will gradually compensate for sensory perceptual deficits.	1. Place patient in multibed environment. 2. Suggest family bring some familiar objects, such as pictures. Keep objects within patient's visual field. 3. Place patient's bed so that people approach from side of intact vision. 4. Teach patient to scan the environment to increase visual fields. 5. Use mirror to teach posture corrections.
Potential for ineffective individual and family coping related to the physical and mental changes from the CVA	Patient and family will adjust to the residual disabilities and make appropriate plans for care after discharge.	1. Provide information about condition and probable progress toward increased function. 2. Explain that emotional lability is part of the disorder and that improvement will be noted. 3. Explain patient's behavior to family/friends and encourage them to visit and interact with patient. 4. Give family/friends opportunities to share their concerns to be more supportive of patient. 5. Encourage family to maintain previous role relationships, as possible. 6. Teach family to support patient's efforts at independence and encourage involvement in outside world. 7. Explore need for assistance from community services.

diagnoses encountered in the thrombotic stroke patient during the rehabilitation phase include:

Impaired physical mobility related to hemiplegia

Feeding, bathing/hygiene, dressing/grooming, or toileting self-care deficit related to hemiplegia and altered thought processes

Impaired verbal communication related to expressive or receptive aphasia

Constipation or bowel incontinence related to interruption of voluntary motor control

Urinary retention or reflex incontinence related to interruption of voluntary motor control

Sensory/perceptual alteration (visual or kinesthetic) related to cerebral hypoxia

Alteration in thought processes related to cerebral hypoxia

Potential for ineffective individual and family coping related to the physical and mental changes resulting from the CVA

Potential for injury related to decreased reflexes and altered sensory input

Expected Outcomes (for Rehabilitative Phase)

Patient will regain independence in the activities of daily living.

Patient will ambulate independently using appropriate assistive devices.

Patient will successfully communicate needs to nursing staff and family.

Patient will reestablish a normal pattern of bowel and bladder elimination and be free of incontinence.

Patient will learn to compensate for sensory perceptual deficits and function safely in the environment.

Patient will participate in decision making and not experience significant mood disorder.

Patient and family will adjust to nature of residual disabilities and plan appropriately for postdischarge care.

Nursing Interventions: Acute Phase

Maintain an open airway:

Keep patient in side-lying position.

Use oral airway and have suction ready for use if needed.

Initiate regular deep breathing. Encourage gentle coughing only as needed to keep airway clear.

Assess and record vital signs and level of consciousness, and do neurologic checks frequently.

Monitor fluid balance accurately:

Keep careful records of intake and output.

Regulate IV carefully. Do not overhydrate.

Maintain fluid intake at 1000 ml/day if ordered.

Turn and position every 2 hours. Promote rest and quiet.

Administer passive range of motion exercises each shift.

Examine and massage skin every 2 hours:

Keep skin clean and dry.

Use pressure relief devices and mattresses.

Apply TED stockings.

Begin oral feedings as ordered:

Put patient in high Fowler's position.

Check for intactness of gag reflex.

Avoid liquids. Offer soft, easily chewed foods.

Record bowel elimination. Institute use of stool softeners and suppositories as needed.

Avoid prolonged use of Foley catheter. Increase fluids as allowed, and offer use of bedpan/urinal frequently.

Support patient and family. Establish effective means of communication.

NOTE: These same basic interventions are appropriate for patients experiencing decreased consciousness from other causes.

Nursing Interventions: Rehabilitative Phase

Mobility:

Implement exercise program designed by physical therapy department. Emphasize full extension of joints and good alignment.

Initiate balance exercise at bedside.

Teach technique for safe transfer to wheelchair or toilet.

Teach use of assistive device for ambulation.

Explore need for sling to prevent shoulder subluxation.

Assist patient to shift self-care activities to unaffected side.

Nutrition:

Teach patient to use unaffected side for feeding.

Provide self-help devices such as rocker knife and plate guards.

Increase fluids and roughage as swallowing improves.

Remind patient to empty and clean paralyzed side of mouth after meals.

Elimination: continue bowel and bladder retraining programs.

Communication:

Establish nature, extent of communication disorder.

BASIC TYPES OF APHASIA

Motor (Expressive): Patient is unable to use the symbols of speech to speak or write words. Muscles of speech are not paralyzed.

Sensory (Receptive): Patient is unable to comprehend the spoken or written word.

Global aphasia: Both motor and sensory problems are present at the same time.

Dysarthria: Weakness in the muscles of speech creates difficulties in pronouncing words or swallowing.

NURSING INTERVENTIONS FOR APHASIA

GENERAL

Establish a relaxed environment.
Encourage persistence and the desire to communicate.
Control and limit the amount of stimuli in environment.

SENSORY (RECEPTIVE)

Sit down and establish eye contact.
Face patient and speak simply and slowly.
Reword the message if misunderstood.
Use appropriate gestures to supplement words.
Allow sufficient time for patient to process words.
Use a normal tone of voice.

MOTOR (EXPRESSIVE)

Avoid interrupting and rushing patient.
Emphasize simple concrete words used for daily care.
Discuss topics of interest to patient.
Encourage use of other means of communication.
Convey acceptance and encourage patient to talk.
Don't speak for the patient.
Keep practice sessions short. Avoid fatigue.

Work with speech therapy department to plan appropriate therapy.
Apply basic principles for aphasic patients (see boxes above and on preceding page).
Share appropriate techniques with family.
Psychological:
Be alert to spatial perceptual difficulties associated with right hemisphere stroke. Patient may have trouble judging position and distance. (See boxes on this page.)
Assist patient to reestablish control over emotion and behavior and set limits.
Assist family to assess patient's capabilities and plan for postdischarge care.
Initiate referrals to appropriate community agencies.

Evaluation

Patient has adapted self-care activities and is independent in the activities of daily living using appropriate self-help devices.
Patient can make safe transfers and ambulate with the use of assistive devices.
Patient is free of immobility-related complications.
Patient is able to communicate needs and desires successfully.
Patient has reestablished bowel and bladder control.
Patient is aware of sensory/perceptual deficits and practices methods to compensate for them.
Patient is able to solve problems effectively and experiences only mild mood swings.
Patient and family have discussed and planned appropriate postdischarge care.

SENSORY/PERCEPTUAL ALTERATIONS

Proprioception: ability to know the position of the body and its parts without looking
Dysesthesia/Paresthesia: abnormalities of touch sensation
Apraxia: inability to perform skilled purposeful movements in the absence of motor problems
Agnosia: inability to recognize objects through use of special senses
Hemianopsia: loss of selected portions of the visual fields

NURSING INTERVENTIONS FOR SENSORY/PERCEPTUAL ALTERATIONS

Keep familiar objects in the patient's environment.
Approach patients from the side of intact vision.
Teach patients to scan to increase their visual fields.
Provide full mirror to assist patient with posture and balance.
Remind patient to care for and protect affected side.
Be alert for incidence of impulsive behavior.

INFECTIONS OF CENTRAL NERVOUS SYSTEM

The nervous system may be attacked by a variety of organisms and viruses as well as suffer from toxic reactions to bacterial and viral disease. The meninges or the brain itself may be affected. If an infection becomes walled off, it may cause an abscess.

MENINGITIS

Meningitis is an acute infection of the meninges that may be caused by a variety of bacteria and viruses. Children are affected more often because of their frequent upper respiratory tract infections.

PATHOPHYSIOLOGY

Organisms that reach the brain disseminate quickly through the meninges and into the ventricles. This dissemination produces the following:
Congestion of the meningeal vessels
Edema of brain tissue
Increased intracranial pressure
Generalized inflammation with white blood cell exudate formation
Hydrocephalus if exudate blocks ventricular passages
Diagnosis is confirmed by the identification of the organism from the cerebrospinal fluid (CSF).

MEDICAL MANAGEMENT

Medical management consists of the following:
Massive doses of antibiotic specific for the causative organism

Steroids and osmotic diuretics if necessary to reduce cerebral edema

Anticonvulsants may be administered to prevent or control seizures

Respiratory isolation for 24 to 48 hours after antibiotics begin

NURSING MANAGEMENT

Assessment

Subjective

History of respiratory infection

History and severity of symptoms: headache, vomiting, stiff neck, fever

Objective

Vital signs (high fever)

Change in level of consciousness and orientation

Signs of meningeal irritation:

Positive Kernig's sign—inability to completely extend the legs without pain

Positive Brudzinski's sign—patient flexes hips and knees when neck is passively flexed

Nursing Diagnoses

Diagnoses will depend on the severity and stage of the disease. The patient initially may be critically ill and completely prostrated. Basic diagnoses include the following:

Pain related to pronounced headache and stiff neck

Fluid volume deficit related to losses from high fever

Potential for injury related to decreased cerebral tissue perfusion

Altered nutrition: less than body requirements, related to severe nausea and vomiting

Hyperthermia related to acute inflammatory response

Expected Outcomes

Patient will experience decreased pain.

Patient will maintain an adequate fluid balance.

Patient will not experience injury.

Patient's nutritional needs will be met and a stable weight will be maintained.

Patient's temperature will return to normal range.

Nursing Interventions

Administer prescribed medications and fluids.

Monitor accurate intake and output; assess skin turgor and mucous membranes.

Offer nutritious semiliquid diet as tolerated.

Keep room darkened; keep sensory stimuli to a minimum. Assess level of consciousness frequently.

Keep side rails up; do not abruptly move or jar patient.

Maintain accurate records of vital signs and neurological checks.

Maintain appropriate isolation procedures.

Observe for signs of inappropriate secretion of antidiuretic hormone (ADH) or diabetes insipidus.

Evaluation

Patient is comfortable and participates actively in self-care.

Patient is well hydrated and has an adequate urinary output.

Patient does not sustain injury or immobility-related complications.

Patient is normothermic.

Patient returns to normal diet and maintains a stable weight.

NOTE: Encephalitis, an inflammation of the brain tissue, is a relatively rare, very serious disease with a high mortality. Treatment is basically supportive and follows that generally outlined above.

HEAD TRAUMA

Craniocerebral trauma causes about 80,000 deaths yearly. It is the major cause of death in individuals aged 1 to 35, but causes death and serious disability in people of all ages. Table 4-5 describes the common types of brain injuries caused by head trauma. The degree of external damage is not necessarily indicative of the extent of brain injury, but compound and depressed skull fractures are associated with serious brain damage.

PATHOPHYSIOLOGY

Craniocerebral trauma may result in injury to the scalp, skull, and/or brain tissues. All head injuries create concern over rising intracranial pressure. The rigid skull leaves little room for expansion. Any alteration in brain mass, blood volume, CSF volume, or intracranial pressure can create hypoxia.

When the head receives a direct blow or injury, the brain moves in the skull and suffers damage of varying degrees, not all of which occurs at the site of direct injury. The brain swells abruptly after injury, and brain edema is a major cause of increased intracranial pressure. The box on the next page reviews the pathologic sequence that occurs as intracranial pressure rises.

MEDICAL MANAGEMENT

Management involves measures to identify and correct the underlying cause of increasing intracranial pressure and cerebral edema. These measures include the following:

Corticosteroids (dexamethasone) to reduce inflammation

Osmotic diuretics (mannitol or urea) to reduce cerebral edema

Fluid restriction and systemic diuretics (furosemide)

Anticonvulsants (Dilantin) to control seizures

TABLE 4-5 Damage of brain tissue due to trauma

Type of Injury	Characteristics	Structural Alteration	Effects
Concussion	Immediate and transitory impairment of neurologic function caused by the mechanical force	No	Possible loss of consciousness that may be instantaneous or delayed—usually is reversible.
Contusion	Likened to bruising with extravasation of blood cells	Yes	Injury may be at site of impact or at opposite site. Often cortex is damaged.
Laceration	Tearing of tissues caused by sharp fragment or a shearing force	Yes	Hemorrhage is a serious complication.
Intracranial hemorrhage	Bleeding into the epidural, subdural, subarachnoid spaces, or into the brain or ventricles	Yes	Effects depend on the site of injury and degree of bleeding
Epidural hematoma	Rupture of a large vessel that lies above the dura mater; tear is usually in an artery (middle meningeal is the most common site)		Signs of rising intracranial pressure develop rapidly with rapid deterioration into full coma.
Subdural hematoma	Usually results from venous bleeding below the dura mater; bleeding may produce acute, subacute, or chronic hematoma formation		Signs of rising intracranial pressure may develop within days, weeks, or even months after the injury.

PATHOLOGIC SEQUENCE OF INCREASING INTRACRANIAL PRESSURE

An increase in brain tissue, vascular tissue and volume, or CSF volume from any cause increases pressure within the cranial cavity. After the brain's compensatory mechanisms have been utilized, the following sequence occurs:

1. Cerebral blood flow decreases, resulting in inadequate perfusion.
2. Inadequate perfusion leads to increasing P_{CO_2} and decreasing P_{O_2} values.
3. Oxygenation changes trigger vasodilation and cerebral edema.
4. Edema further increases intracranial pressure, resulting in a downward spiral of tissue compression and displacement that may be irreversible and fatal.
5. Life-sustaining mechanisms for consciousness, blood pressure, pulse, respiration, and temperature regulation fail.

Barbiturates (Nembutal) to decrease pressure
Surgical repair of fracture or laceration
Airway management with endotracheal tube or tracheostomy
Ventricular puncture or drainage

NURSING MANAGEMENT

Assessment
Subjective
History of the trauma and sequence of symptoms
Patient's complaints of headache, double vision, nausea, or vomiting

SIGNS OF INCREASING INTRACRANIAL PRESSURE

1. Change in level of consciousness
   ALERT: One of the earliest and most sensitive signs of rising intracranial pressure is restlessness.
2. Pupillary signs
   Result from pressure on the oculomotor nerve
   Slower response, pupil inequality, or fixed dilated pupils
3. Blood pressure and pulse
   Increasing systolic pressure with stable or falling diastolic pressure
   Widening pulse pressure
   Slowing of the pulse rate from pressure on the vagus nerve
4. Respirations
   Changes are usually quite late
   Slowing of rate and an irregular breathing pattern
5. Temperature
   Failure of thermoregulatory center occurs late
   High uncontrolled temperature
6. Focal signs
   Muscle weakness or paralysis
   Decreasing response to pain stimulus in comatose patients
   Positive Babinski's sign
   Decerebrate or decorticate posture
7. Decreasing visual acuity; papilledema
8. Headache and vomiting (projectile)

Objective
Vital signs
Level of consciousness
Respiratory status
Signs of rising intracranial pressure (see box above)

Motor strength and equality
Speech difficulties
Bleeding or CSF drainage from ears or nose
Vomiting

Nursing Diagnoses

The diagnoses associated with head injury will depend on the severity and type of the injury. Common diagnoses include the following:

Alteration in cerebral tissue perfusion related to increased intracranial pressure
Alteration in thought processes related to decreasing level of consciousness
Impaired physical mobility related to decreasing level of consciousness and interruption of motor impulses
Potential for injury and infection related to decreasing level of consciousness and head trauma
Alteration in urinary and bowel elimination patterns related to interruption of motor control
Pain related to head trauma
Ineffective airway clearance related to increasing intracranial pressure

Expected Outcomes

Patient will not experience an undetected increase in intracranial pressure.
Patient will remain alert and appropriately oriented to the environment and treatment regimen.
Patient will not experience common complications of immobility during period of bed rest and treatment.
Patient will not experience environmental injury or develop preventable infection.
Patient will maintain regular patterns of urinary and bowel elimination.
Patient will experience manageable levels of discomfort.
Patient will maintain a clear airway for optimal oxygen and carbon dioxide exchange.

Nursing Interventions

Perform accurate neurological checks at frequent intervals including the following:
Vital signs
Level of consciousness using either Glasgow coma scale or hospital-developed continuum (see box at right)
Oculomotor nerve function
Motor and sensory status—hand grips, voluntary movement, sensation.
Administer medications as ordered to reduce or stabilize intracranial pressure.
Maintain bed rest with head of bed slightly elevated as ordered (15 to 30 degrees). Keep environmental stimuli to a minimum.

Use side rails and seizure precautions; avoid neck flexion or sudden movements.
Institute nursing measures or cooling blanket to control temperature. NOTE: Increased temperature dramatically increases brain's metabolic demands.
Observe for signs of hypoxia, such as cyanosis, color changes in nail beds and mucous membranes, restlessness, altered respiratory rate.
Monitor arterial blood gas results.
Observe for bloody or serous drainage from nose or ears.
ALERT: Drainage may indicate tearing of meninges and escape of CSF and precede meningitis. If present:
Do not clean, pack, or obstruct in any way.
Promote gravity drainage onto sterile towel or dressing.
Determine whether serous fluid is CSF or mucus (CSF tests positive for sugar and produces a halo when blotted and dried on gauze).
Change dressings frequently.

LEVEL OF CONSCIOUSNESS RATING SCALES

I. FIVE-POINT LEVEL OF CONSCIOUSNESS SCALE

1. Alert—normal mental activity, aware, mentally functional
2. Obtunded/Drowsy—sleepy, very short attention span, can respond appropriately if aroused.
3. Stupor—apathetic, slow moving, expression blank, staring; aroused only by vigorous stimuli.
4. Light coma—not oriented to time, place, or person. Aroused only by painful stimuli—response is only grunt or grimace or withdrawal from pain
5. Deep coma—no response except decerebrate or decorticate posture to even the most painful stimuli

II. GLASGOW COMA SCALE SCORING

Eyes open	4	spontaneously
	3	on request
	2	to pain stimuli
	1	no opening
Best verbal response	5	oriented to time, place, person
	4	confused but engages in conversation
	3	words spoken but no conversation
	2	incomprehensible sounds, groans
	1	no response
Best motor response	5	obeys commands
	4	localizes pain
	3	flexes either arm
	2	extension of arm to painful stimulus
	1	no response

NOTE: Scores in each category are totaled.

Administer antibiotics as ordered.

Do not suction through the nose.

Monitor intake and output carefully. Fluid intake may be restricted. Check specific gravity hourly. Diabetes insipidus increases urine output while inappropriate antidiuretic hormone (ADH) syndrome decreases it.

Employ bulk cathartics and stool softeners to prevent straining at elimination.

Teach patient to avoid coughing and sneezing if possible. Avoid all isometric contraction.

Institute standard nursing measures for passive range of motion, turning, skin care, and TED stockings to prevent complications of immobility.

Offer support to patient and family to deal with high-anxiety situation with uncertain outcome.

Test all secretions for blood. Administer antacids and cimetidine as ordered to prevent stress ulcers.

NOTE: Many individuals who experience minor head injury are sent home after the initial evaluation. The box below lists specific teaching instructions that should be provided to patients and families.

Evaluation

Patient is free of the effects of increased intracranial pressure.

Patient is alert and oriented and functions at pre-injury cognitive level.

Patient has optimal oxygen and carbon dioxide exchange.

Patient maintains full range of motion, recovers muscle strength, and maintains an intact skin.

Patient is free of injury.

TEACHING INSTRUCTIONS FOR HEAD INJURY PATIENTS AND FAMILIES

Patient should be awakened periodically through the first 24 hours to ensure patient is arousable.

During first 24 to 48 hours, patient and family should watch carefully for the following warning signs:
1. Vomiting—often with force behind it
2. Unusual sleepiness, dizziness, loss of balance, or falling
3. Complaint of double vision, blurring, or jerky eye movements
4. A slight headache is expected—worsening headache or complaints of feeling worse when moving about should be reported
5. Bleeding or discharge from nose or ears
6. Seizures—any twitching or movement of arms or legs that patient cannot stop
7. Any behavior or symptom not normal for the individual

A physician should be called at once if any of these signs are observed. If a physician is unavailable, emergency services should be contacted immediately.

Patient resumes pre-injury patterns of urinary and bowel elimination.

Patient is free of pain.

INTRACRANIAL SURGERY

Cranial surgery may be required for debriding or repairing effects of head trauma, repairing aneurysms, treating abscesses, or excising brain tumors.

BRAIN TUMOR

The box below presents the commonly occurring forms of brain tumor. Symptoms may vary significantly depending on the tumor's location and speed of growth. Surgical intervention is the treatment of choice.

Nursing interventions following craniotomy surgery closely follow those discussed for head injury. The box on the next page describes interventions that relate specifically to the care of the craniotomy patient beyond those previously discussed.

SPINAL CORD INJURY

Spinal cord injury is a significant cause of serious disability and death in the United States. Approximately 10,000 to 12,000 new cases occur annually. Injury typically occurs from fracture or displacement of one or

---

TYPES OF BRAIN TUMORS

GLIOMAS

Gliomas, which account for about one-half of all brain tumors, arise from the brain connective tissue. They tend to be infiltrative, are difficult to excise completely, and grow rapidly. Glioblastomas and medulloblastomas are the most highly malignant and are usually fatal within a matter of months. Astrocytomas and oligodendrogliomas are slower growing, but still frequently fatal in less than a year.

MENINGIOMAS

Meningiomas, which account for 13% to 18% of all primary intracranial tumors, arise from the meningeal coverings of the brain. They vary widely in histologic features and size and are usually benign. They are frequently encapsulated and surgical cure is possible.

ACOUSTIC NEUROMAS

Acoustic neuromas account for about 8% of all primary intracranial tumors. Neuromas may arise from any of the cranial nerves. When the acoustic nerve is affected, the tumor grows from nerve sheath but usually extends to affect the nerve fibers. They are slow growing.

PITUITARY ADENOMAS

Pituitary adenomas may arise from a variety of pituitary tissue types. They are successfully treated by surgery, using either the standard craniotomy or the transsphenoidal approach. Recurrence is possible.

SPECIFIC NURSING INTERVENTIONS FOR THE CRANIOTOMY PATIENT

PREOPERATIVE PERIOD

Assess baseline neurologic and physiologic status.

Encourage patient and family to verbalize fears and concerns.

Provide detailed teaching about procedures, postoperative care, movement and activity restrictions, and equipment to be used.

Prepare family for patient's appearance after the operation:

Head dressing, shaved scalp

Edema and bruising

Temporary decrease in mental status

POSTOPERATIVE PERIOD

Complete or perform nursing interventions for monitoring neurologic status, dealing with rising intracranial pressure, and preventing complications related to immobility. In addition, position patient as follows:

Supratentorial surgery—head of bed elevated 45 degrees. Turn patient only between back and unaffected side if tumor was large, to prevent shift of brain tissue.

Infratentorial surgery—head of bed flat. Avoid positioning patient on back, to prevent shift of brain tissue downward. Avoid neck flexion.

Check urinary output and specific gravity for the following:

Diabetes insipidus—increased output; decreased specific gravity

Inappropriate ADH syndrome—decreased output

Diabetes in response to high-dose steroids—urine sugar and acetone

Prevent coughing and vomiting.

Use Tylenol or codeine to deal with postop discomfort. Avoid use of narcotics and other CNS depressants. Apply ice packs to head for pain and to reduce swelling.

Assist and support patient and family in dealing with residual effects of the tumor or surgery.

---

more vertebrae with damage to the underlying spinal cord and nerve roots. Spinal cord injury primarily affects young males and is associated with vehicular accidents, falls, athletic injuries, and gunshot wounds.

PATHOPHYSIOLOGY

The spinal cord is very tough and is rarely torn or transected by direct trauma. However, even relatively minor compression can have serious results. Significant cord edema occurs, which can extend the level of injury. Actual spinal cord destruction in severe trauma is related to autodestruction. This complex process involves hemorrhage into the gray matter, inflammation, edema, vasospasm, and ischemia, which can lead to irreversible spinal cord necrosis in a matter of hours after the injury.

A complete cord injury is accompanied by total loss

TABLE 4-6 Muscle function after spinal cord injury

Spinal Cord Injury	Muscle Function Remaining	Muscle Function Lost
Cervical		
Above C4	None	All including respiration
C5	Neck	Arms
	Scapular elevation	Chest
		All below chest
C6-C7	Neck	Some arm, fingers
	Some chest movement	Some chest
	Some arm movement	All below chest
Thoracic	Neck	Trunk
	Arms (full)	All below chest
	Some chest	
Lumbosacral	Neck	Legs
	Arms	
	Chest	
	Trunk	

From: Phipps WJ, Long BC, and Woods NF: Medical-surgical nursing: concepts and clinical practice, ed 4, St Louis, 1990, Mosby–Year Book, Inc.

---

of voluntary movement and sensation below the level of the injury. An incomplete injury involves partial destruction of the cord with variable patterns of sensory or motor function loss. Table 4-6 details the muscle functions affected by various levels of spinal cord injury. The period immediately following the injury is called spinal shock (see box below).

MEDICAL MANAGEMENT

Initial interventions are aimed at supporting vital functions and preventing further cord damage through stabilization and realignment. Early surgery may be indicated to decompress or fuse the spinal column, insert rods to stabilize the spine, and correct deformities.

Initial management may involve skeletal traction with the use of Crutchfield or Gardner-Wells tongs and

SPINAL SHOCK

A period immediately following spinal cord injury in which the spinal cord ceases to function. Spinal shock may persist for days or weeks. During this time the patient exhibits:

1. Flaccid paralysis and loss of sensation
2. Urinary and bowel retention
3. Inability to perspire to cool the body
4. Vascular instability with bradycardia and hypotension from loss of sympathetic stimulation

The gradual return of reflexes signals the resolution of spinal shock.

special beds such as the Strkyer frame or kinetic treatment table. The application of halo traction vests allows the patient with a cervical injury to be treated without prolonged immobilization. Fluids and vasoconstrictors may be needed during the period of spinal shock. The use of high-dose steroids to reduce cord edema is under investigation.

NURSING MANAGEMENT (INITIAL CARE AND REHABILITATION)

Assessment

Subjective
Description of the accident or injury
History of loss of consciousness
Absence of sensation—sensory level
Sensory disturbances: pain, paresthesias
Presence of dyspnea

Objective
Respiratory status and quality of respirations
Level of consciousness
Degree and level of motor ability and strength
Baseline vital signs
Body position and alignment
Pain at level of injury that may radiate along nerve pathway
Systems assessment for presence of other injuries

Nursing Diagnoses
Nursing diagnoses will vary depending on the level and severity of the injury and the stage of rehabilitation. Some common diagnoses include the following:
Ineffective breathing pattern or ineffective airway clearance related to weakness or paralysis of intercostal muscles and diaphragm
Constipation related to loss of voluntary muscle control and immobility
Impaired physical mobility related to loss of spinal nerve innervation
Feeding, bathing/hygiene, dressing/grooming, or toileting self-care deficit related to loss of voluntary muscle control
Self-esteem disturbance related to loss of self-care abilities
Sensory/perceptual alteration (tactile) related to loss of sensory innervation
Altered patterns of sexuality related to effects of spinal cord injury.
Potential impairment of skin integrity related to decreased sensory perception and immobility
Alteration in peripheral tissue perfusion related to vasomotor instability
Urinary retention related to loss of voluntary bladder control
Ineffective individual or family coping related to irreversible effects of spinal cord injury and disability

Knowledge deficit related to nature and treatment of spinal cord injury
Body image disturbance related to decreased sensory input and loss of mobility
Dysreflexia related to massive sympathetic response to visceral stimuli

Expected Outcomes
Patient will maintain adequate oxygen and carbon dioxide exchange and not develop atelectasis or pneumonia.
Patient will reestablish a regular pattern of bowel elimination through a bowel-training program.
Patient will not develop complications related to decreased mobility.
Patient will be independent in the activities of daily living to the extent possible with level of injury, using appropriate assistive devices.
Patient will integrate body changes resulting from injury into an altered but positive view of self and have appropriate life goals.
Patient will receive sufficient meaningful stimuli to compensate for sensory/perceptual losses caused by the injury.
Patient will not experience skin breakdown.
Patient will receive counseling concerning sexual gratification within limitations of the injury.
Patient will achieve vascular stability with adequate peripheral tissue perfusion.
Patient will establish a pattern of urinary elimination consistent with the level of spinal damage.
Patient and family will be assisted to develop effective patterns of communicating their fears and frustrations and effectively plan for the future.
Patient and family will be knowledgeable about skills and equipment necessary to handle postdischarge care effectively.
Patient will maintain a stable blood pressure without incidence of dysreflexia.

Nursing Interventions: Immediate Period
Maintain realignment and stabilization of the spinal column, using halo traction, Crutchfield tongs, or other devices.
Avoid any head flexion if cervical injury exists.
Log roll patient to prevent twisting of spine.
Assess tidal volume and respiratory adequacy frequently: provide appropriate care for intubated patient requiring respiratory assistance.
Administer medications as prescribed.
Observe for vasomotor instability (spinal shock):
Assess vital signs frequently.
Assess movement, strength and sensation regularly.
Change positions slowly.

Assess for resolution of paralytic ileus. Resume oral diet slowly.

Begin intermittent catheterization routine or insert Foley catheter, and institute bowel program.

Record accurate intake and output.

Observe for signs of stress ulcer.

Initiate meticulous skin care program.

Begin range of motion exercise if permitted.

Nursing Interventions: Rehabilitative Period

Avoid complications of decreased mobility.

Put TED stockings or Ace bandages on patient to support venous return.

Assess for signs of DVT.

Teach patient pressure release exercises (wheelchair push-ups) and importance of frequent skin inspection. Employ appropriate pressure-relieving devices for bed and wheelchair.

Encourage participation in physical therapy exercise program.

Encourage deep breathing; use incentive spirometer for patients with thoracic and cervical injuries. Assist with coughing.

Institute bowel program.

Provide adequate or increased fluid and roughage in diet.

Use stool softeners, suppositories, digital stimulation. Avoid regular use of laxatives.

Maintain schedule and keep accurate records.

AUTONOMIC DYSREFLEXIA

Autonomic dysreflexia occurs in patients with injuries above T_6, most commonly with cervical damage. It represents a condition in which there are grossly exaggerated autonomic responses to simple visceral stimuli.

SIGNS AND SYMPTOMS

Paroxysmal hypertension to malignant levels
Bradycardia
Severe throbbing headache
Diaphoresis
Gooseflesh

INTERVENTIONS

The most effective intervention is to decrease the stimuli. A full bowel or bladder is the most common stimulus.

Place patient in sitting position if permitted.
Check catheter for patency.
Catheterize if a prolonged interval.
Check rectum for impaction.

If interventions are ineffective, it may be necessary to administer potent vasodilator or ganglionic blocking agent to reduce blood pressure, which can result in CVA or blindness.

Institute bladder retraining if possible.

Teach patient signs of urinary tract infection.

Teach catheterization techniques to patient or family member.

Teach importance of maintaining an acid urine, high fluid intake, and acting promptly if appearance or smell of urine changes. Urinary tract infection is the most common complication of spinal cord injury.

Assist patient to improve self-care capacities.

Teach use of appropriate assistive devices.

Teach transfer techniques and wheelchair safety.

Encourage family involvement in techniques of care.

Be alert to occurrence of autonomic dysreflexia in patients with cervical injury (see box on this page).

Provide patient with accurate information about sexual capacities and fertility specific to level of injury.

Encourage expression of feelings.

Encourage and support all efforts by patient and family to cope with injury and communicate effectively about needs for today and planning for the future.

Support grief resolution.

Initiate contact with appropriate community services.

Evaluation

Patient is free of atelectasis or pneumonia, practices regular deep breathing, and coughs effectively.

Patient maintains a pattern of regular bowel elimination, can insert suppositories, and demonstrates correct digital stimulation.

Patient maintains full range of motion in all joints.

Patient has achieved maximal ability in self-care possible with level of injury.

Patient has integrated body and life-style changes of injury and speaks positively of self and the future.

Patient compensates appropriately for absent sensory stimuli.

Patient maintains an intact skin and utilizes pressure-reducing techniques and devices.

Patient possesses factual data about the impact of the injury on sexual gratification and is able to ventilate feelings.

Patient has stable peripheral perfusion and knows how to recognize, prevent, and correct autonomic dysreflexia.

Patient maintains regular urinary elimination through intermittent catheterization and prevents occurrence of urinary tract infections.

Patient and family are able to express feelings and fears honestly and are making appropriate plans together for future care.

Patient and family are knowledgeable about equipment and skills needed for care and are in touch with appropriate community services.

BIBLIOGRAPHY

Bell J and Hannon J: Pathophysiology involved in autonomic hyperreflexia, J Neurosci Nurs **18:**86-89, 1986.

Boss B: Dysphasia, dyspraxia and dysarthria: distinguishing features, Parts I and II, J Neurosurg Nurs **16:**151-160, 211-216, 1984.

Burns E and Buckwalter K: Pathophysiology and etiology of Alzheimer's disease, Nurs Clin North Am **23:**11-30, 1988.

Chadwick A and Oesting H: Not for specialists only: caring for patients with spinal cord injuries, Nursing 89 **19**(11):52-56, 1989.

Davenport-Fortune P and Dunnum L: Professional nursing care of the patient with increased intracranial pressure: planned or "hit or miss," J Neurosurg Nurs **17:**367-370, 1985.

Francabandera F: Multiple sclerosis rehabilitation: inpatient vs. outpatient, Rehabil Nurs **13:**251-254, 1988.

Hahn K: Left vs. right: what a difference a side makes in stroke, Nursing 87 **17**(9):44-48, 1987.

Hartshorn J and Hartshorn E: Nursing interventions for anticonvulsant drug interactions, J Neurosci Nurs **18:**250-255, 1986.

Hegeman K: A care plan for the family of a brain trauma client, Rehabil Nurs **13:**254-258, 1988.

Keller C and others: Psychological responses to aphasia: theoretical considerations and nursing implications, J Neurosci Nurs **21:**290-294, 1989.

Kelly B: Nursing care of the patient with multiple sclerosis, Rehabil Nurs **13:**238-243, 1988.

MacDonald E: Aneurysmal subarachnoid hemorrhage, J Neurosci Nurs **21:**313-321, 1989.

Morgante L and others: Research and treatment in multiple sclerosis: implications for nursing practice, J Neurosci Nurs **21:**285-289, 1989.

Muwaswes M: Increased intracranial pressure and its systemic effects, J Neurosurg Nurs **17:**238-243, 1985.

Passarella P and Lewis N: Nursing application of Bobath principles in stroke care, J Neurosci Nurs **19:**106-109, 1987.

Vernon G: Parkinson's disease, J Neurosci Nurs **21:**273-284, 1989.

Whitney F: Relationship of laterality of stroke and emotional and functional outcome, J Neurosci Nurs **19:**158-165, 1987.

CHAPTER 5

Disorders of the Eyes and Ears

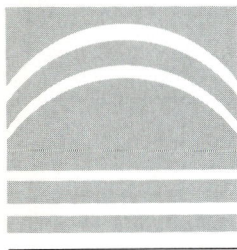

Vision and hearing contribute immeasurably to our understanding and enjoyment of the environment. When the eyes or ears are threatened or impaired, nursing care is directed toward preserving function, helping people meet their basic needs, strengthening support systems, and encouraging effective coping.

The major disorders of the eye affecting adults are infections, glaucoma, cataracts, and retinal detachment. Disorders of the ear are usually classified according to outer, middle, or inner ear problems.

DISORDERS OF THE EYES

EYE INFECTION/INFLAMMATION

Infection and inflammation can occur in any of the eye structures and may be caused by microorganisms, mechanical irritation, or sensitivity to some substance. There are more than 1 million cases of eye inflammation annually, two thirds of which are conjunctivitis. Figure 5-1 shows a horizontal section through the left eyeball. Table 5-1 describes common inflammations involving the eye.

PATHOPHYSIOLOGY

Most eye inflammations are relatively benign, self-limiting disorders that respond promptly to local therapy and antibiotics. They create discomfort and minor interruption of function from the inflammatory response, but resolve without permanent effect. Refer to Table 5-1 for common signs and symptoms.

MEDICAL MANAGEMENT

Standard medical interventions include the application of warm, moist compresses, topical or systemic antibiotics, and patching if eye rest is needed. Refer to Table 5-1 for specific therapies. Table 5-2 lists commonly prescribed ophthalmic drugs and their uses.

NURSING MANAGEMENT

Assessment

Subjective

History and progression of symptoms

Patient's complaints of itching, tearing, pain, or photophobia (light sensitivity)

Objective

Presence of redness or discharge, crusts

Blepharospasm (spasmodic blinking)

Eyelid edema

Nursing Diagnoses

Diagnoses vary slightly based on nature and severity of inflammation but usually include the following:

Pain and itching related to eye irritation

Actual or potential sensory/perceptual alteration (visual) related to presence of infection

Knowledge deficit related to development of infection and treatment plan

Expected Outcomes

Patient will experience increased comfort.

Inflammation will resolve without complications.

Patient's visual perception will return to preinflammation levels.

Patient will follow prescribed treatment plan and take appropriate measures to prevent reinfection.

Nursing Interventions

Apply warm or cold compresses as prescribed:

Warm—comforts, cleanses eye, and promotes healing

Cold—controls itching and edema

The box on p. 70 lists guidelines for the use of eye compresses. Dispose of all used materials carefully if infection is present.

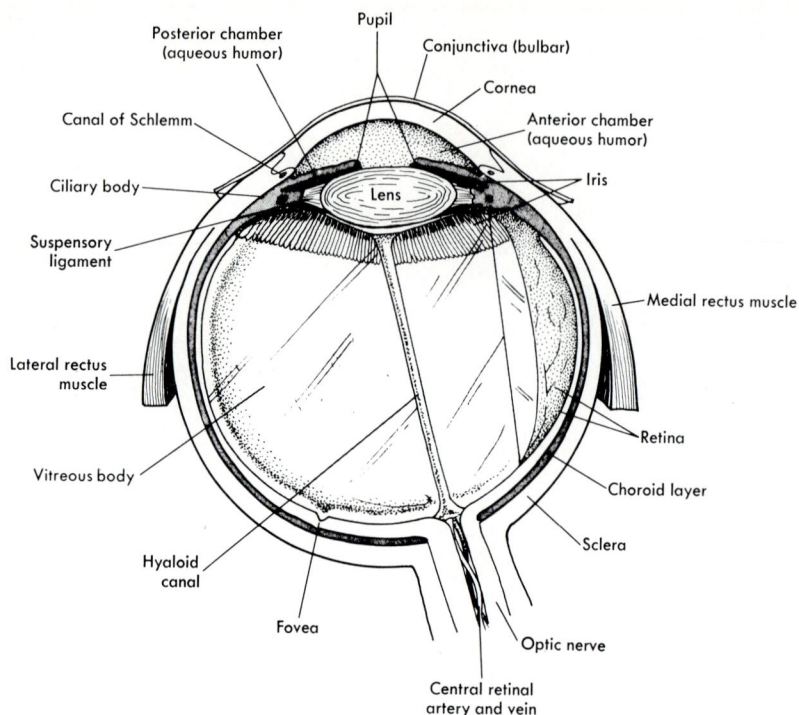

FIGURE 5-1 Horizontal section through left eyeball. (From Long BC and Phipps WJ: Essentials of medical-surgical nursing: a nursing process approach, ed 2, St Louis, 1989, The CV Mosby Co.

TABLE 5-1 Inflammations of the eye

Disorder	Description	Signs and Symptoms	Medical Therapy
Hordeolum (sty)	Staphylococcus infection of gland at eyelid margin	Localized abscess at base of eyelash, edema of lid, pain	Hot compresses to hasten pointing of abscess, topical antibiotic
Chalazion	Cyst from obstruction of sebaceous gland at eyelid margin	Initially, edema and discomfort; later, painless mass in lid	Warm compresses and topical antibiotic initially; surgical removal if cyst becomes large and presses on cornea
Blepharitis	Inflammation of lid margins, usually by staphylococci	Itching, redness, pain of lid, lacrimation, photophobia; crusting ulceration; lids become glued together during sleep	Warm compresses followed by erythromycin or bacitracin eye ointment; steroid eye drops may be prescribed
Conjunctivitis (pink eye)	Inflammation of conjunctiva by viruses, bacteria (highly infectious), allergy, trauma (sunburn)	Redness of conjunctiva, lid edema, crusting discharge on lids and cornea of eye; itching with allergies	Cleansing of lids and lashes, warm compresses; topical antibiotics; steroid eye drops for allergies (contraindicated for herpes simplex virus); no eye patch
Keratitis	Inflammation of cornea by bacteria, herpes simplex virus, allergies, vitamin A deficiency	Severe eye pain, photophobia, tearing, blepharospasm, loss of vision if uncontrolled	Warm compresses; topical antibiotics for bacterial infections; atropine sulfate; Idoxuridine for herpes simplex; eye patch, rest; corneal grafting if cornea is injured
Corneal ulcer	Necrosis of corneal tissue from trauma, inflammation; may be superficial or may penetrate deeper tissue	Pain and blepharospasm may occur; ulcer may be outlined by fluorescein dye	Superficial ulcer: antibiotic eye drops, eye patch. Deep ulcer: topical and systemic antibiotics, atropine sulfate, warm compresses, eye patch; cautery; corneal transplant if necessary

From Long BC and Phipps WJ: Essentials of medical-surgical nursing: a nursing process approach ed 2, St Louis, 1989, The CV Mosby Co.

TABLE 5-2 Commonly used ophthalmic drugs

Drug	Action	Uses
Mydriatics		
Phenylephrine (Neo-Synephrine, Mydfrin) Hydroxyamphetamine (Paredrine)	Dilate pupil	Examination of interior of eye Prevent adhesions of iris with cornea in eye inflammations
Cycloplegics		
Atropine sulfate (Atropisol, Isopto-Atropine) Cyclopentolate (Cyclogyl) Homatropine (Isopto-Homatropine) Scopolamine hydrobromide Tropicamide (Mydriacyl)	Dilate pupil Paralyze ciliary muscle and iris	Decrease pain and photophobia, and provide rest for inflammations of iris and ciliary body and for diseases of cornea Eye examinations
Miotics		
Pilocarpine (Pilocel, Ocusert) Carbachol (Carbacel) Physostigmine (Eserine) Demecarium bromide (Humorsol)	Constrict pupil Permit better drainage of intraocular fluid	Treat glaucoma
Osmotic Agents		
Mannitol (Osmitrol), IV Glycerin (Glyrol, Osmoglyn), PO Urea (Urevert, Ureaphil), IV	Decrease intraocular pressure	Treat acute glaucoma Eye surgery
Carbonic Anhydrase Inhibitors		
Acetazolamide (Diamox) Ethoxzolamide (Cardrase) Dichlorphenamide (Daranide) Methazolamide (Neptazane)	Decrease production of aqueous humor	Treat glaucoma
Beta-Adrenergic Blocker		
Timolol maleate (Timoptic)	Reduce intraocular pressure (mechanism unclear)	Treat glaucoma
Topical Anesthetics		
Proparacaine (Ophthaine, Ophthetic, Alcaine) Lidocaine (Xylocaine)	Decrease sensation (pain)	Surgery, treatments Treat eye inflammations
Topical Antibiotics		
Polymyxin B, bacitracin (Polysporin) Polymyxin B, neomycin, bacitracin (Neosporin) Bacitracin Idoxuridine (IDU) Gentamicin sulfate (Garamycin) Chloramphenicol (Chloromycetin, Chloroptic)	Antiinfective	Treat eye inflammations
Steroids		
Prednisone Prednisolone (Pred Forte) Methylprednisolone (Depo-Medrol) Triamcinolone (Aristocort) Dexamethasone (Decadron, Maxidex) Fluorometholone (FML)	Antiinflammatory	Treat eye inflammations and allergic reactions

Modified from Long BC and Phipps WJ: Essentials of medical-surgical nursing: a nursing process approach, ed 2, St Louis, 1989, The CV Mosby Co, and Phipps WJ, Long BC, and Woods NF: Medical-surgical nursing: concepts and clinical practice, ed 4, St Louis, 1990, Mosby–Year Book, Inc.

GUIDELINES FOR APPLICATION OF MOIST EYE COMPRESSES

GENERAL PRINCIPLES

Use aeseptic technique if infection is present.
If bilateral infection, use separate equipment for each eye.
Wash hands thoroughly before and after soaks.
If bilateral infection, wash hands between treatments of eyes.
Do not exert any pressure on the eye during treatment.

WARM COMPRESSES

Temperature should not exceed 120° F (49° C).
A clean, fresh washcloth is effective for use in the home.
Change compresses frequently over the 10 to 20 minute treatment period.
Never reuse cloth for a second treatment.
Carefully handle and dispose of infected materials.

COLD COMPRESSES

Rubber glove or plastic bag packed with ice chips may be used as disposable compress.

GUIDELINES FOR INSTILLING EYE MEDICATIONS

EYEDROPS

1. Wash hands before touching eyes.
2. Clean eyes before instilling eye drops if crusting or discharge is present.
3. Ask patient to tilt head back and look up.
4. Evert lower lid by pulling down gently on skin below eye.
5. Approach eye by bringing dropper tip in from side, not directly from front.
6. Place drops on *center* of conjunctival sac of lower lid. Avoid touching eye with dropper.
7. Ask patient to close eyes but not tightly squeeze them shut (to prevent loss of medication down cheek).
8. Provide patient with a tissue or cotton ball to absorb excess moisture.

OINTMENT

1. Follow steps 1 through 4 above.
2. Place the ointment from tube directly onto exposed conjunctival sac from the inner to the outer canthus.
3. Avoid touching eye with tube.

GUIDELINES FOR EYE IRRIGATIONS

1. Place patient lying toward one side to prevent fluid from flowing into other eye.
2. Direct the irrigating fluid along the conjunctiva from the *inner* to the outer canthus.
3. Avoid directing a forceful stream onto eyeball or touching any eye structure with the irrigating equipment.
4. A piece of gauze may be wrapped around index finger to raise upper lid for better cleaning if heavy discharge exists.

Provide eye pads if ordered to relieve photophobia and protect the eye. *ALERT:* Eye pads must not be used if bacterial infection is present as they enhance bacterial growth. Keep room lights dim, and recommend the use of dark glasses outdoors.
Administer or teach patient to correctly administer prescribed eye medications. Each patient must have and use own eye drops and ointments to prevent cross-infection; use separate bottles for each eye. The box on this page describes the proper installation of eye drops and ointments.
Administer eye irrigations if prescribed to remove secretions or foreign body. The box on this page describes proper sequence for eye irrigation.
Teach patient to avoid touching either eye while infection is present and to wash hands thoroughly before and after caring for the eye.

Evaluation

Patient's infection resolves without complication or loss of vision.
Patient's discomfort has resolved.
Patient can demonstrate proper technique for applying compresses, irrigating the eye, or instilling eye medications.

GLAUCOMA

The term *glaucoma* refers to an eye disease characterized by increased intraocular pressure associated with progressive loss of peripheral vision. Permanent vision loss is preventable with early detection. Glaucoma occurs in middle-aged and older adults and is the greatest threat to vision in older persons. It is 15 times more common among the black population than among whites.

PATHOPHYSIOLOGY

In the normal eye there is a balance between the production and drainage of aqueous humor, permitting a stable intraocular pressure. In glaucoma, obstruction to the drainage of aqueous humor increases the intraocular pressure and produces damage to the optic nerve.
Chronic simple (wide angle) glaucoma is the primary form of the disease. It takes a slow and insidious course, and results from degenerative changes.
Acute (narrow angle) glaucoma is the result of a change in the angle of the iris against the anterior chamber and causes dramatic symptoms and rapid loss of vision. A congenital form of the disease also exists.

MEDICAL MANAGEMENT

Medical management is aimed at providing better drainage of aqueous humor or decreasing the amount produced. This controls the level of intraocular pressure and helps prevent irreversible vision loss.

Chronic wide angle glaucoma is treated by early detection of the problem and the use of the following:

Miotics such as pilocarpine (see Table 5-2) to constrict the pupil and facilitate drainage

Carbonic anhydrase inhibitors such as acetazolamide to decrease the production of aqueous humor (see Table 5-2)

Beta-adrenergic blockers such as timolol (see Table 5-2), which decrease intraocular pressure by poorly understood mechanisms without causing pupil constriction

Surgery may be indicated if conservative management fails. Trabeculoplasty and trabeculectomy are procedures aimed at improving the outflow and drainage from the anterior chamber.

Acute narrow angle glaucoma can present as an ocular emergency. Pharmacologic treatment may be used, but surgical correction of the position of the iris through iridotomy or iridectomy is frequently required.

NURSING MANAGEMENT

Assessment: Chronic Glaucoma
Subjective
Patient's complaints of the following:
Loss of peripheral vision (tunnel vision)
Dull eye pain, especially in the morning
Difficulty adjusting to dark rooms
Halos seen around lights (late sign)
Objective
Elevated intraocular pressure
Diminished visual fields

Assessment: Acute Glaucoma
Patient's complaints of the following:
Severe eye pain
Nausea and vomiting
Blurred or decreased vision
Acutely increased intraocular pressure
Halos around lights
Enlarged or fixed pupils

Nursing Diagnoses
Diagnoses will depend on the stage and acuity of the disease but commonly include the following:
Pain in eye related to elevated intraocular pressure
Sensory/perceptual alteration (visual) related to decreasing peripheral vision
Knowledge deficit related to the disease process of glaucoma and the drugs used to control it

Expected Outcomes
Patient will be free of eye pain.
Patient will experience no further loss of vision
Patient will understand the disease process of glaucoma

and be able to describe drugs used in its treatment and how to administer them.

Nursing Interventions
Administer prescribed medications.
Teach patient safe and correct use of eye drops and the importance of having spare bottles for travel or office use (refer to box on p. 70).
Teach patient the importance of careful adherence to the medication regimen and need for regular medical follow-up.
If surgery is performed, provide standard postoperative eye surgery care and teaching.

Evaluation
Patient reports no eye pain.
Patient's visual status has stabilized; patient practices safety measures to compensate for diminished peripheral vision.
Patient can discuss long-term irreversible nature of the disease, can discuss purpose and side effects of medications ordered, and can demonstrate safe and correct eye drop administration.

CATARACT

A cataract is a clouding or opacity of the lens that leads to gradual painless blurring of vision and eventual loss of sight. The most common cause of cataracts is aging; 85% of persons over age 80 have some lens clouding. Cataracts are also associated with injury, can be present at birth, and can be secondary to other eye disease.

PATHOPHYSIOLOGY

Cataracts develop as the result of alterations in the metabolism and movement of nutrients within the lens. Persons with diabetes tend to develop cataracts at an earlier age because of an accumulation of sorbitol. As the nuclear portion of the lens becomes increasingly dense, light rays are unable to pass through the opaque lens to the retina.

APPROACHES TO CATARACT REMOVAL

TYPES
Intracapsular extraction—removal of the entire lens
Extracapsular extraction—removal of lens material without disturbing the membrane capsule
TECHNIQUES
Phacoemulsification—insertion of an instrument that uses ultrasonic vibration to break up lens material for removal by irrigation
Cryoextraction—cataract lifted out by adhering lens to a subzero probe

MEDICAL MANAGEMENT

Operative treatment is the only effective management of cataracts, and vision loss can be restored with surgery. Surgeons no longer wait for cataracts to ripen but intervene when visual loss interferes with activities of daily living. There are several approaches to cataract removal, which are summarized in the box on p. 71. Virtually all surgical procedures can be done under local anesthesia. The focusing function of the lens is replaced after surgery by the use of cataract glasses, contact lens, or intraocular lens implants.

NURSING MANAGEMENT

Assessment
Subjective
Patient's report of painless loss of vision occurring over a period of years
Objective
Visible opacity of the lens, unilateral or bilateral

Nursing Diagnoses
Sensory/perceptual alteration (visual) related to decreased stimulus access to the retina
Potential for injury related to decreasing vision

Expected Outcomes
Patient will not experience injury during period of failing vision.
Patient will experience improved vision following surgery.
Patient will not suffer postoperative complications.

Nursing Interventions: Preoperative
Assess patient's vision in unaffected eye.
Ensure that patient understands nature of procedure, use of local anesthesia, and all postoperative care routines.
Encourage patient to discuss fears related to eye surgery.

Nursing Interventions: Postoperative
Avoid activities that increase intraocular pressure:
Squeezing shut the eyelids
Bending over at the waist
Straining for sneezing, coughing, vomiting, defecation
NOTE: Surgeons vary on strictness of activity restrictions.
Maintain a safe environment:
Encourage patient to lie on back or unaffected side.
Use eye shield at night to protect the eye.
Organize self-care articles on unaffected side.
Be alert to complaints of severe pain or pressure that may indicate complications.
Ensure that patient has assistance available for activities of daily living as needed.

Encourage patient to return to normal activities as tolerated. No bending below waist level or heavy lifting are permitted during recovery.
Teach patient about the corrective lens to be used during rehabilitation. See box below

Evaluation
Patient has not been injured during postoperative period.
Patient experiences gradual improvement of vision.
Patient makes successful adaptation to the distortions of cataract lenses and moves about safely in the environment.

RETINAL DETACHMENT

Retinal detachment occurs when the two retinal layers separate because of either fluid accumulation or contraction of the vitreous body. Usually there is no apparent cause, but detachment can be caused by trauma, severe physical exertion, lens loss (as after cataract surgery), degenerative changes of myopia, hemorrhage, or tumor.

PATHOPHYSIOLOGY

Detachment interrupts the transmission of visual images from the retina to the optic nerve, causing progressive loss of vision to complete blindness.

MEDICAL MANAGEMENT

Early surgical intervention is the treatment of choice. Accumulated fluid is drained from the subretinal space, and inflammation is induced by diathermy, photocoagu-

---

VISION CORRECTION FOLLOWING CATARACT SURGERY

INTRAOCULAR LENS IMPLANTS
Method of choice for vision correction.
Can be implanted during or after cataract removal.
Provide near normal vision, minimal magnification.

CATARACT GLASSES
Only central vision is corrected. Peripheral vision remains distorted. Patient must turn head from side to side to compensate.
Objects are magnified about 30%. Distance is distorted and safety issues are of concern—curbs, steps, reaching for objects, driving.
Used only with bilateral surgery or diplopia results.
Extremely heavy if made of glass—irritate nose and ears.

CONTACT LENSES
Can be used after single-eye surgery but not for 2 to 3 months until healing occurs.
Provide good correction and full visual field with about 7% magnification.
Need significant finger dexterity and meticulous care.

NURSING CARE PLAN

PERSON WITH A RETINAL DETACHMENT

Nursing Diagnoses	Expected Patient Outcomes	Nursing Interventions

Sensory/perceptual alteration (visual) related to decreased vision or eye patching	Patients vision will be restored to predetachment level.	1. Maintain prescribed activity restrictions.
		2. Position patient's head during initial period so that retinal tear is at lowest portion of eye.
		3. Assist patient with activities of daily living within the ordered restrictions.
		4. If one eye has decreased vision and patient is restricted in movement:
		  a. Place personal objects within easy reach.
		  b. Provide diversion with radio or conversation.
		5. If total vision is limited by eye patches or blurred vision:
		  a. Orient patient to physical surroundings, time, weather, and news events.
		  b. Speak to patient when approaching and identify yourself.
		  c. Explain activities occurring in room.
		  d. Tell patient when you are leaving.

Potential for injury related to decreased vision	Patient will not experience injury during period of decreased vision.	1. Keep side rails up if binocular patches are used postoperatively or vision is markedly reduced. 2. Keep call button within reach when patient is on bedrest. Orient to immediate physical environment. 3. Assist patient as necessary when ambulating after surgery if vision is still restricted, such as by eye patches. 4. Instruct patient to wear eye shield for sleeping.
Anxiety related to possible loss of vision	Patient will experience manageable levels of anxiety and verbalize concerns about possible visual losses.	1. Give patient opportunities to explore concerns about possible decreased vision. 2. Answer questions honestly. 3. Encourage realistic hope about maintaining vision as described by physician. 4. Explore patient's knowledge of disorder and planned therapy, and correct misunderstandings.
Knowledge deficit related to surgery and postoperative care routines.	Patient accurately describes surgical procedure and postoperative regimen.	1. Teach patient to avoid jerking head (sneezing, coughing, vomiting). 2. Administer antiemetics or cough suppressants if necessary. 3. Teach patient about temporary activity restrictions. Patient may resume normal activities but should restrict active exercise and heavy lifting. 4. Teach patient to report signs of further retinal detachment—eye pain, floaters, or spots.

lation, laser beam, or subfreezing temperatures to cause adhesion formation, which closes the retinal break. Scleral buckling is also used in most cases to push the choroid into contact with the retinal tear during healing.

NURSING MANAGEMENT

Assessment: Subjective
Patient's complaints of the following:
Floating spots or flashing lights
Progressive constriction of vision in one area
Sensation of "curtain being drawn" across the eye (if tear is acute and extensive)

Nursing Diagnoses
Anxiety related to loss of vision and uncertain outcome
Potential for injury related to eye patching or decreased visual acuity
Sensory/perceptual alteration (visual) related to decreased vision or eye patching

Expected Outcomes
Patient will experience manageable levels of anxiety and feel positive about outcomes of surgery.
Patient will not experience injury during period of reduced vision.
Patient's vision will return to predetachment levels.

Nursing Interventions: Preoperative
Maintain patient on bed rest with eyes covered if ordered.
Position head with retinal tear in lowest portion of eyes.
Use side rails; place call bell within easy reach.
Encourage patient to discuss fears and concerns—provide accurate information about surgery and outcomes.
Assist patient to avoid disorientation or sensory deprivation while eyes are patched:
Visit frequently.
Provide radio or TV for time orientation.
Orient to time, weather, and news events regularly.

Nursing Interventions: Postoperative
Position patient in bed as ordered by physician.
Restrict activities as ordered:
Orient to surroundings—personal items, phone, call bell, and so on.
Maintain bed rest for 1 to 2 days.
Avoid jerking movements of head, such as sneezing or coughing.
Assist patient with activities of daily living as indicated by activity restriction.
Maintain safety precautions with side rails.
Provide teaching about gradual resumption of activities over 1 to 2 weeks and about symptoms indicating possible redetachment.

Wear eye shield at night and while resting until healing is complete.
Apply cold compresses as ordered to reduce swelling.
Administer eye medications as ordered.

Evaluation
Patient copes adequately with injury and outcome.
Patient safely completes activities of daily living during period of diminished vision.
Patient's vision improves.
Patient can discuss activity restrictions to be followed in the postdischarge period.

DISORDERS OF THE EARS

Hearing loss is the most common disability in the United States, affecting over 13 million persons, most of whom are over age 65. The range of disability is from difficulty understanding particular words and sounds to complete deafness. Hearing loss may be classified as:
Conductive—any interference with conduction of sound impulses through the external auditory canal, eardrum, or middle ear.
Sensorineural—disease or trauma to the inner ear, neural structures or nerve pathways to the brainstem.
Central deafness—a rare form in which the central nervous system cannot interpret normal auditory signals due to tumor, trauma or CVA.
While some problems may be helped by medicine or surgery, most cannot be effectively treated. Eighty percent of all impairments are caused by sensorineural problems for which there is no known cure.

EAR INFECTION/INFLAMMATION

Ear infections may occur at any age and in any portion of the ear. They are common health problems. The possibility of serious complications following ear infection makes prompt identification and treatment important. Table 5-3 lists common infections of the ear. Figure 5-2 shows the external auditory canal, middle ear, and inner ear.

PATHOPHYSIOLOGY

The pathophysiology of ear infections is related to the specific structures involved and basically results from local tissue inflammatory responses to bacteria or viruses. Pain is a common symptom. External and middle ear infections may cause drainage, itching, and redness. Some diminished hearing frequently accompanies these inflammations. Inner ear problems may affect balance by disturbing the vestibular system.

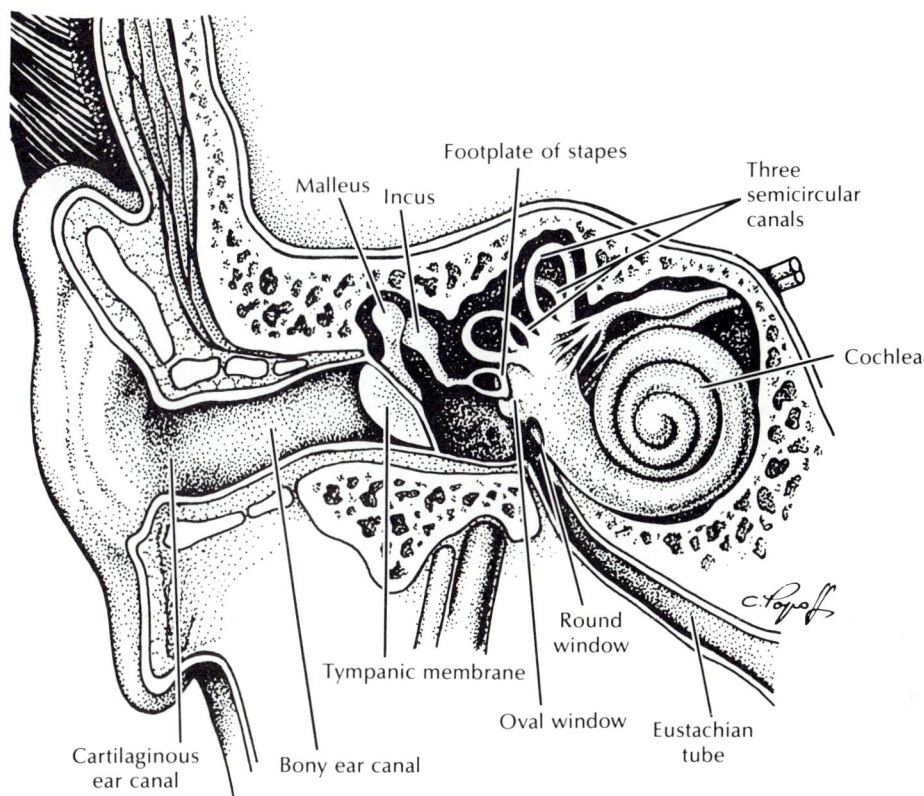

FIGURE 5-2 External auditory canal, middle ear, and inner ear. (From Malasanos L and others: Health assessment, ed 4, 1989, Mosby–Year Book, Inc.).

TABLE 5-3 Inflammations of the ear

Disorder	Description	Signs and Symptoms	Medical Therapy
External otitis	Inflammation of external ear; may be acute or chronic	Pain with movement of auricle, redness, scaling, itching, swelling, watery discharge, crusting of external ear	Cleaning to remove debris; antibiotic drops or ointment; systemic antibiotic if necessary
Serous otitis media	Collection of sterile serum in middle ear; may be acute or chronic	Sense of fullness in ear, hearing loss, low-pitched tinnitus, earache	Removal of eustachian obstruction by aspiration or insertion of tubes for drainage
Acute purulent otitis media	Infection of middle ear, usually by pneumococci, streptococci, staphylococci, or *Haemophilus influenzae*	Sense of fullness in ear, severe throbbing pain, hearing loss, tinnitus, fever	Antibiotics; if severe, bed rest, analgesics, nasal vasoconstrictors; myringotomy if necessary
Chronic otitis media	Chronic inflammation of middle ear; sequela of acute otitis media	Deafness, occasional pain, dizziness, chronic discharge from ear	Local debridement, topical and systemic antibiotics; mastoidectomy and tympanoplasty may be necessary
Chronic mastoiditis	Spread of infection into mastoid from repeated otitis media	Middle ear drainage	Mastoid irrigation; antibiotics; may need mastoidectomy
Labyrinthitis	Inflammation of inner ear	Severe and sudden vertigo, nausea and vomiting, nystagmus, photophobia, headache, ataxic gait	No specific treatment; antibiotics; dimenhydrinate for vertigo; parenteral fluids if nausea and vomiting persist

From Long BC and Phipps WJ: Essentials of medical-surgical nursing: a nursing process approach, ed 2, St Louis, 1989, The CV Mosby Co.

MEDICAL MANAGEMENT

Standard medical interventions include systemic antibiotics and topical ear drops. Surgical intervention includes mastoidectomy, myringotomy, insertion of ventilation tubes, and tympanoplasty.

NURSING MANAGEMENT

Assessment

Subjective

Patient complaints of the following:

Pain or itching in ear

Acute tenderness when pinna pulled or moved

Sense of fullness in ear, blocked ear

Tinnitus (ringing in the ear) or roaring sound

Vertigo

Objective

Decreased hearing

Fever

Redness, drainage, scaling

Nursing Diagnoses

Diagnoses will depend on exact nature and severity of ear inflammation. Common diagnoses include the following:

Pain and itching related to pressure and inflammation in the ear

Potential for injury related to vertigo and diminished hearing

Sensory/perceptual alteration (auditory) related to blockage of auditory conduction

Expected Outcomes

Patient will have decreased pain and discomfort.

Patient will compensate for vertigo and not experience injury.

Patient's hearing will improve.

Nursing Interventions

Administer medications as ordered.

Teach patient correct technique for instilling ear drops (see box on this page).

Perform prescribed ear irrigations (see box on this page and Figure 5-3).

If patient experiences vertigo, keep side rails up and supervise ambulation.

Teach patient about the nature of any planned surgery and the management of common symptoms such as nausea and vertigo.

Teach patient about measures to prevent complications following ear surgery.

Patient should avoid blowing nose or sneezing after surgery.

After healing occurs patient should be taught to blow the nose with both nostrils open and to open the mouth when sneezing.

Patient should avoid flying during healing.

Keep the ear dry for 6 weeks after surgery.

GUIDELINES FOR EAR IRRIGATION

NOTE: Avoid ear irrigation if ear drum is punctured (increases inflammation) or when attempting to remove foreign body (moisture may swell object).

1. Use tap water or normal saline; peroxide may be added to remove wax.
2. Warm solution to body temperature. Dizziness can result from solutions that are too hot or too cold.
3. Straighten ear by pulling pinna up and back.
4. Use a steady stream of solution against roof of auditory canal.
5. Use gentle pressure; do not obstruct outflow with equipment.
6. Have patient lie on affected side after irrigation to promote drainage. Be alert to possibility of vertigo following irrigation.

INSTILLATION OF EAR DROPS

1. Warm solution to body temperature—no more than 100° F (38° C).
2. Have patient tilt head so ear to be treated is up.
3. Straighten ear canal by pulling pinna up and back.
4. Instill drops to run along auditory canal wall.
5. Have patient hold position for 2 to 5 minutes.
6. Gently insert cotton into external auditory canal if desired.
7. Wipe external ear to prevent skin irritation.

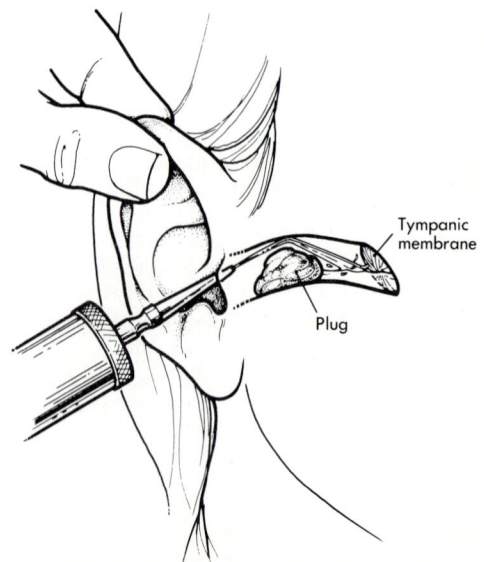

FIGURE 5-3 Irrigation of the external auditory canal.

Evaluation

Patient is free of pain and other annoying symptoms.

Patient has not experienced injury during periods of vertigo.

Patient's hearing has returned to preinfection levels; following surgery, patient's hearing has increased.

Patient can describe postdischarge routine and any measures appropriate for preventing reinfection.

MÉNIÈRE'S DISEASE

Ménière's disease is a disorder of the inner ear that occurs most commonly in women between 50 and 60 years of age. Its cause is unknown. Usually several attacks occur yearly until the disease resolves spontaneously or progresses to complete deafness in the affected ear.

PATHOPHYSIOLOGY

A disturbance in the fluid physiology in the ear, resulting from either increased production or decreased absorption, raises the pressure within the labyrinth of the inner ear. This pressure produces attacks of severe vertigo, tinnitus, and progressive hearing loss. Usually only one ear is involved. The cause is unknown.

MEDICAL MANAGEMENT

No medical treatment is entirely successful. The major goal is to preserve hearing. During the acute phase atropine or diazepam (Valium) may be given to decrease autonomic nervous system function. Benadryl is given for its antihistamine effect in addition to vasodilators.

During remission the patient may receive diuretics to reduce fluid, antihistamines, vasodilators, and a low-salt diet with a fluid restriction. Most patients respond to this regimen, although acute attacks may still occur at unpredictable times. Complete remission usually occurs over 1 to 2 years as a gradual loss of responsiveness occurs from sensory organ degeneration. Some degree of hearing loss is usually permanent. Surgical decompression procedures may also be attempted to preserve hearing.

NURSING MANAGEMENT

Assessment

Subjective

Patient complains of the following:

Episodes of vertigo (described as whirling sensation or room spinning; patient must lie down to keep from falling); attacks are often preceded by a feeling of fullness or tinnitus

Nausea associated with vertigo

Tinnitus (buzzing sounds to painful loud roaring)

History of and patient's knowledge about disorder

Knowledge of circumstances that precipitate attack

Actions taken during attacks and degree of relief they provide

Objective

Unilateral or bilateral hearing loss

Vomiting, diaphoresis, or nystagmus during observed attack

Uncoordinated gait

Nursing Diagnoses

Potential for injury related to severe vertigo

Sensory/perceptual alteration (auditory) related to progressive hearing loss

Self-care deficit related to inability to maintain an upright posture during attacks of vertigo

Knowledge deficit related to course of disease and management of attacks

Anxiety related to symptom reccurrence and potential hearing loss

Expected Outcomes

Patient will not experience injury during vertigo attacks.

Patient will experience sufficient disease control to maintain independence in the activities of daily living.

Patient will not experience disabling anxiety.

Patient's hearing loss will be minimized.

Patient will be knowledgeable concerning factors that precipitate or control attacks.

NURSING CARE PLAN
MÉNIÈRE'S DISEASE

Nursing Diagnoses	Expected Patient Outcomes	Nursing Interventions
Anxiety related to symptoms and possibility of hearing loss	Patient will experience manageable levels of anxiety and verbalize concerns over prognosis.	1. Encourage patient to explore concerns about decreased hearing and dizziness attacks, and to take action related to the concerns. 2. Explore patient's knowledge of the disorder and correct misunderstandings. 3. Encourage realistic hope about expected hearing ability as described by physician. 4. Refer patient to necessary support services, such as social worker or audiologist.

Sensory/perceptual alteration (auditory) related to fluid accumulation in ear	Patient interacts with others accurately and experiences minimal hearing loss.	1. If tinnitus is distressing, increase background sounds such as music.
		2. If hearing is decreased:
		  a. Use measures to facilitate communication with hearing impaired.
		  b. Refer patient to audiologist, if appropriate.

Potential for injury related to severe vertigo	Patient does not experience injury during attacks of vertigo.	1. Keep side rails up when patient with dizziness is in bed. 2. Assist with ambulation as needed. 3. Encourage patient to sit or lie down and to remain immobile if signs of dizziness occur. 4. Encourage patient to move slowly and not turn head suddenly when dizziness is present. 5. Teach patient to stop car at side of road immediately at first signs of dizziness while driving.
Potential self-care deficit related to inability to maintain an upright posture	Patient will maintain independence in the activities of daily living.	1. Provide desired foods and fluids if nausea is present. 2. Assist with hygiene as needed while encouraging independence; place hygiene supplies so that patient does not have to turn head. 3. Provide sufficient time for activities of daily living so patient can move slowly.
Knowledge deficit related to the nature of the disorder and the management of attacks	Patient understands nature of disorder and factors that precipitate or control attacks.	1. Teach patient about the disorder, therapy, and need for medical follow-up. 2. Teach patient ways to protect self from injury and to prevent attacks of dizziness when possible. 3. Help patient to identify avoidable actions that precipitate dizziness attacks.

Nursing Interventions: During Attacks

Instruct patient to lie immobile and not move the head.

Assist patient to meet hygiene needs as required.

Stand in front of patient to foster hearing and prevent head turning.

Encourage regular, slow position changes—try positioning patient on unaffected side.

Avoid use of bright or glaring lights.

Adjust diet to compensate for nausea or anorexia.

Keep side rails up.

Supervise position changes and all ambulation.

Administer medications as prescribed.

Nursing Interventions: Preventing Attacks

Teach use of low-salt diet and fluid limitations.

Patient should avoid reading when any vertigo or tinnitus is present.

Patient should avoid smoking.

Identify factors related to attacks, if possible.

Teach proper actions in case of attack:

If driving, patient should pull over and stop immediately.

If standing, patient should sit or lie down immediately.

Keep medications available at all times.

Reassure patient that disease symptoms are controllable and self-limiting.

Evaluation

Patient successfully avoids injury during attacks.

Patient suffers minimal hearing loss and compensates appropriately for decreased perception.

Patient achieves sufficient disease control to maintain independence in the activities of daily living.

Patient can explain disease and its progress, discuss use of medications and side effects, describe diet and fluid restrictions to prevent attacks, and describe actions to take in case of an attack.

BIBLIOGRAPHY

Boyd-Monk H and Steinmetz CG: Nursing care of the eye, Los Altos, Calif, 1987, Appleton & Lang.

Carver JA: Cataract care made plain, Am J Nurs 87:626-630, 1987.

DeBlase R and Kucler M: Assistive hearing device aids patient-staff communication, Geriatr Nurs 16:223-226, 1986.

DeBlase R and others: Postintraocular lens implant, Geriatr Nurs 9:342-344, 1988.

Fierman P: Newer concepts in otitis media, Hosp Pract 22(3):11-14, 1987.

Hanson CM and others: Glaucoma screening: an important role for N.P.'s, Nurse Pract 12(12):14, 18-21, 1987.

Lawlor MC: Common ocular injuries and disorders, J Emerg Nurs 15(1), 36-43, 1989.

Lent-Wunderlich E and Ott MJ: Helping your patient through eye surgery, RN, 43-45, June 1986.

Soll DB and others: Drugs and glaucoma, Am Fam Physician 34(1):181-185, 1986.

Zavon B and Slater N: A surgical counseling plan for patients undergoing cataract surgery, J Opthal Nurs Technol 7(2):68-71, 1988.

CHAPTER 6

Disorders of the Heart

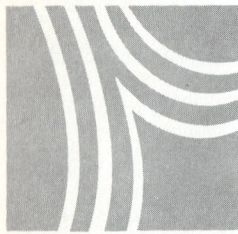

Cardiovascular diseases continue to cause more deaths annually in the United States than all other diseases combined. This fact persists despite a steady rate of decline that has continued over the last decade. Nearly 66 million Americans have some form of cardiovascular disease; about 1½ million suffer a myocardial infarction (MI) each year, and 36% of these result in death.

Heart diseases can be classified into two major groupings—acquired and congenital. This chapter includes discussion of coronary artery disease, congestive heart failure, and inflammatory and valvular heart disease. Figure 6-1 outlines the major structures of the heart and the pattern of blood circulation.

CORONARY ARTERY DISEASE

Coronary artery disease (CAD) is a general term used to describe conditions involving the coronary arteries, the most common of which is atherosclerotic heart disease. Coronary artery disease is recognized as the leading cause of death in the Western world. The dramatic increase in its incidence is attributed to the diet and lifestyle that accompany affluence and prosperity, to increased longevity, and to improved disease identification. Common risk factors for CAD are identified in the box on this page. Nutrition remains one of the key elements in epidemiologic studies. Despite extensive research, the exact cause of CAD remains unknown.

PATHOPHYSIOLOGY

The localized accumulation of lipids and fibrous tissue in the coronary vessels results in arterial narrowing and possible occlusion. Vascular changes gradually inhibit the ability of the arteries to dilate, thereby reducing blood flow to the myocardium. Symptoms are the result of an inadequate supply of oxygen to meet the demand for oxygen by the myocardium. They tend to appear only when the atherosclerotic process is well advanced, usually a greater than 75% occlusion. Myocardial ischemia results in angina, acute myocardial infarction, or sudden cardiac death.

RISK FACTORS ASSOCIATED WITH CORONARY ARTERY DISEASE

NONMODIFIABLE RISK FACTORS
1. *Age*. Mortality from CAD rapidly increases with age.
2. *Sex*. Incidence of CAD in women is very low until after menopause.
3. *Race*. Non-white men and women under 65 years of age have higher mortality rates.
4. *Family history*. A positive family history of CAD in parents or siblings under age 50 increases the risk.

MODIFIABLE RISK FACTORS
*1. *Hyperlipoproteinemia*. Elevated cholesterol, triglyceride, and phospholipid levels are associated with development of CAD.
*2. *Dietary patterns*. A diet chronically high in saturated fats, salt, refined sugar, and cholesterol is linked with CAD.
*3. *Hypertension*. In the presence of hyperlipidemia an elevated systolic or diastolic blood pressure often seems to accelerate atherosclerosis.
*4. *Obesity*. Overweight individuals are more prone to develop associated risk factors. The direct link to CAD is not clear.
*5. *Cigarette smoking*. Relationship is unclear but related to effects of nicotine and carbon monoxide. Risk of death is two to six times greater in heavy smokers.
6. *Personality and life-style*. A sedentary life-style, chronic stress, and low socioeconomic status are often associated with CAD.

NOTE: Asterisks indicate major risk factors.

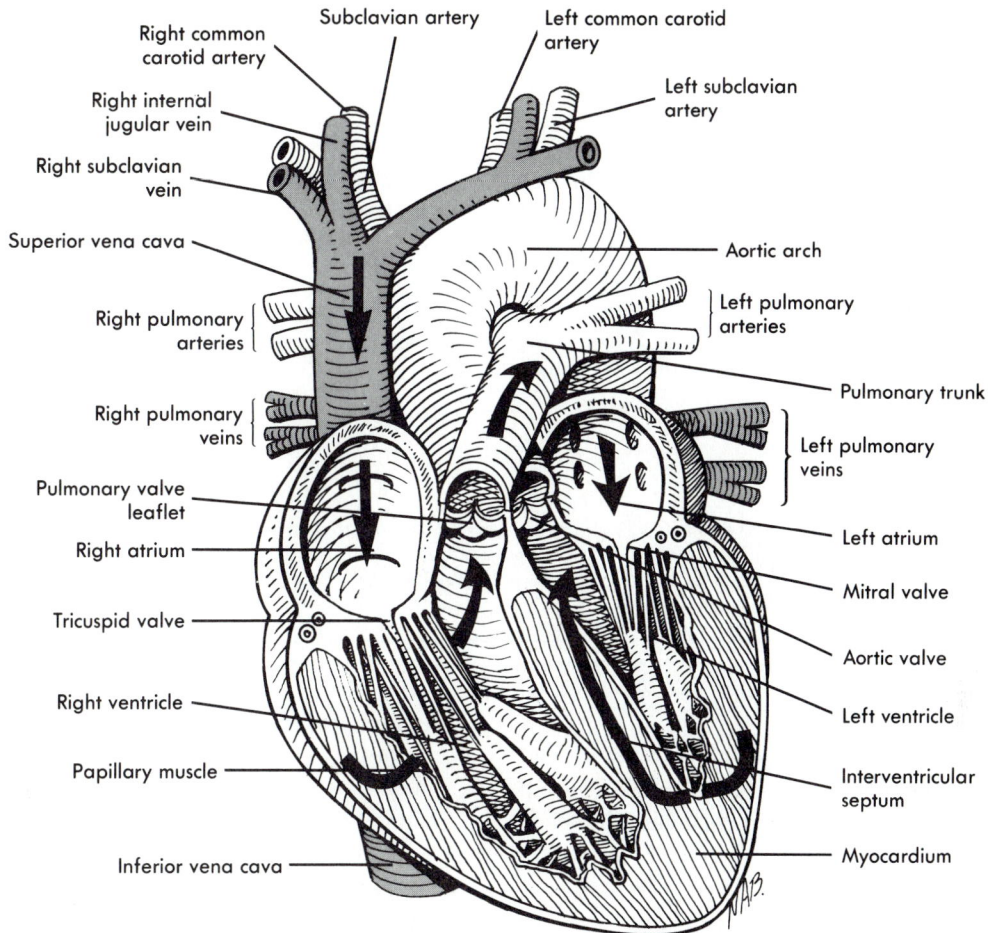

FIGURE 6-1 Major structures of the heart. (From Phipps WJ, Long BC, and Woods NF: Medical surgical nursing: concepts and clinical practice, ed 4, St Louis, 1990, Mosby–Year Book, Inc.)

ANGINA

Angina pectoris occurs when myocardial oxygen demand exceeds the supply. It is characterized by paroxysmal retrosternal or substernal chest pain, which may radiate into the jaw, neck, or shoulder or down the left arm. The pain may be described as heaviness or tightness in the chest and is frequently associated with exertion, exercise, extreme cold, emotion, heavy meals, or anything that increases the work of the heart or myocardial oxygen consumption. The ischemia is temporary and reversible and is usually relieved by rest or vasodilation.

MEDICAL MANAGEMENT

Medical management is aimed at reducing myocardial oxygen demand and includes the following:

Control or elimination of modifiable risk factors

Identification, elimination, or spacing of precipitating factors

Drug therapy with vasodilators, beta-adrenergic blockers, and calcium channel blocking agents (see Table 6-1)

Surgical management options include coronary artery bypass surgery and percutaneous coronary angioplasty. Surgical procedures do not alter the atherosclerotic process, but they do reduce angina and improve activity tolerance.

NURSING MANAGEMENT

Assessment

Subjective

History of the disease and its treatment

Pain pattern, severity, duration

Precipitating and relieving factors

Medications in use, understanding of drugs

Diet and exercise patterns, occupation

Knowledge of disorder, risk factor management

Objective

Baseline vital signs

Weight

Changes in cardiac rhythm

TABLE 6-1 Drugs used in the management of angina

Drugs	Actions	Side Effects
Nitrites/Nitrates		
Nitroglycerin Isosorbide (Isordil) Nitropaste	Dilate coronary arteries and intercoronary collateral vessels Decrease peripheral resistance, systolic blood pressure, and heart workload	Postural hypotension Burning sensation on tongue Throbbing in head, flushing Headache
Beta-Adrenergic Blockers		
Propanolol (Inderal) Nadolol (Corgard) Metoprolol (Lopressor) Atenolol (Tenormin) Esmolol (Brevibloc)	Decrease myocardial oxygen demand by reducing heart rate, blood pressure, and myocardial contractility	Bradycardia (slowed heart beat) Hypotension Gastrointestinal complaints
Calcium Channel Blockers		
Nifedipine (Procardia) Diltiazem (Cardizem) Verapamil (Calan, Isoptin)	Act at the cellular level to block movement of calcium ions, thus reducing cardiac activity and workload of the heart Decrease heart rate and act as potent vasodilators Reduce coronary vasospasm	Bradycardia Hypotension

Nursing Diagnoses

Diagnoses will depend on the severity of the disease but commonly include the following:

Activity intolerance related to occurrence of chest pain with exercise or exertion

Anxiety related to threat of pain and change in health status

Chest pain related to temporary myocardial ischemia

Knowledge deficit related to modification of risk factors, avoidance of precipitating factors, or diet and medications used to control anginal attacks

GUIDELINES FOR USING ANTIANGINAL DRUGS

SUBLINGUAL NITROGLYCERIN

Store tablets in tightly closed dark bottle; keep dry.
Sublingual administration causes burning sensation on the tongue.
Throbbing in head and flushing sensation may be felt.
Make position changes slowly after taking nitroglycerin.
Use tablets prophylactically to avoid pain if known to occur with certain activities.
Take tablet at onset of pain, and repeat every 5 minutes if pain is unrelieved. Call physician if pain is unrelieved after a total of three to four tablets.
Always carry a supply of tablets.
Check expiration date on bottle and be sure to obtain fresh supplies.

NITROGLYCERIN PASTES/OINTMENTS

Apply to any nonhairy area of skin.
Measure dose carefully with ruled papers.
Remove all old cream before applying new dose.

BETA BLOCKERS

Monitor pulse rate. Do not take drug if pulse rate is below 50.
Take drug with meals.
Inform physician of any history of allergy, asthma, or chronic obstructive pulmonary disease (COPD). May induce bronchospasm.

CALCIUM CHANNEL BLOCKERS

Take drug 1 hour before or 1 to 2 hours after meals.

Expected Outcomes

Patient will appropriately space activities to continue preferred life-style without attacks of pain.

Patient will experience decreased anxiety through better control and management of the disease.

Patient will have fewer attacks of pain and will have pain controlled by vasodilator drugs.

Patient will assume knowledgeable control of life-style, will appropriately modify diet patterns and exercise/activity routines, and will be able to discuss drugs used to control symptoms and their side effects.

Nursing Interventions

Teach patient correct use of prescribed medications and their side effects (see Table 6-1 and box on this page).

Discuss with patient elimination of modifiable risk factors:

Plan diet for weight reduction.

Assist patient to reduce salt intake.

Assist patient to modify diet to decrease intake of cholesterol and saturated fats.

Eliminate cigarette smoking.

Maintain adequate control of hypertension if present.

Instruct patient in relaxation and stress management techniques.

Explore modifications of patient's life-style to prevent pain attacks:

Patient should avoid physical and emotional overexertion.

Patient should avoid overeating, especially meals with red meat.

Patient should avoid prolonged exposure to climate extremes, dress appropriately, and avoid extreme cold or hot, humid conditions.

Patient should avoid situations that combine known precipitating factors.

Encourage activity to tolerance but avoid fatigue. Patient should stop activity immediately if pain occurs

Patient should space activities or exercise for shorter periods and should participate in a regularly scheduled exercise regimen if available.

Discuss the use of nitroglycerin *prior* to planned exertion, such as exercise or sexual activity.

Emphasize need for ongoing medical management.

Instruct patient to contact physician if anginal pain pattern changes or worsens.

CARDIOGENIC SHOCK

DEFINITION

Inadequate tissue perfusion of cardiac origin, most commonly caused by myocardial infarction with severe left ventricular failure. Mortality rate is 80 to 90%.

PATHOLOGIC SEQUENCE

1. Cardiac function and output are insufficient to perfuse body cells.
2. Vital organs do not receive nutrients and/or discharge cellular waste, producing metabolic acidosis.
3. Progressive damage occurs in vital organs from prolonged ischemia.
4. Decreased coronary artery perfusion causes progressive ischemia and infarction.

SIGNS AND SYMPTOMS

Hyperventilation—shallow respirations
Falling blood pressure—tachycardia, weak pulse
Decreasing urine output, oliguria (less than 20 ml/hr)
Cool clammy skin, pallor
Restlessness, decreasing level of consciousness, mental confusion, lethargy
Metabolic acidosis

MEDICAL AND NURSING CARE

Monitor arterial lines and pulmonary artery catheters
Drug therapy:
    Vasopressors and cardiotonics
    Dopamine and norepinephrine
Intraaortic balloon pump
Careful fluid replacement
Supplemental oxygen
Support and reassurance to patient and family

Evaluation

Patient is able to space daily activities to maintain lifestyle without occurrence of pain.

Patient reports less anxiety as a result of improved disease control.

Antianginal drugs keep patient free of pain.

Patient can describe effects of drugs, appropriate diet and activity, and signs and symptoms that indicate need to contact physician.

MYOCARDIAL INFARCTION

Myocardial infarction (MI) is caused by a sudden blockage of one of the branches of a coronary artery that interferes with the blood supply to a portion of the myocardium, producing ischemic death of tissue over a period of hours. The location and size of the infarct determine the consequences in terms of contractility and myocardial function. The mortality rate from MI remains high (30 to 40%), with most deaths occurring before the patient reaches the hospital.

PATHOPHYSIOLOGY

Ischemic injury evolves over a period of hours. Ischemia depresses cardiac function and triggers autonomic nervous system responses that worsen the imbalance between oxygen supply and demand. Ischemia that persists longer than 35 to 45 minutes produces irreversible cellular damage to the cardiac muscle, and contractile function in the area is permanently lost. MI may be complicated by the development of dysrhythmias, congestive failure, or cardiogenic shock (see box on this page).

MEDICAL MANAGEMENT

The diagnosis is based on the following symptoms and diagnostic study results:

Severe crushing chest pain unrelieved by rest or nitroglycerin

ECG changes—may include pronounced Q waves, elevated ST segments, T wave abnormalities

Serum enzymes—creatine phosphokinase (CPK), lactic dehydrogenase (LDH), and serum glutamic oxaloacetic transaminase (SGOT) are released into bloodstream from death of tissue

Medical management is directed toward improving oxygenation, relieving pain, improving coronary circulation and preventing complications. Specifics include the following:

Intravenous morphine sulfate for chest pain

Oxygen and beta-adrenergic blockers to reestablish a balance in myocardial supply and demand

Reperfusion efforts with thrombolytic agents (see box on next page)

Percutaneous transluminal coronary angioplasty

Bypass surgery after initial recovery period

Staged cardiac rehabilitation begins as soon as the patient is stable.

USE OF THROMBOLYTICS IN TREATMENT OF MI

PURPOSE
Used to restore blood flow and preserve injured myocardial tissue to limit area of infarction.

ACTION
Thrombolytics accelerate the natural fibrinolytic process by activating plasminogen, thereby lysing the clot

AGENTS USED
Streptokinase—Activates all circulating plasminogen creating, a systemic lysis state.

Tissue plasminogen activator (t-PA)—Activates only fibrin-bound plasminogen and is more clot specific. Causes less systemic risk and is associated with greater effectiveness in reperfusion

Heparin—Used in continuous infusion to help prevent reocclusion from new thrombus formation

CONCERNS
Must be given within 4 to 6 hours of onset of MI

Contraindicated in presence of bleeding disorders, severe hypertension, or history of CVA

Used cautiously if at all in patients of advanced age or with recent history of trauma or surgery

All patients are at risk for bleeding and/or reocclusion

NURSING MANAGEMENT

Assessment (Acute Phase)
Subjective
Character of pain (there may be none in the elderly)

History of onset, treatment attempted, prior CAD history

Dyspnea

Objective
Vital signs (signs of shock), increased pulse, decreased blood pressure

Diaphoresis (perspiration), skin temperature

Skin color, cyanosis

Arrhythmias

Intense anxiety and apprehension

Presence of nausea/vomiting

Nursing Diagnoses
Diagnoses will depend on the severity of the MI and the stage of recovery. Common diagnoses include the following.

Acute phase
Extreme anxiety related to intense pain and fear of death

Chest pain related to severe myocardial ischemia

Altered tissue perfusion (cardiopulmonary) related to myocardial ischemia

Decreased cardiac output related to loss of myocardial contractility

Rehabilitative phase
Activity intolerance related to decreased myocardial function

Potential for ineffective individual and family coping related to life-style changes mandated by the MI

Knowledge deficit related to progressive cardiac rehabilitation following MI

Altered role performance related to life-style modifications resulting from MI

Expected Outcomes: Acute Phase
Patient will not experience disabling anxiety.

Patient's pain will be significantly reduced.

Vital functions will be supported and preserved.

Patient's metabolic demands will be reduced to the lowest possible level.

Expected Outcomes: Rehabilitative Phase
Patient will have sufficient energy to participate in a program of progressive activity.

Patient and family will receive ongoing support and education about MI and be encouraged to openly discuss their feelings and fears.

Patient will discuss the elements of the cardiac rehabilitation program—drug, diet, and exercise therapy.

Patient will successfully return to prior roles—familial, social, sexual, and occupational.

Nursing Interventions: Acute Phase
Attach monitoring devices and observe for arrhythmias.

Provide additional oxygen by nasal cannula.

Monitor vital signs—check intake and output balance carefully.

Position patient in semi-Fowler's position.

Administer drugs as prescribed:
IV morphine for relief of pain and anxiety

Valium to reduce anxiety and restlessness if ordered

Prophylactic lidocaine to prevent arrhythmias

IV heparin to prevent thromboembolism

Reduce activity to absolute minimum.

Maintain a calm environment.

Provide physical comfort measures.

Promote rest and reassure the patient.

Caution patient to avoid straining and the Valsalva maneuver. Administer stool softeners.

Take time for patient's family—offer support.

Explain all equipment and procedures.

Nursing Interventions: Rehabilitative Phase
Maintain strict bedrest for 24 to 48 hours.

Add activities gradually on the basis of metabolic demands. Monitor patient's response. (See box on p. 87.)

Add lying and sitting exercises as ordered.

Teach patient to take and monitor own pulse.

MYOCARDIAL INFARCTION—ACUTE PHASE

Nursing Diagnoses	Expected Patient Outcomes	Nursing Interventions
Anxiety related to intense pain and fear of death	Patient will not experience disabling anxiety.	1. Assure patient that the most dangerous stage of MI has passed. 2. Give family opportunities to discuss their concerns, and keep them informed of patient's progress. 3. Provide a calm unhurried environment. 4. Be sure patient understands that the function of the continuous ECG is to monitor, not to keep the heart beating. 5. Give prescribed tranquilizers or sedatives as needed.
Chest pain related to myocardial ischemia	Patient's pain will be significantly reduced or relieved.	1. Monitor degree of pain and effectiveness of interventions. 2. Give prescribed analgesics as needed, IV morphine and other drugs as prescribed. 3. Stay with patient and offer reassurance. 4. Administer prescribed oxygen by nasal cannula.

Altered tissue perfusion (cardiopulmonary) related to coronary artery obstruction	Patient's vital functions will be preserved.
	ECG monitor shows normal sinus rhythm.
		1. Monitor vital signs for signs of shock and irregular pulse.
		2. Monitor ECG continuously for arrhythmias.
		  a. Record strips every 4 hours.
		  b. Notify physician if premature ventricular contractions occur.
		  c. Give prescribed lidocaine.
		3. Monitor breath sounds for respiratory congestion.
		4. Place patient in semi-Fowler's position.
		5. Encourage fluids but avoid overhydration.
		6. Give anticoagulant, if prescribed.

Decreased cardiac output related to loss of myocardial contractility	Patient's metabolic demands will be reduced to minimal.	1. Monitor vital signs for signs of shock. 2. Use measures to decrease anxiety. 3. Provide absolute rest. 4. Assist with all activities of daily living. 5. Teach patient to avoid Valsalva maneuvers.

NURSING CARE PLAN

MYOCARDIAL INFARCTION—REHABILITATIVE PHASE

Nursing Diagnoses	Expected Patient Outcomes	Nursing Interventions

Activity intolerance related to decreased myocardial function	Patient will have sufficient energy to gradually resume self-care activities.	1. Space activities with rest.
		2. After 24 to 48 hours encourage a gradual increase in self-care activities.
		3. Decrease mealtime fatigue:
		  a. Offer small, frequent meals.
		  b. Avoid very hot or very cold foods.
		  c. Allow sufficient time for meals.
		4. Begin rehabilitation teaching early, so patient has sense of expected recovery.
		5. Encourage and supervise an increased activity schedule:
		  a. Start with lying and sitting exercises.
		  b. Increase length of ambulation gradually.
		  c. Encourage exercises for 20 minutes twice a day.
		6. Assess for signs of activity intolerance (chest pain, dyspnea, change in vital signs or monitor ECG).
		7. Teach patient to monitor pulse during exercises and to stop exercise if pulse does not increase or if it increases >20 over resting pulse.
		8. Reinforce plans for home activity program.

Potential for sexual dysfunction related to fears of recurrent MI	Patient will gradually resume preillness pattern of sexuality.	1. Give patient opportunities to explore concerns about own sexuality and resumption of sexual activity (usually after 6 weeks). 2. Correct misunderstandings about effect of coitus after infarction. 3. Encourage patient and partner to identify coital positions that are less stressful to patient. 4. Suggest that coitus be delayed until 3 hours after a heavy meal or excessive alcohol intake. 5. Teach patient symptoms occurring during coitus that need to be reported to physician.

Knowledge deficit related to the regimen of progressive cardiac rehabilitation	Patient will be knowledgeable about treatment regimen and able to describe drug, diet, and exercise restrictions.	1. Teach the patient:
		  a. Nature of MI and rationale for prescribed therapies.
		  b. Measures to prevent future MIs.
		  c. Effect of stressors and methods to relieve stress.
		  d. Benefits of a regular planned activity program.
		  e. Principles of sodium- and cholesterol-restricted diet.
		  f. Action and side effects of all prescribed medications.

Potential for ineffective family coping related to lifestyle changes required by the MI	Patient and family will receive ongoing support and education and be encouraged to discuss their feelings and fears.	1. Provide patient and family with teaching and reteaching as needed. 2. Clarify misconceptions and misunderstandings. 3. Discuss return to employment and leisure patterns. 4. Refer for counseling follow-up if appropriate.

COMMON ACTIVITIES CATEGORIZED BY ENERGY EXPENDITURE

VERY LIGHT ACTIVITY

Eating, dressing, bathing
Driving, walking ≤2 mph
Cooking

Bowling
Golfing (cart use)

LIGHT ACTIVITY

Use of commode or bedpan
Housework
Stair climbing (one flight)
Sexual activity
Fitness walking ≤4 mph

Gardening
Dancing
Cycling <8 mph
Lawn mowing (power-mower)

MODERATE ACTIVITY

Jogging
Snow shoveling
Tennis
Skiing

Swimming
Skating
Basketball

HEAVY ACTIVITY

Handball
Jump rope
Cross country skiing

Lifting >75 lb
Carrying loads upstairs
Wet snow shoveling

Adapted from Beare PG and Myers JL: Principles and practice of adult health nursing, St Louis, 1990, The CV Mosby Co.

Terminate exercise if patient has chest pain or pulse rate greater than 100.

Teach patient and family about MI and its physical effects.

Patient can be discharged within 10 to 14 days if no complications arise.

Teach principles of diet modification:
Avoid extremely hot or cold food initially.
Plan weight control.
Restrict excess salt intake.
Reduce cholesterol and saturated fats.

Discuss patient's resumption of sexual activity after 4 to 6 weeks.

Help patient give up smoking.

Refer patient to structured cardiac rehabilitation program if available.

Evaluation: Acute Phase

Patient reports decrease of pain and anxiety.
Patient does not experience complications.
Patient's cardiac workload is reduced to minimal levels.

Evaluation: Rehabilitative Phase

Patient engages in progressive cardiac rehabilitation program and gradually resumes former activities.

Patient and family participate in cardiac education program.

Patient can describe dietary restrictions, medications to be taken, and exercise plan to follow at home.

PACEMAKERS

DEFINITION

A battery-powered pulse generator attached to a pacing wire that delivers an electronic stimulus to the heart's atrial and/or ventricular conduction system to control the heart rate. The pacing unit initiates and maintains the heart rate when the natural pacemakers are unable to do so.

TYPES

Fixed rate—Pacemaker fires electrical stimuli at a preset rate regardless of heart's inherent rhythm.
Demand—An electrode at the tip of pacing wire senses the patient's own heart beat and produces a stimulus only when the heart rate drops below a preset level.

ASSOCIATED NURSING CARE

External pacemaker
Monitor patient's heart rate—observe for pacing stimulus on monitor and ensure that it is not below the preset rate.
Ensure catheter terminals are securely connected
Ensure that pacemaker is adequately secured to patient so accidental dislodgement is prevented.
Monitor patient for signs of infection or inflammation at insertion site
Internal pacemaker
Teach patient to do the following:
Monitor pulse daily if ordered by physician.
Resume normal physical activity.
Use only electrical equipment in good working order.
Carry pacemaker ID card specifying type.
Have pacemaker function monitored monthly at center or over telephone.
Report symptoms of dizziness or fatigue.
Show pacemaker card at airport security checks.

Patient can describe symptoms indicative of need for immediate physician attention.

Patient successfully resumes occupational, familial, and sexual roles.

NOTE: Pacemakers are occasionally needed by patients whose cardiac damage is such that they are unable to sustain a stable cardiac rhythm. The box above outlines basic data about pacemakers and associated nursing care. Patients may also be candidates for implantable defibrillator units.

CONGESTIVE HEART FAILURE

Congestive heart failure (CHF) represents a state in which the heart is no longer able to pump an adequate supply of blood to meet the demands of the body. The failure may be acute or chronic. The chronic form develops gradually and generally produces milder symptoms. Congestive heart failure is caused by two types of conditions:

1. Conditions resulting in direct heart damage, such as MI

2. Conditions that produce ventricular overload
   a. Preload—Amount of blood in ventricle at end of diastole is increased as in fluid overload or valvular and septal defects.
   b. Afterload—Force that the ventricle must exert to eject blood into the circulatory system is increased as with valvular stenosis, or pulmonary or systemic hypertension.

PATHOPHYSIOLOGY

The overt symptoms of CHF appear as the heart's compensatory mechanisms are first set in motion and then exhausted. Symptoms include the following:

Tachycardia—Heart rate increases to increase cardiac output but diastole is shortened and inadequate filling time is present.

Ventricular dilation—Myocardial fibers stretch to provide more forceful contractions.

Myocardial hypertrophy—Increased muscle mass causes more efficient contraction. Muscle mass can outgrow the blood supply and cause hypoxia.

As the mechanisms of cardiac compensation become inadequate additional homeostatic mechanisms are triggered:

Sympathetic stimulation with release of norepinephrine causes general vasoconstriction.

Glomerular filtration is reduced and aldosterone secretion causes retention of sodium and water.

Hepatic congestion decreases clearance of aldosterone and antidiuretic hormone (ADH), worsening the fluid overload.

Congestive heart failure may be classified in a variety of ways. The mechanisms of left and right ventricular failure are described in the box on this page. Excess fluid retention by the body results in venous stasis, an increase in venous pressure, and congestion in either the pulmonary system or systemic venous circulation.

MEDICAL MANAGEMENT

Primary goals of treatment are aimed at decreasing oxygen requirements, optimizing cardiac output, removing excess fluid, and restoring the balance between the supply of and demand for blood by body tissue. Major approaches include the following:

Providing supplemental oxygen, usually by nasal cannula

Reducing body's need for oxygen

Restricting sodium and fluid intake

Administering medications

Digitalis to improve strength and force of contractions

Diuretics to reduce circulatory volume

CONGESTIVE HEART FAILURE

LEFT-SIDED FAILURE

Left ventricle cannot pump all the blood coming from the lungs. The symptoms are primarily the result of lung congestion.

Blood backs up into pulmonary bed.

Increased hydrostatic pressure causes fluid to accumulate in the pulmonary tissues.

Blood flow is decreased to brain, kidneys, and systemic cells.

Symptoms

Severe dyspnea, orthopnea, rales, cough productive of frothy blood-tinged sputum

Severe anxiety, restlessness, confusion

Severe weakness, fatigue

Oliguria

RIGHT-SIDED FAILURE

Right ventricle cannot pump all the blood coming from the right atria; right atria cannot accept all the blood coming from the systemic circulation. Rarely seen alone—usually occurs with left-sided failure.

Blood backs up into systemic circulation.

Increased hydrostatic pressure causes peripheral and dependent pitting edema. Fluid may weep from edematous tissues.

Venous congestion in kidneys, liver, and gastrointestinal tract.

Symptoms

Peripheral and dependent edema—pitting type

Distended neck veins

Anorexia, nausea, bloating

NURSING MANAGEMENT

Assessment

Subjective

History and development of symptoms, history of heart disease

Shortness of breath, degree of orthopnea

Recent abrupt weight gain

Ankle swelling

Increasing fatigue, loss of appetite, dizziness

Exercise intolerance

Objective

Visible dyspnea, presence of cough, nature and quantity of sputum

Edema: site, degree

Abdominal distention

Neck vein distention

Baseline vital signs

Baseline weight, daily weights

Presence of adventitious breath sounds

Level of consciousness

Nursing Diagnoses

Diagnoses will vary based on the severity of the disorder but common diagnoses include the following:

Activity intolerance related to decreased muscle oxygenation

Anxiety related to severe dyspnea and fear of death

Decreased cardiac output related to excess fluid level

Fluid volume excess related to decreased cardiac output

Potential impairment of skin integrity related to tissue edema

Impaired gas exchange related to ventricular perfusion imbalance

Knowledge deficit related to the control of and management of CHF

Sleep pattern disturbance related to nighttime orthopnea

Expected Outcomes

Patient will gradually resume self-care activities without excessive fatigue.

Patient will breathe freely without supplemental oxygen and experience decreased anxiety.

Patient's oxygen and carbon dioxide exchange in the lungs will improve.

Patient's cardiac output will improve.

Patient will gradually excrete excess fluid.

Patient will maintain an intact skin.

Patient will be knowledgeable about the treatment regimen and prevention of CHF.

Patient will experience uninterrupted restful sleep.

Nursing Interventions

Ensure rest by providing support and anticipating needs. Assist with activities of daily living as needed to avoid dyspnea. Reinforce importance of conserving energy.

Place patient in semi-Fowler's or high Fowler's position.

Provide oxygen at 2 to 6 L by nasal cannula as ordered.

Position patient with pillow on overbed table to facilitate breathing during acute phase. Elevate feet when out of bed.

Reassure patient and assist to control breathing pattern.

Administer prescribed medications and teach patient about desired effects and side effects (see Table 6-2 and box on next page.)

Explain all care routines fully.

Monitor vital signs frequently.

Monitor daily weight; assess status of edema.

Maintain accurate intake and output records. Restrict fluids if ordered.

Teach patient principles of restricted sodium diet.
Teach patients to read labels carefully.

Teach patient principles of potassium enrichment in diet.

Prevent constipation and straining through use of stool softeners and bulk-forming cathartics.

Monitor skin and prevent skin breakdown:
Wash and dry skin frequently and gently.
Use antipressure devices on bed.
Change patient's position frequently.
Pay special attention to sacrum; avoid abrasion and shearing force.

Increase patient's self-care activities slowly as condition improves. Monitor for exercise intolerance.

TABLE 6-2 Diuretics used in the treatment of heart failure

Type	Example	Onset/Peak/Duration	Side Effects
Thiazide	Chlorothiazide (Diuril)	2 hr/4 hr/6-12 hr	Gastrointestinal upsets (can be minimized by taking medication with meals); hypokalemia; hyperglycemia
	Hydrochlorothiazide (Esidrix, HydroDIURIL)	2 hr/4 hr/6-12 hr	
Loop	Furosemide (Lasix)	1 hr/1-2 hr/6-8 hr	Similar to thiazide diuretics; also ototoxicity and blood dyscrasias
	Ethacrynic acid (Edecrin)	30 min/2 hr/6 hr	
	Bumetanide (Bumex)	Oral: 30-60 min/1-2 hr/4-6 hr IV: within minutes/15-30 min/3-6 hr	
Potassium sparing	Spironolactone (Aldactone)	Gradual/3 days/2-3 days after therapy discontinued	Gastrointestinal irritation; hyperkalemia
	Triamterene (Dyrenium)	Rapid/7-9 hr/12-16 hr	

From Phipps WJ, Long BC, and Woods NF: Medical-surgical nursing: concepts and clinical practice, ed 4, St Louis, 1990, Mosby–Year Book, Inc.

NURSING ACTIONS RELATED TO ADMINISTRATION OF DIGITALIS

ADMINISTERING DIGITALIS

Take apical pulse before administering digitalis preparations; withhold medication and notify physician if pulse is below 60 or above 120.

If giving digoxin intramuscularly, inject it deeply and massage area well since drug is a tissue irritant.

Monitor serum potassium blood levels. Hypokalemia potentiates the effects of digoxin and the heart becomes more excitable. Hypokalemia is the most common cause of digitalis toxicity.

Give potassium supplements (if prescribed) and instruct patient in potassium-rich food sources.

MONITORING PATIENT FOR DIGITALIS TOXICITY

Cardiovascular effects
  Bradycardia
  Tachycardia
  Bigeminy (double beats)
  Ectopic beats
  Pulse deficit (difference between apical and radial pulse)

Gastrointestinal effects
  Anorexia
  Nausea and vomiting
  Abdominal pain
  Diarrhea

Neurologic effects
  Headache
  Double, blurred, or colored vision
  Drowsiness, confusion
  Restlessness, irritability
  Muscle weakness

Adapted from Phipps WJ, Long BC, and Woods NF: Medical-surgical nursing: concepts and clinical practice, ed 4, St Louis, 1990, Mosby–Year Book, Inc.

Teach patient and family the signs and symptoms of incipient failure and the importance of planning and spacing activities to avoid fatigue and stress. Report any sudden weight gain of 2 to 3 lb over 1 to 2 days.

Evaluation

Patient's energy level increases; patient moves toward independent self-care.

Patient is able to breathe freely and experiences no dyspnea.

Improved oxygen and carbon dioxide exchange increases patient's energy level, kidney function, and appetite.

MANAGEMENT OF PULMONARY EDEMA

SYMPTOMS

Profound dyspnea and pallor
Cough that produces large quantities of blood-tinged frothy sputum
Audible wheezing
Tachycardia
Acute anxiety and restlessness

MANAGEMENT

Administer medications as ordered:
  Morphine IV to decrease anxiety and lower left atrial pressure
  Aminophylline IV to dilate the bronchial tree and increase urine output
  Digitalis to strengthen cardiac contractions
  Diuretics to reduce fluid load
  Vasodilators

Place patient in high Fowler's position.

Give 40% to 70% humidified oxygen by face mask.

Monitor serum potassium, as large amounts will be excreted with treatment.

Administer rotating tourniquets, if preceding regimen fails, to trap blood in the extremities, reducing cardiac overload:
  Place tourniquets high up toward axilla or groin.
  Tourniquets should be tight enough to occlude veins, but pulses must remain palpable.
  Tourniquets should be on three extremities at a time; rotate in a clockwise manner every 15 minutes. Each extremity is occluded for 45 minutes each hour.
  When treatment ends, remove one tourniquet at a time at 15 minute intervals to prevent a sudden increase in venous return.

Patient's cardiac output improves; lungs are clear.

Patient is without edema and maintains a stable weight.

Patient's skin is intact.

Patient is able to sleep at night without episodes of dyspnea.

Patient and family can accurately describe the activity restrictions, diet modifications, and medication schedule to follow for successful home maintenance.

NOTE: Pulmonary edema is a medical emergency that may be associated with left-sided congestive heart failure. It results from the rapid effusion of serous fluid from the pulmonary vasculature into the interstitial tissue and alveoli. Gas exchange fails and the patient begins to drown in pulmonary secretions. The box on this page describes the major symptoms and management.

NURSING CARE PLAN
CONGESTIVE HEART FAILURE

Nursing Diagnoses	Expected Patient Outcomes	Nursing Interventions
Decreased cardiac output related to excess fluid load	Patient will experience an improvement in cardiac output.	1. Monitor respirations q4h for increased effort and rate, and pulse for tachycardia or for rate <60. 2. Monitor heart sounds q4h for presence of S_3 or gallop rhythm. 3. Give prescribed digitalis preparations or vasodilators. Monitor patient's response. 4. Teach patient to avoid Valsalva maneuver.
Impaired gas exchange related to pulmonary congestion	The exchange of O_2 and CO_2 in the lungs will improve. Patient will not need supplemental oxygen.	1. Assess for evidence of hypoxia. 2. Monitor for adventitious breath sounds q4h. 3. Assess neck vein distention q4h (presence, degree). 4. Provide oxygen by nasal cannula or face mask at 2 to 6 L/min as prescribed during early period. 5. Place patient in well-supported high Fowler's or semi-Fowler's position; elevate feet if sitting in chair.
Anxiety related to severe dyspnea	Patient will breathe freely and experience decreased anxiety.	1. Give patient opportunities to explore feelings about effect of illness on life-style. 2. Assist patient to identify personal strengths. 3. Give medications to reduce anxiety, if prescribed. 4. Teach measures to control heart failure and reduce stress.
Potential impairment of skin integrity related to tissue edema	Patient's skin remains intact.	1. Keep patient's legs elevated when sitting in chair. 2. Encourage frequent position changes when lying in bed. 3. Keep skin soft and supple with special attention to sacrum and heels. 4. Use additional measures, as necessary, to protect skin from pressure. Avoid abrasion or shearing force.

Knowledge deficit related to the management of congestive heart failure	Patient understands nature and management of CHF and how to prevent recurrence.	1. Teach patient:
		  a. Nature of CHF and rationale for therapy.
		  b. Self-monitoring for recurring signs of CHF.
		  c. How to be active yet avoid fatigue.
		  d. Management of prescribed sodium-restricted diet.
		  e. Need for follow-up care.
		  f. Importance of weighing daily and reporting any abrupt weight gain of 2 to 3 lb in 1 to 2 days.

Activity intolerance related to decreased tissue oxygenation	Patient will gradually resume self-care activities without excessive fatigue.	1. Plan rest periods. Space activity and rest. 2. Encourage gradually increasing activity within prescribed restrictions; monitor for intolerance. 3. Assist with activities of daily living as necessary; encourage self-care as tolerated. 4. Provide small frequent feedings. Prevent constipation.
Fluid volume excess related to decreased cardiac output	Patient will gradually excrete excess fluid.	1. Assess extremities for edema (site, degree of pitting) and coolness of skin q4h. 2. Maintain an accurate intake and output. 3. Weigh daily. 4. Give prescribed diuretics. 5. Give sodium-restricted diet as prescribed.

INFLAMMATORY HEART DISEASE

Bacterial, viral, and fungal disorders, as well as inflammatory reactions, may produce inflammatory heart disease. Any layer of the heart muscle may be involved. The process may be acute and life threatening or mild and relatively asymptomatic. It may cause no residual damage or trigger serious problems in later years. A description of the major forms of inflammatory heart disease is presented in Table 6-3. Infective endocarditis is described in the text as a model.

INFECTIVE ENDOCARDITIS (ACUTE ENDOCARDITIS, SUBACUTE BACTERIAL ENDOCARDITIS)

Infective endocarditis is an infection of the endocardium, usually involving the heart valves. Acute endocarditis often develops on normal valves, has a rapid onset, and can cause death within days or weeks even with treatment. Subacute endocarditis develops more slowly, usually on previously damaged valves, and responds well to treatment. The disease may also be classified according to causative organism. Viridans (alpha) streptococci, staphylococci, and enterococci are the major infective agents.

PATHOPHYSIOLOGY

Patients who experience intrusive procedures, mainline drugs, or have cardiac anomalies and faulty valves that increase blood turbulence are at high risk for endocarditis. The infecting organisms are carried in the bloodstream and deposited on heart valves or other portions of the endocardium. The organisms bombard the valves and become embedded. The hallmark of the disease is the platelet-fibrin-bacteria mass termed a vegetation that develops and then scars and perforates the valve leaflets. The growths may also break off as emboli.

MEDICAL MANAGEMENT

Medical management includes intravenous antibiotic therapy specific to cultured organism (usually a penicillin). Therapy is continued even after symptom cessation to eliminate all microorganisms from the vegetations and prevent complications. Heart action is reduced and supported as needed.

NURSING MANAGEMENT

Assessment
Subjective
History of heart or valvular disease
Recent history of intrusive procedure, such as dental

TABLE 6-3 Pericarditis, myocarditis, and rheumatic heart disease

Disorder	Etiology	Signs and Symptoms	Medical Management
Pericarditis	Inflammation of the sac that contains the heart, as a result of trauma, neoplasm, systemic disease, or infection—fluid accumulates in the pericardial space (acute); fibrous thickening of pericardial layers occurs; follows both an acute and a chronic course	Severe chest pain, aggravated by deep breathing. Pain is precordial, radiates to left shoulder, and is relieved by sitting up and leaning forward. Pericardial friction rub Fever; increased white blood cells Signs of CHF (chronic) Cardiac tamponade (acute): excess fluid impairs diastolic filling and cardiac output	Treatment of underlying condition or organism if known Pericardiocentesis if large effusion or tamponade Fenestration or pericardectomy for severe cases Symptomatic treatment for pain and fever
Myocarditis	Inflammation of heart muscle—may occur alone or with systemic illnesses, especially infectious ones; may develop secondary to endocarditis or pericarditis	May be nonspecific, such as fever, fatigue, dyspnea, flulike symptoms Signs of CHF Pericardial pain, arrhythmia	Identification and treatment of underlying condition Supportive CHF therapy, digoxin General comfort measures Possible use of immunosuppressives
Rheumatic heart disease	Inflammatory disease involving all three heart layers—residual damage through scarring and deformity of heart valves occurs in 10%; seen in conjunction with beta-hemolytic streptococcal infections; autoimmune response causes antibody formation	Joint pain, recurrent heart murmur, friction rub Follows upper respiratory infection by 1 to 4 weeks May advance to signs of arrhythmias, CHF	Parenteral antibiotics Antiinflammatory drugs Comfort measures Symptom management Prophylactic antibiotic use for years

work, minor surgery, Foley catheters, or cystoscopy

History of IV drug abuse

Malaise, fatigue, joint pain

Anorexia

Objective

Presence of fever (low grade or high grade)

Dyspnea

Edema

Weight loss

New murmur over cardiac valves or change in quality of existing murmur

Anemia and petechiae

Nursing Diagnoses

Diagnoses will depend on the severity of the disease.
Common diagnoses include the following:

Activity intolerance related to systemic illness and
decreased tissue oxygenation

Knowledge deficit related to treatment regimen and
prevention of future episodes

Decreased cardiac output related to failing valvular
function

Fatigue related to decreased tissue oxygenation

Expected Outcomes

Patient's energy level will gradually increase until patient can resume normal activity pattern.

Patient will be knowledgeable about the disease: its origins, treatment regimen, and prevention of future attacks.

Patient's cardiac function will return to normal with effective antibiotic therapy.

Patient will gradually resume normal activity without
incidence of pain or dyspnea.

Nursing Interventions

Administer prescribed IV antibiotics.

Teach patient role of antibiotics in controlling the disease. Prolonged antibiotic treatment is essential.

Monitor vital signs frequently.

Assess temperature patterns.

Provide for adequate rest, but strict bed rest is not necessary. Gradually increase activity as cardiac status
improves.

Be alert for complications, such as signs of CHF or emboli.

Provide comfort measures for fever and joint aches.

Encourage well-balanced diet. Encourage adequate fluids while febrile.

Assist patient to find adequate diversionary activities.

Teach patient about need for prophylactic antibiotics in
the future, especially before dental work. Strict adherence is essential.

Teach patient importance of scrupulous oral hygiene
and regular dental care.

Teach patient to follow healthy heart diet, eating foods
that contain cholesterol, saturated fat, and sodium in
moderation.

Evaluation

Patient resumes normal activities and experiences no
unusual fatigue.

Patient can discuss origins of disease, purposes and
goals of treatment regimen, and measures to follow to
prevent reoccurrence.

Patient's cardiac function returns to preillness levels or
patient is scheduled for surgical replacement of damaged heart valves.

NOTE: The major features of pericarditis, myocarditis,
and rheumatic heart disease are summarized in Table
6-3.

VALVULAR HEART DISEASE

Valvular heart disease may occur congenitally or as a se-
quela of the inflammatory disorders previously discussed. Rheumatic heart disease is one of the most
common precipitating disorders. Diseased or impaired
heart valves may become stenosed and obstruct the normal flow of blood through the heart or become insufficient and cause regurgitation and backflow of blood.
Initially the heart compensates through gradual myocardial hypertrophy, but as the condition worsens CHF
eventually develops and may necessitate valve replacement or repair.

PATHOPHYSIOLOGY

Initially the heart is able to compensate for the diseased
valves through myocardial hypertrophy. Effective medical treatment may extend the compensatory period by
years. If the condition worsens, CHF will develop. Table
6-4 describes the specific forms of valvular dysfunction.

MEDICAL MANAGEMENT

Initial treatment is conservative and is aimed at reducing circulatory congestion and decreasing the cardiac
workload. Surgical repair or replacement is typically delayed until the symptoms are significantly impairing the
patient's activities of daily living.

NURSING MANAGEMENT

Assessment (Preoperative)

Subjective

History and course of disease

Current medical treatment

Diet and activity

Medications

TABLE 6-4 Valvular heart disorders

Disorder	Etiology	Signs and Symptoms	Medical Management
Mitral insufficiency	Papillary muscle dysfunction allows valve to flap in direction of atria during systole. Caused by rheumatic heart disease, congenital factors, bacterial endocarditis. Primarily affects males.	Fatigue and weakness Right-sided heart failure Frequently accompanied by atrial fibrillation Blowing, high-pitched systolic murmur Third heart sound	Restricted activity Low-sodium diet Diuretics Cardiac glycosides to augment left ventricular output Surgical valve repair or replacement when symptoms are advanced
Mitral stenosis	Valve leaflets become thickened and calcified and eventually fuse, resulting in progressively narrowed and immobile valve. Caused by rheumatic heart disease, congenital factors. Two thirds of patients are female.	Fatigue Dyspnea Pulmonary hypertension Right-sided failure Atrial fibrillation with pooled blood in atria, causing thrombus Low-pitched, rumbling presystolic murmur Snapping, loud first heart sound May be asymptomatic for 20 or more years	Low-sodium diet Diuretics Cardioversion or drug treatment for atrial fibrillation Surgical valve repair or replacement when activity is significantly impaired
Aortic insufficiency	Deforming of the valve leaflets causes them to close improperly, allowing blood to backflow. Caused by rheumatic heart disease, congenital factors. Primarily affects males.	Symptoms are rare until left ventricular failure is imminent Palpitations, exertional dyspnea Angina at rest or with exertion Soft blowing aortic diastolic murmur Widened pulse pressure	Cardiac glycosides Low-sodium diet Diuretics Nitroglycerin Surgical valve replacement is usually necessary
Aortic stenosis	Aortic valve becomes stenosed, obstructing left ventricular outflow during systole. Caused by congenital valvular problem (most common cause), rheumatic heart disease, atherosclerosis in elderly. Eighty percent of patients are male.	Exertional dyspnea Angina Exertional syncope (loss of consciousness) Harsh, rough midsystolic murmur Systolic thrill over aortic area	Rest Cardiac glycosides Diuretics Low-sodium diet Nitroglycerin if angina is present Surgical valve replacement as severity of symptoms worsens
Tricuspid insufficiency	Rare disorder since the normal valve leaflets are very small and play less of a role in valve closure. Impaired valve allows backflow of blood into right atrium. Caused by rheumatic heart disease (rare), congenital factors. Primarily affects females.	Symptoms of right-sided heart failure Hepatomegaly, jugular vein distention	Cardiac glycosides Low-sodium diet Diuretics Surgical valve repair or replacement
Tricuspid stenosis	Rare disorder in which shortening and fusion of the commissures cause orifice to narrow and block blood returning to the heart. Caused by rheumatic heart disease. Usually occurs with mitral or aortic stenosis. Primarily affects females.	Symptoms of right-sided heart failure Hepatomegaly, jugular vein distention	Cardiac glycosides Low-sodium diet Diuretics Surgical valve repair or replacement

CARDIAC CATHETERIZATION

RIGHT-SIDED
Purpose
Confirm presence of congenital or acquired valvular disease.
Procedure
1. Cutdown is made in large vein, such as the medial, cubital, or brachial.
2. Catheter is threaded through superior vena cava, right atrium and ventricle, pulmonary artery, and capillaries.
3. Blood samples are taken and pressures recorded to assess oxygen saturation and content.

LEFT-SIDED
Purpose
Evaluate pressures in left side of heart, valve competency, left ventricular function, and selective coronary angiography.
Procedure
1. Cutdown is made in large artery, such as femoral or brachial.
2. Catheter is threaded through the aorta and aortic valve, and into left ventricle or coronary arteries.
3. Blood samples and pressure gradient measurements are taken, and contrast medium is inserted to outline the coronary circulation.

GENERAL CONSIDERATIONS
Procedure is performed under local anesthetic.
Procedure lasts from 1 to 3 hours; patient must lie still.
Right-sided catheterization produces little discomfort.
Left-sided catheterization may produce the following:
  Warm flushing sensation when contrast medium injected
  Nausea
  Fluttering sensation (ectopic beats) from catheter irritation
  Transient chest pain when contrast media is injected

Knowledge and attitude about proposed surgery
Patient's complaints:
  Fatigue
  Dyspnea on exertion, orthopnea, or paroxysmal nocturnal dyspnea
  Angina
  Palpitations or syncope (fainting with drop in blood pressure)
Objective
Activity and energy level
Respiratory rate and quality—breath sounds
Baseline vital signs
Presence of abnormal heart sounds
Presence of edema, pitting or nonpitting
Prominent neck veins
Peripheral oxygenation—nail beds, skin tone, temperature, pulses, and capillary refill
NOTE: Diagnostic workup usually involves cardiac catheterization. The boxes on this page outline the two major

NURSING CARE ASSOCIATED WITH CARDIAC CATHETERIZATION

PRETEST CARE
Reinforce teaching provided by the physician as needed. Encourage patient to ask questions.
Give nothing by mouth prior to test—IV is generally started.
Explore any history of allergy to drugs, contrast media, iodine, or shellfish.

POSTTEST CARE
Monitor patient by prescribed routine, which usually includes the following:
  Vital signs (blood pressure taken on nonoperative arm every 15 min for 1 hr, every 30 min for 3 hr)
  Peripheral pulses distal to insertion site
  Color and sensation on operative side
  Site for evidence of bleeding, swelling, or hematoma (sandbag, pressure dressing, or ice bag may be used); apply firm direct pressure if any bleeding occurs
  Intake and output; encourage fluids if cardiac status is stable
Femoral approach necessitates bed rest for 12 to 24 hr; head of bed should be elevated no more than 30 degrees, and leg should be kept straight.
Brachial approach necessitates keeping arm straight for several hours; patient may be out of bed when vital signs are stable.
ALERT: Procedure may cause vessel spasm or thrombus, arrhythmia, hypotensive reaction to contrast material, and significant diuresis from contrast material.

procedures and give basic nursing care associated with this procedure.

Nursing Diagnoses
Diagnoses will be variable and are based on the severity of the disorder, but commonly include:
  Activity intolerance related to insufficient cardiac output
  Ineffective breathing pattern related to fluid accumulation in lung spaces
  Decreased cardiac output related to failing valves and cardiac pumping mechanism
  Anxiety related to seriousness of open heart surgery and uncertainty of prognosis
  Knowledge deficit related to post heart surgery routines and procedures
  Fluid volume excess related to retained extracellular fluids
  Fatigue related to decreased tissue oxygenation
  Sleep pattern disturbance related to dyspnea in recumbent position

Expected Outcomes
Patient will modify activities as needed to adjust to fluctuating energy levels.

Patient will experience optimum oxygen and carbon dioxide exchange in lungs.

Patient will steadily improve cardiac output after surgery.

Patient will experience only manageable levels of anxiety over anticipated surgical procedure.

Patient will be knowledgeable about proposed surgery and the postoperative treatment regimen to be followed.

Patient will have normal fluid volume as cardiac function improves.

Patient will reestablish a pattern of restful sleep.

Nursing Interventions

Patient care during the extended period of medical management is similar to that received by the patient with CHF and focuses on patient teaching for adherence to diet and medication protocols and strategies for balancing activity and rest. The following items relate to the patient undergoing surgery.

Preoperative

Explain and discuss planned surgical procedure.

Describe and, if possible, take patient to visit intensive care unit.

Discuss expected tubes and equipment and their purposes:

Venous and arterial lines

Monitors

Chest tubes

Intubation tube/ventilator

Urinary catheter

Teach patient bed exercises and breathing exercises to be performed after the operation.

Assist in stabilizing medical condition:

Administer medications as prescribed.

Monitor cardiopulmonary status.

Establish baseline perfusion, pulses.

Foster balance of rest and activity.

Monitor intake and output and daily weights carefully.

Postoperative

Position patient in semi-Fowler's to high Fowler's position.

Provide supplemental oxygen as ordered.

Maintain turn, coughing, and deep breathing schedule. Suction as necessary.

Provide cough pillow for adequate splinting.

Monitor lung sounds, blood gases.

Maintain patency of water seal drainage.

Assess for fluid overload and CHF. Be alert for symptoms of pulmonary congestion.

Check daily weights and for signs of peripheral edema and dyspnea.

Assess peripheral pulses, skin color and temperature, and capillary refill.

Encourage patient to begin progressive activity and ambulation. Provide adequate analgesia.

Provide for periods of uninterrupted rest. Assess for signs of confusion or disorientation, occurrence of nightmares.

Provide TED stockings and encourage leg exercises.

Administer anticoagulants as ordered. Assess for signs of thrombus or embolus.

Instruct patient in importance of long-term anticoagulation with

Warfarin sodium (Coumadin)

Dipyridamole (Persantine)

Reinforce the importance of regular medical follow-up.

Refer patient to structured cardiac rehabilitation program as appropriate.

Evaluation

Patient returns to normal occupational and recreational patterns, and has increased activity tolerance.

Patient has effective respiratory pattern; lungs are clear to auscultation.

Patient is without systemic signs of cardiac failure.

Patient is knowledgeable about postdischarge diet and activity patterns; can state purpose and side effects of all medications.

Patient maintains a normal fluid balance.

Patient can state signs that indicate need for immediate medical follow-up.

Patient's incisions heal without complications.

BIBLIOGRAPHY

Alpert JS: The pharmacologic management of coronary artery disease in 1986, Heart Lung **15**:558-561, 1986.

American Heart Association: AHA Heart Facts 1988, Dallas, 1988, The Association.

Andreoli KG and others: Comprehensive cardiac care: a text for nurses, physicians, and other health practitioners, ed 6, St Louis, 1987, The CV Mosby Co.

Curran CC and Mathewson M: Use of cardiac glycosides in the critically ill, Crit Care Nurse **7**(6):31, 1987.

Deans K and Hartshorn J: Use of antithrombotic agents in valvular heart disease, J Cardiovasc Nurs **1**(3):65-69, 1987.

Fardy P and others: Cardiac rehabilitation, adult fitness and exercise testing, Philadelphia, 1988, Lea & Febiger.

Fletcher GF: Exercise and exercise testing: current state of the art, Heart Lung **13**:5-6, 1984.

Guzzetta CE and Dossey BM: Cardiovascular nursing—body-mind tapestry. St Louis, 1984, CV Mosby.

Kern K: Advances in the surgical treatment of coronary artery disease, J Cardiovasc Nurs **1**(1):1-14, 1986.

Kleven MR: Comparison of thrombolytic agents and mechanisms of action, efficacy and safety, Heart Lung **17**:750-755, 1988.

Marrie TJ: Infective endocarditis: a serious and changing disease, Crit Care Nurse **7**(2):31-46, 1987.

Misenski M: Pathophysiology of acute myocardial infarction: a rationale for thrombolytic therapy, Heart Lung **17:**743-750, 1988.

Miracle V: Anatomy of a murmur, Nursing **16**(7):26, 1986.

Purcell JA and Burrows SG: A pacemaker primer, Am J Nurs **85:**553-568, 1985.

Riegel B, editor: Advances in treatment for CAD, J Cardiovasc Nurs, **1:**15-21, 1986.

Seifert P: Surgery for acquired valvular heart disease, J Cardiovasc Nurs **3**:26-40, 1989.

CHAPTER 7

Disorders of the Vascular System

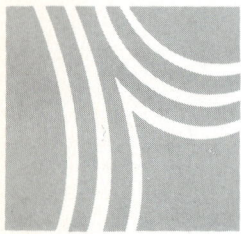

Vascular diseases include a number of disease entities affecting either the arteries or the veins outside the heart. The signs and symptoms of these diseases are frequently the result of interference with the blood supply to the tissues or of structural abnormalities. Figure 7-1 outlines the anatomical structure of the cardiovascular system.

HYPERTENSION

Hypertension is defined as a consistent elevation of blood pressure above 140/90 mm Hg or a consistent elevation of diastolic pressure above 90 mm Hg on an average of two or more readings. The disorder affects some 58 million people, occurring slightly more often in males. It is theorized that millions more are affected but neither diagnosed nor treated. The incidence of hypertension increases with age, and it is twice as prevalent among the black population, who also typically have more severe forms of the disease.

Hypertension is commonly classified into two types: primary and secondary. The cause of primary or essential hypertension, which accounts for 90% of all cases, is basically unknown. Secondary hypertension results from a known cause such as glomerulonephritis, Cushing's disease, or renal stenosis.

PATHOPHYSIOLOGY

Blood pressure is determined by the following:
- Volume of blood flow and strength, rate, and rhythm of the heart
- Peripheral vascular resistance as determined by the diameter of blood vessels and the viscosity of the blood

Increased peripheral resistance from narrowing of the arterioles is the single most common characteristic of hypertension. This peripheral resistance is influenced by renal regulation of the renin angiotensin network and by stimulation of the sympathetic system and release of catecholamines.

With prolonged hypertension, the elastic tissue of arterioles is replaced by fibrous collagen tissue, making the arteriole walls less distensible. As resistance increases, so does the ventricular workload, leading to possible congestive heart failure. The process of atherosclerosis also appears to be accelerated. Inadequate blood supply to the coronary arteries can lead to angina and myocardial infarction. Permanent damage may occur in the kidney and cerebral vessels.

MEDICAL MANAGEMENT

Medical management of hypertension is directed at control of the disease and prevention of associated diseases and complications. Nonpharmacologic strategies include risk factor reduction through weight loss, regular aerobic exercise, stress management, reduction of dietary sodium, and smoking cessation. These strategies are frequently employed first and are often successful at initial control, although drug therapy is usually necessary eventually. A wide range of drugs exists. Some of the commonly prescribed drugs are described in Table 7-1. Initial therapy frequently begins with a diuretic, beta blocking agent, or calcium channel antagonist. A small dose of the least potent drug is prescribed, and additions or substitutions are made on the basis of the patient's response.

NURSING MANAGEMENT

Assessment
Subjective
Knowledge of hypertension and its treatment
Compliance with previous drug or life-style therapy
ALERT: Early hypertension is usually completely asymptomatic.
Headaches (occipital and present in the morning)

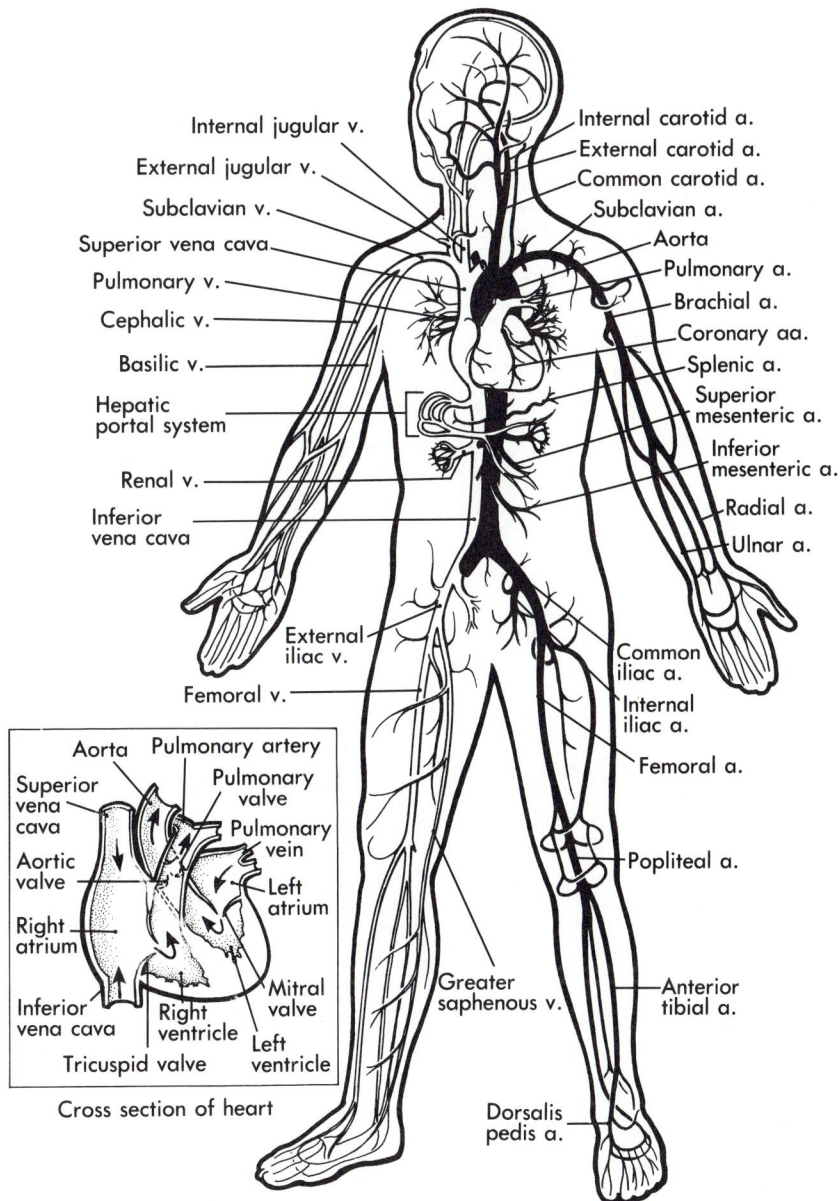

Internal jugular v.
External jugular v.
Subclavian v.
Superior vena cava
Pulmonary v.
Cephalic v.
Basilic v.
Hepatic portal system
Renal v.
Inferior vena cava

Internal carotid a.
External carotid a.
Common carotid a.
Subclavian a.
Aorta
Pulmonary a.
Brachial a.
Coronary aa.
Splenic a.
Superior mesenteric a.
Inferior mesenteric a.
Radial a.
Ulnar a.

External iliac v.
Femoral v.

Common iliac a.
Internal iliac a.
Femoral a.

Popliteal a.

Greater saphenous v.

Anterior tibial a.

Dorsalis pedis a.

Aorta   Pulmonary artery
Superior vena cava
Pulmonary valve
Pulmonary vein
Aortic valve
Left atrium
Right atrium
Inferior vena cava
Right ventricle
Mitral valve
Left ventricle
Tricuspid valve

Cross section of heart

FIGURE 7-1 Cardiovascular system.

Flushing of face
History of nose bleeds
Occupation and life-style
Usual dietary patterns
Presence of risk factors: obesity, smoking, alcohol use, sedentary life-style, stress, family history
Objective
Vital signs
Body weight
Increased cholesterol and lipid levels

Nursing Diagnoses
Diagnoses may be variable but commonly include the following:

Knowledge deficit related to treatment of hypertension, side effects of medications, principles of diet control, and seriousness of complications
Noncompliance with medication and diet regimen prescribed for hypertension

Expected Outcomes
Patient will be knowledgeable about nature of hypertension and its physiologic effects.
Patient will be able to state action and side effects of prescribed medications and measures to control their side effects.
Patient will modify diet to meet prescribed restrictions.

TABLE 7-1 Drugs commonly used to treat hypertension

Type	Action	Side Effects
Diuretics		
Thiazide/thiazide-like diuretics Chlorothiazide (Diuril) Hydrochlorothiazide (HydroDIURIL) Quinethazone (Hydromox) Chlorthalidone (Hygroton) Metolazone (Zaroxolyn)	Block sodium reabsorption in tubules; water is excreted with sodium	Decreased potassium, increased glucose and uric acid, hypovolemia, dehydration, anorexia, nausea
Loop diuretics Bumetanide (Bumex) Ethacrynic acid (Edecrin) Furosemide (Lasix)	Block sodium and water reabsorption in tubules; cause rapid volume depletion	Decreased potassium, postural hypotension, nausea
Potassium-sparing diuretics Spironolactone (Aldactone) Triamterene (Dyrenium)	Antagonize effect of aldosterone; sodium is excreted in exchange for potassium	Hyperkalemia, diarrhea, drowsiness, confusion
Adrenergic Inhibitors		
Beta-adrenergic blockers Atenolol (Tenormin) Metoprolol (Lopressor) Nadolol (Corgard) Propranolol (Inderal)	Decrease heart rate and blood pressure by blocking beta-adrenergic receptors of sympathetic nervous system	Bradycardia, fatigue, bronchospasm, sexual dysfunction
Centrally acting alpha blockers Clonidine (Catapres) Guanabenz (Wytensin) Methyldopa (Aldomet)	Activate central receptors that suppress vasomotor and cardiac centers, causing a decrease in peripheral resistance	Drowsiness, sedation, dry mouth, fatigue, sexual dysfunction, orthostatic hypotension
Peripheral acting adrenergic antagonists Guanethidine (Ismelin) Reserpine (Serpasil)	Deplete catecholamines in peripheral postganglionic fibers; block norepinephrine release from nerve endings	Lethargy, depression, nasal congestion, orthostatic hypotension, sexual dysfunction
Alpha-1-adrenergic blockers Prazosin (Minipress) Terazosin (Vasocard)	Block receptors that regulate vasomotor tone Dilate arterioles and venules	Orthostatic hypotension, weakness, dizziness
Vasodilators		
Hydralazine (Apresoline) Minoxidil (Loniten)	Dilate peripheral blood vessels by relaxing smooth muscle	Headache, dizziness, tachycardia, palpitations, edema
Angiotensin-converting Enzyme (ACE) Inhibitors		
Captopril (Capoten) Enalapril (Vasotec) Lisinopril (Prinivil)	Inhibit conversion of angiotensin to angiotensin II, thus blocking release of aldosterone	First-dose hypotension, headache, dizziness, fatigue, increased potassium
Calcium Antagonists		
Diltiazem (Cardizem) Nifedipine (Procardia) Verapamil (Calan)	Inhibit influx of calcium into muscle cells; act on vascular smooth muscles to reduce spasm and promote vasodilation	Dizziness, fatigue, nausea, headache, edema

Patient will express desire to maintain treatment regimen and control effects of the disease.

Nursing Interventions

Assist patient to reduce weight and maintain desired weight.

Teach patient principles of modified fat and sodium diets.

Assist patient to explore and reduce factors contributing to personal and occupational stress. Patient should:

Balance rest, recreation, and activity.

Plan regular exercise patterns.

Use relaxation techniques.

Help patient reduce or stop smoking.

Teach patient about prescribed medications. Provide written materials.

Teach patient how to manage side effects of medications. Patient should:

Take diuretics early in the day.

Maintain adequate intake of potassium in diet.

Recognize symptoms of hypovolemia.

Prevent or control orthostatic hypotension by avoiding alcohol use and hot baths and making position changes slowly.

Sit immediately if faintness is felt.

Avoid prolonged periods of standing.

Be alert for symptoms of depression or impotence.

Explore adjustment of drugs or doses with physician.

Monitor lying, sitting, and standing blood pressures.

Teach patient to accurately monitor own blood pressure.

Support patient's adjustment to long-term management of the disease. Explore obstacles to compliance.

Encourage patient to report changes in sexual functioning (libido, erection, or decreased ejaculation), as changes in drug regimen are possible. Sexual problems are common with alpha and beta blockers.

Evaluation

Patient can discuss effects and complications of hypertension.

Patient can discuss action and expected side effects of prescribed medications.

Patient employs measures to counteract expected side effects of medications.

Patient lowers fat and sodium intake in diet and maintains desired weight.

Patient employs relaxation techniques and modifies lifestyle to reduce stress; engages in regular exercise.

Patient exhibits compliance with diet and drug regimens.

ANEURYSMS

An aneurysm is a localized or diffuse enlargement of an artery at some point along its course. Aneurysms occur when the vessel wall becomes weakened by trauma, congenital disease, infection, or atherosclerosis. They can occur virtually anywhere, but the most common site is along the course of the aorta, particularly in the abdominal segment.

PATHOPHYSIOLOGY

Once an aneurysm develops and the middle arterial layer is damaged, there is a tendency toward progressive dilatation and degeneration, with a risk of rupture. There are three major types of aneurysms:

saccular Involving only part of the artery's circumference. They take the form of a sac or pouch attached to the side of the vessel.

fusiform A spindle-shaped defect involving the entire circumference of the arterial wall.

dissecting Produced when there is hemorrhage into a vessel wall that splits and dissects the wall, causing it to widen. They are usually caused by a degenerative defect.

MEDICAL MANAGEMENT

After angiographic studies to determine the location, size, and extent of the aneurysm, surgery is usually performed to resect it and replace the diseased section with a Teflon or Dacron graft. Surgical approaches vary, depending on the site and extent of the aneurysm.

NURSING MANAGEMENT

Assessment

Subjective

History of disease and symptoms (aneurysms are often discovered on routine examination and are asymptomatic)

Knowledge and fears about planned surgery

General health status

Objective

Baseline vital signs

Peripheral circulation, pulses, color, temperature, and capillary refill

Baseline intake and output

Nursing Diagnoses

Diagnoses vary and are based on the location and severity of the disorder. Common diagnoses include the following:

Anxiety related to seriousness of surgery and uncertainty of outcome

Pain related to pressure of the aneurysm or postoperative tissue trauma

Knowledge deficit related to proposed surgical procedure and the postoperative care

Potential alteration in urinary elimination related to inadequate postsurgical renal perfusion

Expected Outcomes

Patient will have only manageable levels of anxiety concerning the impending surgery.

Patient will experience only manageable levels of pain.

Patient will be knowledgeable about proposed surgery and the associated postoperative care.

Patient will maintain a normal urine output.

Nursing Interventions: Preoperative

Teach patient about surgery and postoperative care routines, special care environment.

Take patient on tour of intensive care unit if permitted.

Assess and mark peripheral pulses and baseline vital signs.

Nursing Interventions: Postoperative

Monitor vital signs and central venous, pulmonary artery, and pulmonary capillary wedge pressures per routine.

Observe color, temperature of extremities, capillary refill, and peripheral pulses.

Report occurrence of pale or mottled color, cold numb extremities.

Monitor peripheral sensation and movement.

Monitor urine output hourly (at least 30-50 ml/hr).

Position flat in bed; avoid hip flexion.

Turn side to side; encourage flexion and extension of feet.

Provide TED stockings; check Homans' sign.

Use abdominal binder and pillow splinting for coughing and deep breathing. Encourage hourly deep breathing.

Provide adequate pain medication.

Monitor nasogastric tube if ileus is present.

Encourage patient to ambulate as permitted to prevent thrombophlebitis.

Encourage patient to dorsiflex and extend feet and perform other leg exercises until out of bed.

Monitor chest tube output; patient may be autotransfused.

Assess level of consciousness; be alert to incidence of disorientation, hallucinations or nightmares.

Assist patient in progressive return to activity.

Evaluation

Patient has minimal discomfort and is able to do coughing and deep breathing effectively.

Patient maintains a normal urinary output.

Patient understands postoperative care regimen and postdischarge activity restrictions.

Patient has adequate peripheral blood flow, palpable peripheral pulses, and negative Homans' sign.

SHOCK

Shock is a syndrome characterized by inadequate tissue perfusion at the cellular level. Any condition that prevents cells from receiving an adequate blood supply can produce shock. Shock is commonly classified as follows:

hypovolemic   Related to an inadequate volume within the vascular compartment. It is the most common form of shock and will serve as the model for discussion.

cardiogenic   Related to inability of the heart to pump sufficient blood to perfuse the body. Myocardial infarction is the most common cause (see Chapter 6).

neurogenic/vasogenic   Related to massive dilation of the blood vessels caused by interference with the sympathetic nervous system, as occurs with spinal cord injury (see Chapter 4); release of vasoactive substances during an allergic response or anaphylaxis; or release of endotoxins from gram-negative organisms, which trigger release of numerous vasoactive substances in sepsis.

Common causes of each type of shock are summarized in the box on this page.

COMMON CAUSES OF SHOCK

HYPOVOLEMIC SHOCK

Excessive blood loss from trauma, gastrointestinal bleeding, surgery, or coagulation disorders

Loss of body fluids other than blood—vomiting and diarrhea, ketoacidosis

Movement of fluids from the vascular to the interstitial compartment or peritoneal cavity, as in burns or complete bowel obstruction

CARDIOGENIC SHOCK

Myocardial infarction
Pulmonary embolism
Cardiac tamponade
Dysrhythmia

NEUROGENIC/VASOGENIC SHOCK

Spinal cord injury
Anaphylactic response to drugs, toxins, dyes
Gram-negative sepsis, particularly involving the urinary tract and prostate

PATHOPHYSIOLOGY

In the early stages of shock the body's compensatory mechanisms are able to sustain adequate blood flow to the tissues. The mechanisms are primarily mediated by the sympathetic nervous system and include the following:

Tachycardia and tachypnea to increase oxygen delivery

Vasoconstriction of skin and abdominal organs

In addition, the kidney secretes renin to support vasoconstriction and aldosterone to sustain fluid volume.

As shock progresses, however, blood flow to all body tissues becomes impaired. Anaerobic metabolism takes over and adenosine triphosphate production is severely impaired. Acid metabolites accumulate and cause dilation at the arteriole end of the capillaries. Fluid shifts to the interstitium and decreases blood volume. Decreased flow to the kidney results in oliguria and anuria, with accumulation of metabolic wastes. Ischemia of the abdominal organs causes release of a myocardial depressant factor from the pancreas, which compromises cardiac contractibility. Beyond a certain point the cycle of shock becomes irreversible. At this point the patient is vulnerable to tubular necrosis and renal failure, paralytic ileus and stress ulcers, falling cardiac output and dysrhythmias, adult respiratory distress system (ARDS), sepsis, and disseminated intravascular coagulation (DIC). The classic symptoms are summarized in the box on the next page.

MEDICAL MANAGEMENT

Medical management is determined by the stage of shock and the patient's unique condition. Strategies in-

SIGNS AND SYMPTOMS OF SHOCK

EARLY SHOCK
Tachycardia, tachypnea
Blood pressure normal or slightly lowered, decreased pulse pressure
Decreased urine output, increased specific gravity, thirst
Alert, restless, nonspecific anxiety

PROGRESSIVE SHOCK
Tachycardia
Decreased blood pressure
Rapid shallow respirations
Oliguria or anuria
Cool clammy skin
Decreased bowel sounds, ileus
Petechiae, spontaneous bleeding
Lethargy, coma

clude fluid replacement with crystalloid, colloid, and blood solutions; vasoactive drugs to sustain blood pressure; antibiotics; and supplemental oxygen. An intraaortic balloon may be inserted to support the action of a failing left ventricle.

Commonly employed drugs in shock states include the following:
  Mixed alpha- and beta-adrenergics—dopamine, dobutamine, epinephrine
  Beta-adrenergics—isoproteronol
  Vasodilators—nitroprusside, nitroglycerin

NURSING MANAGEMENT

Assessment
  ##### Subjective
  History of surgery, trauma, infection
  Level of consciousness—presence of confusion
  Sense of anxiety or restlessness
  Nausea or thirst
  ##### Objective
  Vital signs—lying and sitting if possible
  Central venous pressure, other hemodynamic monitoring as available
  Respiratory rate, depth, pattern; breath sounds
  Blood gases
  Intake and output, urine specific gravity
  Bowel sounds
  Skin temperature, moisture

Nursing Diagnoses
Diagnoses will vary somewhat based on the severity of the shock state. Common diagnoses include the following:
  Fluid volume deficit related to fluid shifts or direct losses
  Decreased cardiac output related to hypoxia and effects of depressant factors

Altered tissue perfusion (renal, cerebral, and peripheral) related to state of hypovolemia
Impaired gas exchange related to decreased lung compliance and interstitial edema
Potential for infection related to decreased immune response and insertion of monitoring devices
Anxiety related to seriousness of condition and uncertainty of outcomes

Expected Outcomes
Patient will receive sufficient blood and fluid replacement to restore a normal fluid balance.
Patient will regain a normal range of cardiac output.
Patient will sustain sufficient perfusion to vital organs and tissues to prevent metabolic acidosis.
Patient will maintain a satisfactory exchange of oxygen and carbon dioxide.
Patient will remain free of local and systemic infection.
Patient will feel supported and able to control anxiety.

Nursing Interventions
Administer blood or fluid replacement as ordered.
Administer vasoactive drugs as ordered.
  Always use IV pump to control flow.
  Monitor vital signs continuously every 5 to 15 minutes.
  Maintain patency of infusions—drugs are very irritating to tissue.
  Follow hemodynamic parameters if available.
Administer prescribed supplemental oxygen.
NOTE: Patient will need to be intubated if symptoms of adult respiratory distress syndrome (ARDS) develop.
Auscultate bowel sounds—maintain NPO status if ileus is present. Provide mouth care.
Protect patient from injury if restless or confused.
Maintain strict aseptic technique for inserting all monitoring lines, suctioning, and so forth. Monitor carefully for signs of infection.
Place patient flat in bed with legs slightly elevated. Change positions frequently.
Encourage deep breathing—actively prevent complications related to immobility.
Monitor frequently for petechiae or signs of bleeding.
Keep patient at absolute rest. Maintain a neutral environmental temperature to conserve energy.
Support and reassure patient and family frequently. Assist to remain quiet and relaxed if possible.
Administer antacids or histamine H_2 receptor blockers as ordered.

Evaluation
Patient's fluid and electrolyte status is within normal limits.
Patient's cardiac output level is restored to normal range.

Patient's tissue perfusion is adequate to sustain normal metabolic functions.

Patient's blood gases show normal level of oxygen and carbon dioxide.

Patient is free of infection or injury.

Patient no longer experiences anxiety regarding condition.

ARTERIAL DISEASE

The symptoms of arterial disease are the result of disturbances in the delivery of blood and oxygen to the tissues. The severity of the symptoms reflects the degree of circulatory deprivation, which is influenced by blood pressure and degree of collateral circulation. Many of the specific disorders are related to the development of atherosclerosis and arteriosclerosis in the peripheral tissues. Table 7-2 describes some of the more common arterial disorders. Arteriosclerosis obliterans is discussed as a model.

ARTERIOSCLEROSIS OBLITERANS

Arteriosclerosis obliterans is the most common cause of arterial occlusive disease in individuals over 30. It affects men more commonly than women, with clinical symptoms typically appearing between ages 50 and 70.

The lower extremity is usually involved. Risk factors include the following:

Cigarette smoking (extremely important)
Obesity
Hypertension and hyperlipidemia
Diabetes mellitus

Symptoms are the result of tissue ischemia and may progress to ulceration, necrosis, and gangrene.

PATHOPHYSIOLOGY

Arteriosclerosis obliterans occurs when there is segmented arteriosclerotic narrowing or obstruction of the intimal and medial layers of the artery. The primary lesion is plaque formation that causes partial or complete occlusion. Calcification of the medial layer with loss of elasticity further weakens the arterial walls and predisposes to aneurysm and thrombus formation. Symptoms appear when the vessels can no longer provide enough blood to supply oxygen and nutrients and remove metabolic wastes from the tissues.

MEDICAL MANAGEMENT

Medical management is directed toward preventing occlusion and includes comfort measures, carefully planned exercise programs, vasodilating medications, and preventive measures.

TABLE 7-2 Peripheral arterial disorders

Disorder	Etiology	Signs and Symptoms	Medical Management
Thromboangiitis obliterans (Buerger's disease)	Obstructive inflammatory process in small arteries and veins Strongly associated with cigarette smoking Appears in males aged 20 to 40 and slightly more often in semitic and oriental persons	Pain: intermittent claudication, pain at rest, or general aching; cold sensitivity Numbness and tingling Superficial thrombophlebitis	Stopping smoking (may be enough to reverse symptoms) Sympathectomy if unresponsive to conservative measures May require amputation of affected digits Preventive measures
Raynaud's phenomenon or disease	Episodes of arterial spasm—most often in the hands May appear alone or secondary to another disease process Occurs primarily in women aged 20 to 40	Cold, numbness, and pain in one or more fingers or toes Bilateral process, affects both hands Fingers appear white or mottled Cold aggravates spasms Intense redness and throbbing follows the spasms	Avoiding cold Stopping smoking Calcium antagonists or muscle relaxants Sympathectomy if unresponsive to conservative measures May require amputation of affected digits
Arterial embolism	Blood clots floating in arterial blood usually originate in the heart and tend to lodge in bifurcation of an artery, severely impairing blood flow	Symptoms depend on size and location. Abrupt onset of severe pain and burning, loss of distal pulses, and a cold, pale, numb extremity	Bedrest and anticoagulants or fibrinolytics Surgery—embolectomy or endarterectomy within 6 to 10 hours

Surgery to improve blood supply may be indicated in severe cases where ischemic changes are present or pain severely limits activity. Options include bypass grafts, endarterectomy, angioplasty, or amputation in the face of gangrene or sepsis (see Chapter 3).

NURSING MANAGEMENT

Assessment

Subjective

History of disease and its treatment

History of pain and intermittent claudication (cramping pain, usually in calf, that develops with exercise and lessens with rest)

    Type and severity, location

    Relationship to exercise and rest

Healing of simple cuts and abrasions

Usual diet, life-style, occupation, and exercise habits

Smoking history; presence of related risk factors

Objective

Presence, strength, and equality of peripheral pulses

Prolonged or absent capillary refill

Skin

    Temperature, color, hair growth

    Texture changes, appearance of nails

    Presence of ulcers or skin breakdown

Diminished sensation, paresthesias

Results of Doppler ultrasonography

Nursing Diagnoses

Diagnoses will vary slightly depending on the severity of the disease. Common diagnoses include the following:

Activity intolerance related to the onset of ischemic pain with exercise

Pain related to ischemic changes and spasms in extremities

Potential for injury related to decreased sensory awareness in extremities

Knowledge deficit related to preventive and comfort measures appropriate with peripheral vascular disease

Potential impairment of skin integrity related to lack of nutrients to peripheral tissue.

Altered tissue perfusion (peripheral) related to arterial obstruction

Expected Outcomes

Patient will increase tolerance for exercise with treatment.

Patient will balance rest and activity and be able to perform activities of daily living without pain.

Patient will not have tissue injury from heat, cold, pressure, or trauma.

Patient will be knowledgeable about the components of the treatment regimen.

Patient will maintain intact skin over legs, feet, and hands.

Patient will have increased peripheral tissue perfusion.

Nursing Interventions

Assist patient to develop an exercise plan that carefully balances rest and activity. *Moderate* regular exercise improves arterial circulation by stimulating development of collateral circulation.

ALERT: Too much exercise puts excess metabolic demand on the circulation. Walking is ideal exercise.

Teach patient to observe the following precautions:

    Avoid sitting or standing in one position for too long.

    Arrange frequent rest periods when traveling.

    Avoid crossing legs while sitting.

    Ensure that chairs do not impair circulation.

    Wear comfortable protective shoes at all times.

    Trim nails carefully, soaking feet first. Trim straight across.

    Seek professional help for care of corns, blisters, and ingrown toe nails.

    Cleanse feet daily and lubricate with moisturizing lotion. Avoid use of rubbing alcohol.

    Use clean cotton socks and change daily.

    Assess condition of skin daily.

    Rest with legs in slightly dependent position.

    Avoid constricting clothing and exposure to cold.

    Avoid use of direct heat to extremities.

    Avoid trauma and pressure to extremities.

    Refrain from massaging legs.

Reinforce to patient importance of giving up smoking.

Administer vasodilator, anticoagulant medications as prescribed.

Assist patient to reduce weight and dietary cholesterol and fat.

If acute obstruction is present, perform the following:

    Monitor limb distal to affected site for changes in color, temperature. NOTE: initially pale and cool, bluish in color; if obstruction becomes complete, tissue will become necrotic and black.

    Assess peripheral pulses manually or with Doppler probe.

    Place bed cradle to protect limb from pressure of linens.

    Monitor for edema.

Evaluation

Patient is able to maintain a normal activity pattern without experiencing claudication.

Patient effectively spaces activities throughout the day to remain free of pain.

Patient maintains skin integrity in the extremities and does not experience injury.

Patient is knowledgeable about the disease process and measures to increase comfort and perfusion.

Patient maintains desired body weight.

Patient adjusts diet to decrease cholesterol and fat intake.

Patient successfully quits smoking.

VENOUS DISEASE

Venous problems develop when there is an alteration in the transport of blood from the capillary beds back to the heart. Valves may malfunction or muscle and connective tissue can make the veins less distensible.

THROMBOPHLEBITIS/DEEP VEIN THROMBOSIS

Thrombophlebitis and deep vein thrombosis (DVT) are common venous disorders characterized by vein inflammation and clot formation. They are associated with venous stasis, endothelial damage, and hypercoagulability of the blood and may occur in both the deep and superficial veins of the lower extremities. These conditions are more common in women, increase in incidence with age, and are a serious potential complication of major surgery and any illness requiring immobilization.

PATHOPHYSIOLOGY

Thrombi form as a result of the accumulation of platelets, fibrin, and white and red blood cells. DVT tends to occur at the bifurcations of deep veins. An inflammatory response may be triggered in the vein and can be severe and produce swelling, warmth, and tenderness along the course of the vein. Superficial veins may feel hard and thready. The development of an embolus is a major risk during the acute period.

MEDICAL MANAGEMENT

Superficial thrombophlebitis is treated by bed rest and the use of anticoagulants. Warm, moist heat may be used in treatment, although some physicians feel that heat increases the risk of emboli. Thrombectomy or placement of a vena caval filter may be performed when the risk of emboli is extremely high.

NURSING MANAGEMENT

Assessment

Subjective

History of precipitating activity

Immobility, especially prolonged sitting while riding

Minor trauma to leg

Pattern and severity of pain

Objective

Unilateral swelling of calf or thigh

Redness and heat in affected leg

Positive Homans' sign

ALERT: Homans' sign should not be elicited once the diagnosis is established as it increases the risk of embolization.

Nursing Diagnoses

Associated diagnoses commonly include the following:

Pain related to inflammation and ischemia

Knowledge deficit related to prevention and treatment of venous disease

Impaired physical mobility related to bed rest for treatment of thrombophlebitis

Potential for injury or bleeding related to anticoagulant therapy

Expected Outcomes

Patient's pain will decrease.

Patient will be knowledgeable about the development, treatment, and prevention of thrombophlebitis.

Patient will not develop complications from bed rest.

Patient will not experience bleeding while receiving anticoagulant therapy.

Nursing Interventions

Maintain patient on bed rest or activity restriction as prescribed with affected leg elevated.

Apply warm, moist heat or cold packs as ordered.

Administer anticoagulants and/or fibrinolytics as ordered and check for signs of bleeding. Avoid rectal temperature and intramuscular injections.

Administer heparin IV or deep subcutaneously with a fine-gauge needle, using a 90 degree angle into lower abdomen.

Do not aspirate or massage site.

Have protamine sulfate available to reverse effects of heparin.

Monitor patient's partial thromboplastin time (PTT).

Hold all venipuncture sites firmly for 3 to 5 minutes.

Teach patient to avoid products containing aspirin.

Hematest urine, emesis, and stools.

Examine skin for petechiae or ecchymoses.

Teach patient to use soft toothbrushes and avoid use of straight razors.

Observe for signs of pulmonary embolism, such as sudden sharp chest pain or dyspnea.

Measure calf or thigh circumference daily.

Assess adequacy of peripheral circulation.

Apply TED stockings. Measure leg carefully for correct fit. Teach patient proper use for home care—put on before getting out of bed in morning.

Teach patient general principles of leg and foot care.

Elevate legs above the heart at intervals throughout the day.

Perform ankle flexion and extension exercises frequently when standing or sitting.

Engage in regular aerobic exercise.

Avoid constricting clothing around the knee or calf.

Wear support hose/TED stockings, particularly during periods of enforced immobility such as long car or plane trips.

Evaluation

Patient is able to resume normal activities without discomfort.

Patient can discuss treatment plan and outline preventive measures to prevent recurrence.

Patient maintains intact skin, full range of motion and muscle strength, clear lungs, and adequate bowel and bladder function.

Patient manages anticoagulation therapy without incidence of spontaneous bleeding.

VARICOSE VEINS

Varicose veins are abnormally dilated veins with incompetent valves. They affect 20% of the population and occur most often in the lower extremities and lower trunk, usually in the great and small saphenous veins. Congenitally defective valves, prolonged standing, and systemic conditions that interfere with venous return such as pregnancy or ascites all contribute to the development of varicose veins.

PATHOPHYSIOLOGY

The primary pathologic factor is weakening of the vein wall. Weakened vein walls do not adequately withstand normal pressure and dilate with blood pooling. Dilation increases the valve stretching and worsens the condition.

MEDICAL MANAGEMENT

Mild problems with varicosities may be treated by teaching patients to elevate their legs at regular intervals throughout the day, to avoid constriction and stasis, and to wear support stockings.

Surgical treatment involves ligation and removal of varicosed vein and is performed in the presence of chronic pain or leg ulcers.

NURSING MANAGEMENT

Assessment (Preoperative)

Subjective

History of the problem and patient management

Obstetrical history if patient is female

Patient's occupation and leisure time activities

Patient's complaints of the following:

Dull aching, muscle cramping

Fatigue

Feeling of pressure or heaviness in legs

Swelling

Objective

Visible evidence of varicosities

Presence and severity of edema and degree of pitting

Nursing Diagnoses

Common diagnoses include the following:

Pain related to cramping in legs

Activity intolerance related to edema and feelings of fatigue in legs

Potential impaired skin integrity related to chronic edema in ankles and feet

Expected Outcomes

Patient's discomfort will decrease.

Patient will be able to complete usual occupational and leisure activities without developing fatigue or leg edema.

Patient will maintain intact skin over ankles and feet.

Patient will be knowledgeable about measures to prevent reoccurrence of varicosities.

Nursing Interventions: Preoperative

Teach patient about surgical procedure and regimen for postoperative positioning and activity.

Nursing Interventions: Postoperative

Elevate foot of bed for first 24 hours. Keep head of bed flat for first 4 to 6 hours.

Provide adequate analgesia.

Initiate early ambulation and encourage frequent walking. Assist patient with walking and transferring if needed.

Monitor incisions for bleeding. Keep bandages intact and free of wrinkles.

Teach patient how to prevent recurrence of varicosities (see general measures under Thrombophlebitis/Deep Vein Thrombosis in this chapter).

Evaluation

Patient is free of cramping, pain, swelling, and fatigue.

Patient resumes desired activity pattern without reoccurrence of symptoms.

Patient is able to discuss measures to help prevent recurrence of varicosities.

BIBLIOGRAPHY

Beaver BM: Health education and the patient with peripheral vascular disease, Nurs Clin North Am **21**:265-272, 1986.

Cunningham SG: Nonpharmacologic management of blood pressure, J Cardiovasc Nurs **2**(4):18-22, 1987.

Daeschner SA: Action stat—pulmonary embolism, Nursing 88 **18**(9):33, 1988.

Doyle JE: Treatment modalities in peripheral vascular disease, Nurs Clin North Am **21**:241-253, 1986.

Ekers MA: Psychosocial considerations in peripheral vascular disease: cause or effect?, Nurs Clin North Am **21**:255-263, 1986.

Hancock BG and Eberhard NK: The pharmacological management of shock, Crit Care Nurs Q **11**(1):19-29, 1988.

Hill MN and Cunningham SG: The latest words for high blood pressure, Am J Nurs **89**:504-509, 1989.

Kirkpatrick MK: Self-care guide for hypertension risk reduction, Am Assoc Occup Health Nurs J **35**:254, 1987.

Littleton MT: Pathophysiology and assessment of sepsis and septic shock, Crit Care Nurs Q **11**(2):30-47, 1988.

McCord MA: Compliance: self-care or compromise, Top Clin Nurs **7**:1, 1986.

McMahan BE: Why deep vein thrombosis is so dangerous, RN **51**:20-23, 1987.

Moore LD and Pulliam CB: An on the spot guide to antihypertensive drugs, Nursing 86 **16**(1):54-57, 1986.

Perry AG: Shock complications: recognition and management, Crit Care Nurs Q **11**(1):1-8, 1988.

Powers M and Jalowiec A: Profile of the well controlled, well adjusted hypertensive patient, Nurs Res **36**:106-110, 1987.

Swithers CM: Tools for teaching about anticoagulants, RN **51**(1):57-58, 1988.

Turner JA: Nursing interventions in patients with peripheral vascular disease, Nurs Clin North Am **21**:233-240, 1986.

CHAPTER 8

Disorders of the Blood and Blood-forming Organs

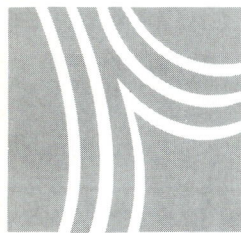

Diseases associated with the blood and blood-forming organs involve the development and functioning of red blood cells, white blood cells and platelets, as well as the mechanism of coagulation. They vary widely in pathology, overt symptoms, and response to treatment. The nursing care associated with major problems of each type is discussed in this chapter.

DISORDERS OF THE RED BLOOD CELLS

Red blood cells (RBCs) are produced in the bone marrow and circulate in the blood for about 120 days, transporting oxygen and carbon dioxide and maintaining the normal pH of the blood through a series of intracellular buffers. The major health problems associated with the RBCs are the anemias and polycythemia. Anemia is a broad category of disorders involving a deficiency in RBCs as reflected in the hemoglobin, hematocrit, or RBC count. The anemias may be classified by examining the size of the cell and the amount of hemoglobin it contains. Table 8-1 summarizes the various changes in red cell morphology that occur in anemia and typical causes of each. Table 8-2 describes the most common types of anemia grouped by cause. The general body responses to different types of anemia are quite similar. Specific symptoms characteristic of each type of anemia and the associated medical management are also summarized in Table 8-2.

PATHOPHYSIOLOGY

Regardless of the cause, anemia interferes with the RBC function of transporting oxygen to the tissues. This leads to tissue hypoxia. The body responds by increasing the speed of blood circulation and the rate of respiration. These compensatory mechanisms keep the individual quite asymptomatic until the severity of the anemia worsens. The heart and lungs bear the brunt of the compensatory efforts and usually exhibit the most distinct symptoms, up to and including cardiac failure.

MEDICAL MANAGEMENT

General medical treatment is aimed at decreasing demands on the body and replacing RBCs while treating the deficiency. Treatment may include giving iron and vitamins to support RBC production, preventing or halting conditions causing hemolysis, or replacing volume and cells through blood transfusion. Treatments for specific anemias are outlined in Table 8-2.

NURSING MANAGEMENT (IRON DEFICIENCY ANEMIA)

Assessment
Subjective
History and progression of symptoms
Menstrual history, if female

TABLE 8-1 Common anemias classified by red blood cell morphology

Anemia	Cause
Normocytic (normal cell size) Normochromic (normal hemoglobin content)	Acute blood loss, most hemolytic processes
Microcytic (small cell size) Normochromic (normal hemoglobin content)	Tumor, infection, chronic illness
Microcytic (small cell size) Hypochromic (decreased hemoglobin content)	Iron deficiency
Macrocytic (abnormally large cell size) Normochromic (normal hemoglobin content)	Folic acid deficiency, vitamin B_{12} deficiency

TABLE 8-2 The anemias classified by common causes

Disorder	Etiology	Signs and Symptoms	Medical Management
I. Blood loss A. Acute	Hemorrhage (trauma, gastrointestinal [GI] bleeding)	Physiological signs of shock: Restlessness or irritability Cool, moist skin; pallor Increased pulse; decreased blood pressure	Stop source of bleeding; restore losses with IV fluid, whole blood, or packed cell transfusions. Treat shock. Support vital functions with oxygen, vasopressors.
B. Chronic	Slow GI loss (malignancy, peptic ulcers) Vaginal bleeding (menstrual disorders) Hemorrhoids	Patient may remain asymptomatic with RBC and hemoglobin at significantly depressed levels, then have chronic fatigue, weakness, elevated pulse, exertional dyspnea, pallor of skin and mucous membranes	Stop source of blood loss. Promote proper nutrition; give supplemental iron.
II. Impaired production A. Aplastic anemia (depression or cessation of *all* blood-forming elements)	Bone marrow depression from drugs, chemicals, virus, radiation; unidentified causes in 50% of cases Special attention to: Chloramphenicol Anticonvulsants Sulfonamides Butazolidine Definitive diagnosis is made by bone marrow biopsy	Symptoms as with chronic blood loss; problem often affects white cells and platelets as well; infection; petechiae, spontaneous GI, genitourinary (GU), or CNS bleeding	Remove causative agent if possible. Provide supportive care until bone marrow regeneration is possible: transfusions of RBCs, platelets; laminar air flow to protect from infection. Bone marrow transplant if suitable donor available; immunosuppressive therapy.

III. Increased destruction of RBCs (hemolysis)
   A. Congenital
      1. Sickle cell disease (hemoglobinopathy)
	Hereditary abnormality in hemoglobin protein that occurs primarily in black population; intermolecular rearrangement causes hemoglobin S to be formed, which tends to sickle in shape during lowered oxygen tension, slowing circulation and increasing cellular hypoxia and infarcts. RBC lifespan is shortened	General symptoms of anemia plus painful episodes of vasoocclusive crisis: acute-onset severe pain (generalized, localized, or migratory bone or joint pain), low-grade fever.
		Crisis may be precipitated by any condition increasing body's need for oxygen: infection, overexertion, alcohol, smoking.
			No specific therapy.
			Treat symptoms with analgesics, oxygen, IV hydration.
			Provide supportive care during exacerbations.
			Provide genetic counseling.
			Prevent imbalance in oxygen needs.

2. Thalassemia	Inherited disorder of decreased synthesis of hemoglobin and malformation of RBCs that increases their hemolysis; occurs primarily in Orientals or persons of Mediterranean heritage	Thalassemia minor—usually asymptomatic or symptoms of mild anemia Thalassemia major—severe anemia, enlarged spleen, jaundice, growth failure	No therapy usually needed. Transfusions for severe form to maintain patient in relatively symptom-free state; usually fatal in young adulthood.
3. Enzyme deficiency (G-6-PD, glucose-6-phosphate dehydrogenase)	Inherited deficiency of enzyme in pathways that metabolize glucose and generate ATP, leading to premature RBC destruction	General symptoms of anemia are produced through acute hemolysis occurring when cells are exposed to oxidant drugs such as aspirin or sulfonamides, usually in response to infection	Diagnose condition and remove the drug stimulus.

Continued.

TABLE 8-2 The anemias classified by common causes—cont'd

Disorder	Etiology	Signs and Symptoms	Medical Management
B. Acquired hemolytic	Most often drug-induced or autoimmune; antibodies are produced that cause premature destruction of the RBCs	General symptoms of anemia reflecting severity of the disorder	Attempt to suppress the antigen-antibody reactions through administration of corticosteroids. Beneficial in about 50% of cases.
IV. Nutritional deficiency			
A. Iron deficiency	Deficiency of iron leads to synthesis of RBCs with a decreased amount of hemoglobin; eventually leads to decreased number of cells	Few overt clinical signs in early stages, then gradual development of fatigue and exertional dyspnea, plus: Brittle concave nails Shiny, bright red, smooth tongue Cracks in corner of mouth	Determine cause and correct. Provide adequate balanced diet (rarely a major factor). Administer ferrous sulfate orally or parenterally if GI absorption is insufficient.
B. Megaloblastic anemia			
1. Vitamin B_{12} deficiency (pernicious)	Insufficient amount of B_{12} absorbed from intestine (B_{12} is essential for synthesis of RBCs); malabsorption syndrome and loss of intrinsic factor following gastric surgery are possible causes	General signs of anemia plus: Peripheral neuropathy Ataxia	Administer vitamin B_{12} parenterally weekly or monthly.
2. Folic acid deficiency	Often occurs with chronic alcoholism, or malabsorption syndromes (folic acid is essential for synthesis of RBCs)	General signs of anemia plus symptoms of underlying disease	Administer oral folic acid and a well-balanced diet. Treat underlying disorder.

Prior medication or treatment
Usual dietary pattern
Associated health problems
Occupational exposure to drugs and chemicals
Patient's complaints of the following:
   Fatigue and malaise, activity intolerance
   Cold intolerance
Complaints of paresthesias
Joint/bone pain
Objective
Vital signs—orthostatic blood pressure and pulse
Evidence of dyspnea
Skin color, temperature, presence of cyanosis/jaundice
Oral mucous membranes
Laboratory results

Nursing Diagnoses
Diagnoses will depend on the specific type of anemia and degree of severity. Common diagnoses include the following:
   Activity intolerance related to chronic tissue hypoxia
   Potential for injury related to systemic weakness and dizziness
   Altered nutrition: less than body requirements, related to inadequate ingestion or absorption of needed nutrients

Expected Outcomes
Patient will gradually be able to resume normal occupational and leisure activity pattern without incidence of fatigue.
Patient will not experience injury during ambulation or position changes.
Patient will be able to identify foods rich in iron and vitamins and adapt diet to increase intake of needed nutrients.

Nursing Interventions
Balance rest and activity.
   Assist patient with activities of daily living as needed.
   Keep outside stimulation at a controlled level.
   Monitor pulse rate and assess for dyspnea during activity.
Supervise weak patient to prevent injury.
   Avoid abrupt changes of position.
   Check orthostatic blood pressure.
   Avoid use of hot baths and showers.
Administer supplemental oxygen as needed.
   Provide extra pillows; keep head of bed elevated.

Monitor for exertional dyspnea.
Turn and change position every 2 hours.
  Offer skin care and massage.
  Provide blankets if patient feels cold.
Teach patient about balanced diet and iron-rich foods.
Administer and teach patient about prescribed medications.
Administer blood transfusions if prescribed.
Observe and monitor patient for signs of transfusion reaction.
NOTE: The box on p. 113 discusses nursing care during RBC transfusion.

Evaluation
Patient performs self-care and resumes normal activities without fatigue, weakness, or onset of dyspnea.
Patient discusses elements essential to balanced diet and selects and eats iron-rich foods.
Patient can discuss purpose and side effects of medications.
Patient does not experience injury or complications of treatment regimen.

DISORDERS OF THE PLATELETS

Platelets are nonnucleated cell fragments formed in the bone marrow that serve as the body's first barrier to blood loss through vessel injury. They have the ability to aggregate and adhere at the site of vessel injury, thus plugging small leaks. Platelets also release thromboplastin as the first step in the coagulation cascade. Two thirds of the body's platelets are in circulation. The remainder are usually held in the spleen as a reserve pool. Their normal life span is only 10 days. Platelet production is suppressed by most of the same drugs and chemicals that suppress RBC production. Aspirin is the primary drug known to have active antiplatelet activity.

THROMBOCYTOPENIA

By definition, thrombocytopenia exists when a lower than normal number (150,000 to 400,000/mm^3) of circulating platelets exists as a result of decreased production, decreased survival, or increased destruction. Thrombocytopenia may be idiopathic or occur as a secondary effect of drugs, chemicals, malignant disease, and radiation. Idiopathic thrombocytopenia purpura is a primary disorder of young adults in which an autoantibody is produced against a platelet antigen.

PATHOPHYSIOLOGY

The decreased number of circulating platelets interferes with hemostasis, producing excessive and spontaneous bleeding, often reflected in purpuric lesions and visible bruising on the skin. Petechiae occur *only* in platelet disorders.

MEDICAL MANAGEMENT

Attempts are made to isolate and remove the cause of platelet depression if possible. A splenectomy may be indicated to remove the organ primarily involved in the destruction and removal of circulating platelets. Steroids may be administered to decrease antibody production and reduce phagocytosis of circulating platelets. Direct platelet transfusions may be given if the patient is experiencing thrombocytopenic bleeding. Transfusions must be given at least twice weekly because platelets are destroyed so rapidly.

NURSING MANAGEMENT
Assessment
Subjective
History and pattern of symptoms
Medications used, including over the counter drugs
Occupational exposure to drugs and chemicals
Patient's reports of the following:
  Recent viral infections
  Alcohol use
  Bleeding from gums or nose
  Excessive menstrual flow
  Blood in stool or urine
Objective
Presence of visible bruises, petechiae
Positive urine hematest
Positive guaiac test of stool
Evidence of gingivitis
Laboratory reports of depressed platelets

Nursing Diagnoses
Potential for injury related to easy bruising and interrupted or delayed clotting
Knowledge deficit related to measures to be used to prevent bleeding

Expected Outcomes
Patient will be knowledgeable about safety precautions to follow to avoid bleeding and bruising.
Patient will not experience preventable bleeding.

Nursing Interventions
Monitor patient for new bruising or extension of existing bruises.
Institute and teach patient about bleeding precautions:
  Test urine and stool for blood.
  Avoid taking rectal temperature.
  Avoid all injections if possible.

NURSING CARE DURING BLOOD TRANSFUSIONS

BEFORE TRANSFUSION

Take baseline set of vital signs.

Keep blood refrigerated in the blood bank until ready for use.

Use two nurses to check blood bag data and ensure positive identification. Verify data with patient ID band before starting blood.

Prime tubing with normal saline solution—IV should have 18-gauge needle.

ALERT: Never hang blood products with glucose solutions as they induce RBC hemolysis and clumping.

Tell patient to immediately report signs of reactions (see below).

DURING TRANSFUSION

Stay with patient during first 15 minutes of transfusion to observe for reaction. Run blood slowly during first 15 minutes. Compare serial vital signs.

Administer remainder of unit in less than 4 hours. If whole blood is used, watch for signs of fluid overload.

Monitor vital signs at regular intervals throughout transfusion.

Monitor for signs of delayed transfusion reactions (see below).

SIGNS OF ACUTE HEMOLYTIC REACTION (USUALLY OCCUR IMMEDIATELY)

Burning sensation along the vein

Flushed face, abrupt fever and chills

Chest pain, labored breathing

Headache, backache, flank pain

Nursing Interventions

Stop transfusion immediately—run saline.

Call physician immediately.

Collect urine samples.

Send urine specimens, unused blood, and identifying tags to laboratory for analysis.

SIGNS OF ALLERGIC REACTION (USUALLY OCCUR WITHIN 30 MINUTES):

Hives and itching

Facial edema

Dyspnea, wheezing, anaphylaxis

Nursing Interventions

Stop transfusion immediately—run saline.

Notify physician.

Administer antihistamine as prescribed.

Transfusion may be continued under close observation if reaction is mild.

SIGNS OF PYROGENIC REACTIONS (USUALLY OCCUR WITHIN 1 TO 1½ HOURS)

Chills and fever

Headache and tachycardia

Palpitations or abdominal pain

Nursing Interventions

Stop transfusion immediately—run saline.

Notify physician.

Treat symptomatically as prescribed.

Monitor patient status closely.

Apply at least 5 minutes of pressure to all venipuncture sites.

Avoid use of straight razors.

Patient should use soft toothbrush or Water Pik for oral hygiene.

Patient should avoid trauma—no contact sports, no anal sex.

Patient should avoid use of any product containing aspirin.

Teach patient to contact physician with any sign of worsening of bruising or overt bleeding.

Teach patient about all medications prescribed.

Administer platelet transfusions if prescribed.

Teach patient importance of informing all physicians and particularly dentists of condition.

ALERT: Serious bleeding from relatively minor injury is likely when platelet count is below 60,000/ml; spontaneous hemorrhage is a life-threatening possibility below 20,000/ml.

Evaluation

Patient can describe signs indicative of increased bleeding.

Patient can describe safety measures to employ while platelet level is low.

Patient does not experience preventable bleeding.

DISORDERS OF COAGULATION

In addition to the role of the platelets, coagulation of blood results from the interaction of a number of clotting factors in a complex series of events called the coagulation cascade. Coagulation disorders may result from the depletion or absence of one or more of these clotting factors and may be either congenital or acquired. The bleeding problem may be mild or severe.

HEMOPHILIA

Both hemophilia A (factor VIII) and hemophilia B (factor IX) are hereditary sex-linked recessive disorders that are almost exclusively limited to males. The diagnosis is usually made in infancy or early childhood on the basis of a history of persistent bleeding.

PATHOPHYSIOLOGY

Patients with hemophilia have life-long histories of bleeding, either spontaneous or following trauma. Complications are the direct result of the bleeding tendency:

Joint deformities from repeated spontaneous bleeds

Life-threatening bleeding into soft tissue areas such as intracranial or retroperitoneal areas

MEDICAL MANAGEMENT

Treatment consists of replacement of deficient clotting factors if bleeding episodes do not respond to local treatment such as local pressure and application of ice. Transfusions of cryoprecipitate or concentrates of other deficient factors are given. Concentrated factors restore blood levels without volume overload. Desmopressin acetate (DDAVP) has been shown to increase levels of factor VIII in persons with mild hemophilia A. Ambulatory and home administration programs have dramatically increased the quality of life in persons with hemophilia.

NURSING MANAGEMENT

Assessment

Subjective

History and pattern of disease and treatment

Treatment regimen: side effects, costs, impact

Pain: type, location, severity

Life-style adaptations required by disease

General knowledge base concerning genetic transmission of the disease

Objective

Presence of active visible bleeding site or pattern of bruising

Joint limitation or deformity

Nursing Diagnoses

Diagnoses will depend on the severity and control of the disease but may include the following:

Pain related to bleeding into joints and tissues

Knowledge deficit related to self-control and mastery of the disease

Ineffective individual or family coping related to chronic nature of disease and the ongoing cost of treatment

Potential for injury related to spontaneous bleeding developing from minor injury

Expected Outcomes

Patient will maintain close control of disease process and experience minimal pain.

Patient will understand disease symptoms and scope and limitations of treatment regimen.

Patient and family will receive available community assistance for dealing with the financial and psychic hardship associated with the disease.

Patient will maintain effective control and not experience spontaneous bleeding.

Nursing Interventions

Teach patient about clotting factor replacement therapy used to control the disease.

Teach patient and family the technique of home administration of clotting factors if feasible.

Teach patient appropriate preventive measures. Patient should do the following:

Avoid trauma and minor injury.

Carry Medic Alert information at all times.

Know first-stage first aid for minor bleeding.

Provide patient and family with information about local agencies that can provide support or financial assistance and about the National Hemophilia Foundation.

Provide patient and family with accurate information concerning the genetic patterns of the disease.

Evaluation

Patient maintains knowledgeable control of hemophilia and is free of pain.

Patient can discuss disease, treatment regimen, and appropriate life-style modifications.

Patient and family maintain optimistic outlook and are assisted in coping with financial costs of treatment.

Patient adjusts activities to avoid injury.

DISSEMINATED INTRAVASCULAR COAGULATION

Disseminated intravascular coagulation (DIC) is a complicated and potentially fatal process characterized initially by widespread clotting and then by hemorrhage. It

---

MANAGEMENT OF DISSEMINATED INTRAVASCULAR COAGULATION

ASSOCIATED DISEASE STATES

Endothelial cell wall damage: factor XII formation

Sepsis	Anaphylaxis
Burns	Acidosis
Anoxia	Transfusion reaction

Tissue thromboplastin release: factor VII activation

Carcinoma/leukemia	Abruptio placenta
Blunt trauma	Retained dead fetus
Sepsis	Amniotic fluid embolus

Activation of factors X and II

Snake venom

Pancreatitis

Liver disease

EARLY SIGNS

Bleeding into mucous membranes and tissues

Prolonged prothrombin time (PT) and partial thromboplastin time (PTT)

Decreased platelets and fibrinogen

MEDICAL MANAGEMENT

Control or eliminate underlying disease.

Administer blood or blood products to replace depleted factors:

Platelets

Packed cells

Cryoprecipitate

The use of heparin to inhibit the underlying thrombolytic process is extremely controversial.

NURSING INTERVENTIONS

Administer medical plan.

Observe and test for evidence of new bleeding.

Provide symptomatic comfort and support for critically ill patient and family.

Assess for symptoms of fluid overload.

is a pathophysiologic response to a variety of diseases and injuries. A primary disease causes initiation of the clotting process that occurs throughout the vascular system. Fibrinolytic processes are stimulated and clotting factors become depleted, leading to severe hemorrhage. The box on p. 114 outlines common primary diseases that may trigger DIC and basic principles of management of this complex clinical disorder.

DISORDERS OF THE WHITE BLOOD CELLS

The primary function of the white blood cells (WBCs) is to provide for humoral and cellular response to infection. Any compromise in the integrity of the WBC system leaves the individual extremely susceptible to infection.

Neutrophils are primarily responsible for phagocytosis and destruction of bacteria and other infectious organisms. Lymphocytes are the principal cells of immunity involved in the production of antibodies.

Chemotherapy drugs, exposure to other drugs and chemicals, and radiation may all suppress white cell function, but the most common disorders involve malignant disease.

LEUKEMIA

The leukemias are malignant disorders involving the bone marrow and lymph nodes and are characterized by uncontrolled proliferation of WBCs and their precursors. Table 8-3 lists the common leukemias and their characteristics. The leukemias are classified as either acute or chronic and then further divided according to cell type and degree of cell maturity.

PATHOPHYSIOLOGY

Large numbers of WBCs accumulate first at the site of origin and then spread to hematopoietic organs, causing enlargement. The proliferation of one type of cell interferes with production of other blood components. Immature cells decrease immunocompetence and increase susceptibility to infection. Peripheral WBC count may show an increase or decrease in numbers. The cause of leukemia remains unknown.

MEDICAL MANAGEMENT

Medical management is specific to the particular type of leukemia (see Table 8-3), but utilizes aggressive chemotherapy as its base. Dramatic increases in survival have been achieved for some forms of the disease,

TABLE 8-3 Leukemias

Leukemia	Peak Age	Prognosis	Symptoms	Medical Management
Acute Leukemias				
Acute lymphocytic leukemia (ALL)	2-4 yr (80% are children)	Good response to treatment; over 50% of patients under 15 achieve 5-year survival	Fever, respiratory infections, anemia, bleeding mucous membranes, lymphadenopathy, fatigue and weakness, tendency to infection	Combined chemotherapy Drugs: Vincristine Prednisone 6-Mercaptopurine Methotrexate
Acute myelogenous leukemia (AML)	12-20 yr, after 55	High mortality from infection and hemorrhage; an initial remission is possible in 50-75% but 5-yr survival is poor	Same symptoms as ALL, but less lymphadenopathy	Chemotherapy: Cytosine arabinoside Thioguanine Adriamycin Daunorubicin Bone marrow transplant
Chronic Leukemias				
Chronic lymphocytic leukemia (CLL)	50-70 yr but can occur at any age; three times more common in men	Most patients do quite well; survive 10 or more years with disease	Insidious onset; weakness, fatigue, massive lymphadenopathy, pruritic vesicular skin lesions, anemia, thrombocytopenia	Chemotherapy: Alkylating agents— chlorambucil and glucocorticoids Treated only when symptomatic
Chronic myelogenous leukemia (CML)	30-50 yr	Death usually occurs in less than 5 years from infection and hemorrhage	Weakness, fatigue, anorexia, weight loss, splenomegaly, anemia, thrombocytopenia, fever; can have fulminant stage	Chemotherapy with same agents used with AML; also vincristine, busulfan, hydroxyurea Bone marrow transplant

particularly acute lymphocytic leukemia (ALL). Combination drug therapy, coupled with maintenance therapy while disease is in remission, is a normal protocol. Therapy is intense and rigorous, often demanding extensive hospitalization and intensive nursing care to sustain the patient. Prophylactic treatment of the central nervous system has dramatically decreased reoccurrences.

NURSING MANAGEMENT

Assessment

Subjective
History and duration of symptoms
History of prior treatment, if any
Patient's complaint of fatigue and weakness
History of frequent infection
Possible weight loss or anorexia
Family's response to symptoms and diagnosis
Medications in current use

Objective
Fever
Presence of anemia, thrombocytopenia
Bruising, petechiae
Lymphadenopathy
Bleeding or ulceration on mucous membranes
General systems assessment

Nursing Diagnoses
Diagnoses will depend on the disease type and severity and the nature of the treatment. Common diagnoses include the following:

Activity intolerance related to severe fatigue and weakness

Ineffective individual or family coping related to the treatment regimen and prognosis of the disease

Pain related to blast crisis in marrow

Potential for injury and infection related to the disease symptoms and side effects of the treatment regimen

Altered nutrition: less than body requirements, related to anorexia and gastrointestinal side effects of chemotherapy

Potential for altered oral mucous membranes related to side effects of chemotherapy

Knowledge deficit related to the management of the side effects of chemotherapy

Anxiety related to the side effects of treatment and fear of death

Expected Outcomes
Patient will maintain sufficient energy to remain independent in the activities of daily living.

Patient and family will receive support and honestly share their feelings and fears about the disease.

Patient will remain comfortable during treatment.

Patient will be protected from bleeding and infection during chemotherapy.

Patient will maintain an adequate nutrient intake to meet minimal body requirements.

Patient's mucous membranes will remain intact to allow for oral nutrition.

Patient will be knowledgeable about treatment regimen, expected side effects, and their management.

Patient will experience only manageable anxiety.

Nursing Interventions
Administer combined chemotherapy, if covered by hospital policy. Ensure patency of vascular access (see Chapter 2 for specific interventions for IV administration of chemotherapy).

Institute bleeding precautions.
  See discussion under thrombocytopenia.
  Monitor for signs of bleeding.

Administer blood and blood products as ordered.

Assist patient to space activity to conserve energy.

Assist patient with activities of daily living as needed.

Protect patient against nosocomial infection.
  Promote scrupulous hygiene, particularly oral.
  Insist on rigorous handwashing by staff.
  Prep skin thoroughly before skin puncture.
  Monitor for early signs of infection.
  Establish protective isolation if indicated: laminar air flow rooms may be needed to preserve life in severely leukopenic patients.

Employ nursing measures to counter anorexia and nausea (see Chapter 2 for specific nutrition interventions for chemotherapy).

Teach patient and family about treatment regimen including the following:
  Purposes of combination drug therapy
  Expected side effects of drugs
  Management of side effects
  Purpose of isolation
  Measures to prevent infection or bleeding
  Symptoms indicating complications

Provide emotional support to patient and family.
  Ensure adequate time for questions; encourage expression of fears and concerns.
  Include family in all aspects of care.
  Explore community agencies that can provide patient and family with support and specific assistance.

Promptly report the incidence of petechiae, ecchymoses, and gingival bleeding.

Evaluation
Patient rests at frequent intervals but is able to maintain independence in activities of daily living.

Patient and family openly discuss disease, treatment, and prognosis, and actively deal with fears and frustrations.

Patient experiences minimal discomfort.

Patient maintains adequate blood levels and does not experience spontaneous bleeding or acquired infection.

Patient maintains a stable body weight and adjusts diet to ensure intake of minimal nutritional requirements while receiving chemotherapy.

Patient does not develop extensive mouth ulceration and is able to comfortably ingest food and fluid orally.

Patient can describe purpose and side effects of treatment regimens; plans with nurse to adjust diet, hygiene, and activity to minimize the side effects of treatment.

Patient feels comfortable and optimistic about the future.

DISORDERS ASSOCIATED WITH THE LYMPH SYSTEM

The chief functions of the lymph nodes and lymph system are to assist in phagocytosis of cellular debris and to provide an immune response to antigens received from the structures drained by the lymph node. Lymph nodes are not normally palpable but enlarge in the presence of a wide variety of infectious processes. Infectious mononucleosis is the best known primary disorder and is summarized in the box on this page. Most of the other disorders of the lymph system are malignant in nature.

LYMPHOMA

The category of lymphoma includes a variety of malignant disorders in which the lymph tissue is infiltrated with malignant cells and the affected nodes enlarge. The disease then spreads to lymph tissue of other nodes such as the liver or spleen. Lymphomas usually follow a pattern of exacerbation and remission.

INFECTIOUS MONONUCLEOSIS

Infectious mononucleosis is an acute self-limiting disease caused by the Epstein-Barr virus. It is more common in young persons and is usually a benign disease with a good prognosis.

The symptoms are variable:
Malaise—usual early complaint
Flulike symptoms—fever, sore throat, generalized aches, enlarged lymph nodes
Moderate spleen enlargement

MEDICAL AND NURSING CARE

Most persons recover spontaneously within a few weeks.
Promote rest and comfort.
Avoid stress and strain.
Prepare patient for persistent fatigue.

PATHOPHYSIOLOGY

Lymphomas are generally classified as follows:
1. *Hodgkin's disease:* potentially curable disease characterized by presence of Reed-Sternberg cells in affected nodes. Treatment plans and prognosis are closely tied to accurate disease staging.
2. *Non-Hodgkin's lymphoma:* broad spectrum of lymphoid malignancies with different histologic features and prognoses. Treatment again is closely tied to accurate histologic identification, disease staging, and responses to treatment.

Table 8-4 compares the major aspects and treatment of Hodgkin's disease and non-Hodgkin's lymphoma.

MEDICAL MANAGEMENT

Treatment for all lymphomas is carefully tied to accurate identification of cell types and degree of disease spread. Successful treatment protocols have been well defined for Hodgkin's disease in particular. Repetitive courses of combined chemotherapy are the basis of re-

TABLE 8-4 Disorders of the lymph system

Disorder	Etiology	Signs and Symptoms	Medical Management
Hodgkin's disease	Unknown, viruses possibly implicated Affects primarily young adults	Lymph node enlargement (firm, nontender, painless), fever, weight loss, night sweats, pruritus (itching), fatigue and weakness, presence of Reed-Sternberg cells, enlarged liver and spleen	Radiotherapy for early stages; combination chemotherapy for middle and late stages MOPP regimen most commonly used: nitrogen mustard, vincristine, procarbazine, and prednisone
Non-Hodgkin's lymphoma	Unknown, viruses implicated Affects 50 to 70 year olds	Nontender "bulky" lymphadenopathy, moderate hepatomegaly and splenomegaly; patient may experience unexplained weight loss, fever, night sweats	Radiotherapy for initial treatment for localized disease Combination chemotherapy is the mainstay of treatment for diffuse disease; a variety of drug combinations are employed

mission induction and maintenance. Treatment may be augmented by radiation, particularly for the early stages of non-Hodgkin's lymphoma. Surgery is used to facilitate the staging and diagnosis.

NURSING MANAGEMENT

Assessment

  Subjective

  History, duration, and severity of symptoms
  Knowledge of disorder
  Prior treatment and response if appropriate
  Patient's complaints of the following:
      Fever
      Weakness
      Anorexia
      Night sweats
      General pruritus (itching)
  Effect of fatigue on self-care capabilities

  Objective

  Nontender enlarged lymph nodes
  Weight loss
  Fever
  Nutritional status
  Enlarged liver and spleen
  Positive lymph node biopsy or lymphangiogram
  Condition of skin

Nursing Diagnoses

Diagnoses will vary according to the severity and stage of the disease. Common diagnoses include the following:

  Activity intolerance related to systemic fatigue and fever
  Potential alteration in skin integrity related to pruritis, fever, and night sweats
  Knowledge deficit related to treatment regimen and side effects of chemotherapy
  Altered nutrition: less than body requirements, related to side effects of chemotherapy
  Potential ineffective individual coping related to disease exacerbations and treatment side effects

Expected Outcomes

Patient will maintain sufficient energy to be independent in self-care.

Patient will maintain an intact skin.
Patient will be knowledgeable of the treatment regimen and the management of the side effects of drugs.
Patient will maintain an adequate nutritional intake and stabilize body weight.
Patient will cope effectively with unpredictability of the disease.

Nursing Interventions

Assist patient to deal with the side effects of chemotherapy and radiation (see Chapter 2 for specific interventions).
Help patient to arrange activities to conserve energy.
Provide comfort measures appropriate to symptoms.
    Keep bedding and linen fresh and dry.
    Offer baths and skin care.
    Administer antipyretic and antipruritic medication as prescribed.
Plan with patient to adjust diet to insure adequate nutritional intake and fluids.
Teach patient about treatment regimen and measures to control side effects.
Explain importance of detailed diagnostic workup.
Provide teaching about the effects of broad field radiation and chemotherapy on reproductive capacities.
    Males are frequently sterile and should consider sperm banking.
    Females usually regain fertility in time; may have ovaries relocated outside radiation treatment zone.
Provide ongoing support to patient and family.

Evaluation

Patient has sufficient energy to maintain self-care independence.
Patient maintains an intact skin.
Patient is knowledgeable about disease, treatment regimen, and the treatment of side effects.
Patient maintains stable weight and eats a diet that contains the minimal nutritional requirements.
Patient copes with disease and treatment regimen with minimal disruption in family or occupational roles.

NURSING CARE PLAN

SICKLE CELL CRISIS

Nursing Diagnoses	Expected Patient Outcomes	Nursing Interventions
Pain related to imbalance in oxygen supply and demand	Patient's pain is managed effectively.	1. Perform good pain assessment. 2. Give prescribed analgesics as needed and evaluate effectiveness of medication. 3. Explore the use of patient-controlled analgesia for pain control. 4. Identify measures patient has found helpful and include these measures in the care. 5. Support joints gently when assisting patient to do ROM exercises. 6. Use moist heat or massage, if helpful. 7. Use other pain-relieving measures; person with frequent crises may benefit from learning special techniques such as biofeedback or self-hypnosis. 8. Assist patient in avoiding habituation and dependence on narcotics if possible.
Altered tissue perfusion (peripheral) related to blockage in small arterioles and capillaries	Patient does not develop thrombosis, skin ulcerations, or retinal infarction.	1. Administer prescribed intravenous fluids; because large amounts may be given, monitor patient for fluid overload. 2. Encourage oral fluids, if permitted. 3. Monitor for signs of thrombosis (pain in chest or abdomen, headache, decreased vision, oliguria or low urinary specific gravity). 4. Assess legs, especially medial malleoli, for signs of skin breakdown; use measures to prevent skin dryness or injury from trauma. 5. Provide prescribed oxygen. 6. Reduce activity to lower body's metabolic needs.
Potential ineffective individual coping related to disease exacerbations	Patient utilizes positive coping strategies to deal with illness-related problems.	1. Provide opportunities for patient to discuss feelings about inability to fulfill expected roles. 2. Assist patient to identify personal strengths. 3. Identify and support all positive coping strategies. 4. Suggest joining a support group or obtaining counseling to minimize dependency behaviors.
Activity intolerance related to pain and decreased tissue oxygenation	Patient will have sufficient energy to remain independent in the activities of daily living.	1. Space daily activities and encourage frequent rest periods. 2. Assist with activities of daily living as needed. 3. Assist with gentle ROM exercise each shift.

Knowledge deficit related to disease origins and treatment and genetic implications	Patient/family understand the nature of the disorder and its treatment and receive appropriate genetic testing and counseling.	1. Assess patient's knowledge of sickle cell anemia and correct misunderstandings.
		2. Teach patient the basis of sickle cell disease and genetic effects.
		3. Provide resources for family planning and genetic counseling.
		4. Teach patient to avoid situations that cause crises.
		  a. Infection, dehydration, and overexertion
		  b. Smoking and alcohol use
		5. Reinforce importance of folic acid supplement to support RBC formation.
		6. Teach patient to drink 4 to 6 quarts fluid daily.
		7. Discuss genetic counseling and contraceptive methods if patient is concerned about transmitting disease.

BIBLIOGRAPHY

Freedman SL: An overview of bone marrow transplantation, Semin Oncol Nurs **4**(1):3-8, 1988.

Froberg J: The anemias: causes and courses of action, RN **52**(1):24-29, 1989.

Huckstadt A: Hemophilia: the person, family and nurse, Rehabil Nurs **11**(3):225-228, 1986.

Lakhani AK: Current management of acute leukemias, Nursing 88 **3:**755-758, 1987.

Lamb C: Managing sickle cell emergencies, Patient Care **19**(1):92-95, 1985.

Simonson GM: Caring for patients with acute myelocytic leukemia, Am J Nurs **88:**304-309, 1988.

Terry BA: Hodgkin's disease and non-Hodgkin's lymphoma, Nurs Clin North Am **20:**207-217, 1985.

CHAPTER 9

Disorders of the Respiratory System

Disorders of the respiratory system are numerous and varied. They range from transient infectious processes to chronic degenerative and malignant problems. This chapter separates respiratory disorders into two major categories: disorders of the upper airway and disorders of the lower airway. Figure 9-1 shows the anatomical structure of the respiratory system.

DISORDERS OF THE UPPER AIRWAY

Disorders of the upper airway include problems of the nose, sinuses, pharynx, tonsils, and larynx. They are very common health problems and include infections, structural defects, and problems of cosmetic appearance.

NOSE AND SINUSES

Disorders of the nose and sinuses include a variety of allergic, infectious, and obstructive problems. Uncomplicated cases of rhinitis, allergic rhinitis, and sinusitis are frequently treated with over-the-counter decongestants, antihistamines, and antibiotics. Nasal obstructions from structural abnormalities, tumors, or trauma are usually surgically treated. Common surgeries include the submucous resection, rhinoplasty, and nasal polypectomy. The box on this page outlines basic principles of care for a patient experiencing nasal surgery.

PHARYNX AND TONSILS

The most common disorders affecting the pharynx or tonsils in adults are acute infections that may be relieved by symptomatic care or antibiotics if indicated. Surgical interventions through tonsillectomy and adenoidectomy are usually more serious procedures in the adult patient than in the child. The box on p. 123 outlines basic principles for a patient with a tonsillectomy.

LARYNX

Disorders involving the larynx range from relatively benign laryngitis to cancer of the larynx. Cancer of the larynx is a relatively uncommon disorder that occurs most frequently in men over 60 years of age. It may be confined to the vocal cords where it grows slowly or extend rapidly to the deep lymph nodes of the neck. Its development appears to be related to heavy smoking, alcohol abuse, chronic laryngitis, and vocal abuse.

PATHOPHYSIOLOGY

Tumor growth prevents the free vibration of the vocal cords. This produces the classic early sign of hoarseness of a progressive nature. More advanced disease may

CARE OF THE PATIENT WITH NASAL SURGERY

PREOPERATIVE CARE
Teach patient about procedure and type of anesthesia (general or local) to be used.
Teach patient about necessity for mouth breathing after surgery as a result of nasal packing.
Teach patient about anticipated swelling and discoloration.

POSTOPERATIVE CARE
Monitor vital signs regularly.
Monitor for signs of bleeding:
    Observe for excessive swallowing and hematemesis.
    Assess bleeding through nasal drip pad.
Change drip pad under nose as needed.
Place patient in mid-Fowler's position—apply ice over nose for 24 hours.
Encourage fluid intake.
Provide oral mouth care frequently.
Provide adequate analgesia and relief for nausea if indicated.
Maintain or provide adequate room humidity.
Inform patient that first stools may be tarry from swallowing blood.

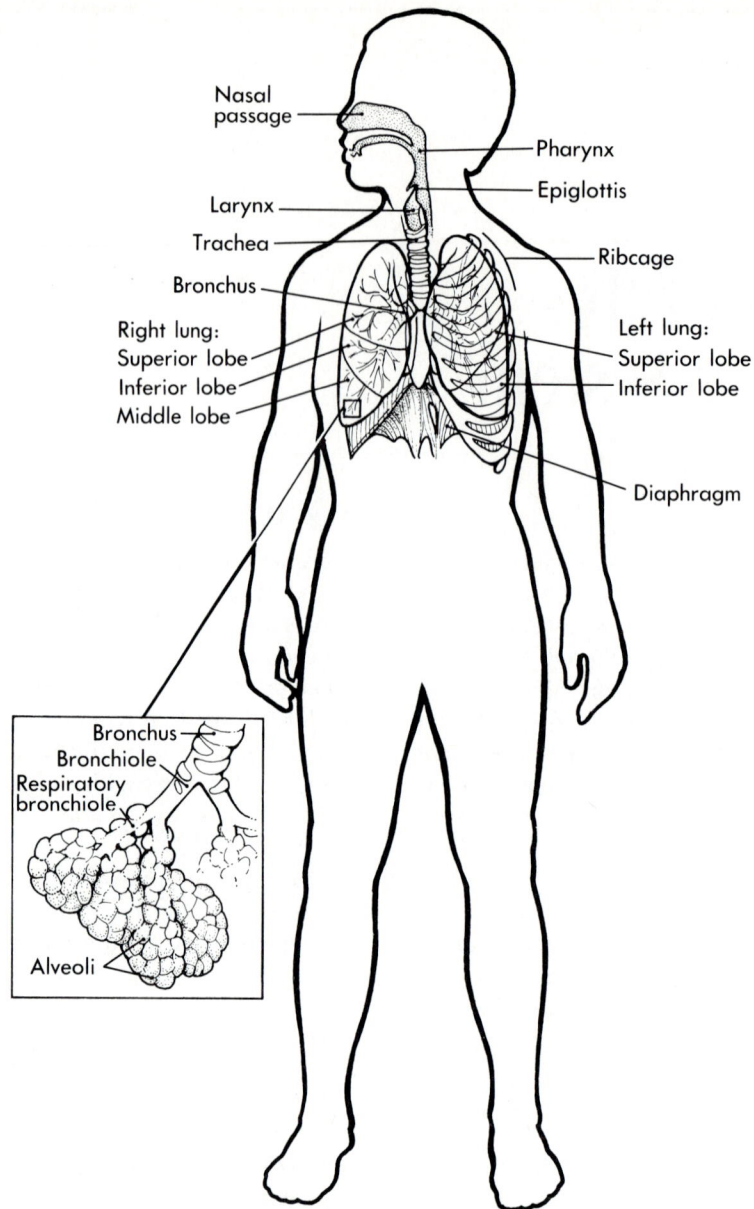

FIGURE 9-1 Respiratory system.

produce signs of dysphagia, a feeling of a "lump in the throat," or pain in the region of the Adam's apple.

MEDICAL MANAGEMENT

In patients diagnosed very early, radiation therapy may be feasible, but the treatment of choice is usually surgical. A variety of procedures are available, depending on the exact location and extent of the disease. Partial laryngectomy preserves the voice but does impair swallowing. Total laryngectomy usually also necessitates radical neck dissection and results in significant alterations in both structure and the patient's appearance. Surgery also removes the cervical lymph nodes and may

sacrifice the sternocleidomastoid muscle, internal jugular vein, and accessory nerve because the risk of neck metastases is high.

NURSING MANAGEMENT

Assessment (Preoperative)

Subjective

History and severity of symptoms

Patient's history of smoking, alcohol use, or voice abuse

Patient's knowledge of surgical procedure and outcomes

Patient's response to potential loss of vocal function

CARE OF THE PATIENT WITH TONSILLECTOMY

PREOPERATIVE CARE
Teach patient about the surgical procedure and type of anesthesia planned.
Teach patient about diet and analgesia after surgery.

POSTOPERATIVE CARE
Position patient on side until fully awake and alert.
Use Fowler's position once patient is awake.
Provide adequate analgesia. Avoid use of aspirin.
Apply ice collar if prescribed.
Observe for bleeding:
  Teach patient not to cough or attempt to clear throat for 1 to 2 weeks.
  Observe patient for frequent swallowing.
  Prevent vomiting if possible; observe for blood.
Offer ice cold fluids and soft bland diet when patient is stable:
  Avoid use of straw as it creates throat suction.
  Suggest patient use large swallows since they hurt less.
  Cold items are better tolerated.
  Avoid irritating foods until healing is complete.
Keep fluid intake high, at least 2 to 3 liters.
Patient should avoid rigorous activity and exercise during first 3 to 5 days but can resume normal activity.
Teach patient to expect worsening of pain between days 4 and 8 when the membrane separates over the incision.

Assessment of past coping mechanisms
Occupation and leisure activities
Objective
General health status, especially respiratory system
Degree of hoarseness
Difficulty with swallowing, pain

Nursing Diagnoses
Common postoperative nursing diagnoses include the following:
  Ineffective airway clearance related to edema around surgical area and increased volume of secretions
  Impaired verbal communication related to loss of vocal mechanism
  Potential for ineffective individual coping related to loss of verbal communication and its impact on social and family roles
  Knowledge deficit related to artificial airway management and mechanisms of speech rehabilitation
  Body image disturbance related to neck stoma and effects of surgery

Expected Outcomes
Patient will maintain a clear airway through appropriate use of positioning and suctioning.
Patient will effectively communicate needs to nursing staff.

Patient will begin to resolve grief over vocal loss and receive appropriate support from family and staff.
Patient will learn how to manage artificial airway and will be knowledgeable about rehabilitation options.
Patient will begin to incorporate body changes into a revised but positive body image and continue presurgical social and family roles.

Nursing Interventions: Preoperative
Prepare patient for surgery and postoperative care. Explain the following:
  Presence and appearance of stoma and nature of neck breathing
  Hemovac or other wound drainage if planned
  Technique of suctioning and equipment
  Devices to deliver humidity
  Presence of nasogastric tube for tube feeding
Encourage patient and family to ask questions and discuss fears and concerns about surgery and rehabilitation.
Discuss loss of normal speech
Discuss with patient the communication device to be used after the operation, such as magic slate, chalkboard, or pad and pencil.
Present options of speech rehabilitation:
  Assess patient for readiness for visit from a rehabilitated patient.
  Establish location of nearest Lost Chord or New Voice Club.
  Put family in touch with services of the American Cancer Society.

Nursing Interventions: Postoperative
Suction tracheostomy frequently to clear airway (see box on next page for suctioning procedure).
ALERT: Suctioning may be needed every 5 minutes during the first few hours.
Maintain humidity to stoma.
Encourage frequent deep breathing and coughing.
Keep head of bed elevated.
Auscultate lungs.
Have call bell within easy reach—answer immediately.
Ensure that agreed-upon communication device is at bedside.
Avoid using patient's writing arm for IV tubes.
Monitor wound drainage including Hemovac.
Provide skin care around stoma as needed.
Provide frequent mouth care.
Provide nasogastric tube feedings (usually for about 10 days); ensure adequate hydration.
Begin feedings by mouth cautiously; keep head of bed elevated.
  Provide support and reassure patient that aspiration cannot occur. A sensation of choking is common.
Teach patient to support head when changing positions.

TRACHEOSTOMY CARE AND SUCTIONING

TRACHEOSTOMY SUCTIONING

Explain the procedure to patient.
Wash hands before the procedure.
Auscultate lungs before the procedure.
Suction oropharnyx before suctioning the tracheostomy.
Prepare sterile equipment needed, using strict sterile technique.
   Use sterile gloves and catheter.
   Use sterile container and water.
Have patient take five to six deep breaths of 100% oxygen before the procedure. Use Ambu bag and administer breaths if patient is unable to cooperate.
Lubricate catheter with sterile water or water-soluble lubricant before insertion.
Insert catheter *without suction* about 8 inches, or deep enough to produce an effective cough.
Apply intermittent suction and withdraw catheter slowly, rotating while withdrawing. Suction for no longer than 10 to 15 seconds at one time.
Rinse catheter in sterile water between insertions.
Hyperoxygenate again between insertions. Allow patient to rest for 1 to 3 minutes between suctionings.
Repeat procedure if needed.
Monitor for signs of hypoxia, bradycardia, or dysrhythmia.
Auscultate lungs at conclusion to ensure effectiveness.
Clean inner cannula (if present) every 4 hours or as necessary.

TRACHEOSTOMY CARE

After suctioning, unlock and remove inner cannula if present.
Immerse in H_2O_2 and cleanse with brush.
Rinse in sterile water or saline, shake dry, reinsert, and lock in place.
Cleanse around stoma with H_2O_2 and saline on applicators or 4 × 4 inch gauze pads.
Apply Betadine solution or ointment around tracheostomy if part of hospital protocol.
Change tracheostomy dressing as needed.
Change ties as needed.
   Insert ties through slits to secure to outer cannula.
   Tie tapes with double knot at side of neck.
   ALERT: Tracheostomy tube should be manually secured in place whenever tapes are not in place.
   Tapes should be snug but allow passage of fingertips beneath them when tied.

GENERAL CARE

Provide constant airway humidification.
Change all respiratory equipment every 24 hours.
Provide frequent mouth care.
Establish communication and minimize sensory deprivation.

Nursing Interventions: Rehabilitative Phase

Teach patient self-care of tube if permanent stoma has not been created (suctioning is rarely needed after discharge).
Encourage supportive visits from family and friends.
Encourage contacts with volunteer groups.

Assist patient to plan the following life-style modifications that will be necessary after discharge:
   Prevent water and foreign objects from entering stoma.
   Adjust hygiene routines—take precautions when bathing or showering and when shaving (avoid use of talc).
   Make clothing adjustments such as scarf or collar of porous material to cover stoma.
   Make recreational adjustments—swimming and water sports are contraindicated.
Teach patient signs of complications:
   Increased or purulent secretions
   Fever and cough
Support patient in all appropriate expressions of coping.
Arrange for follow-up with a speech pathologist. Options for rehabilitation include the following:
   Tracheoesophageal speech—formation of a fistula for silicone prothesis insertion that allows speech when air is diverted from the trachea to the esophagus
   Esophageal speech—speech produced by expelling swallowed air
   Electrolarynx—electronic device that assists in producing the sounds of speech
Refer patient to services of the Association for Laryngectomies.

Evaluation

Patient's airway is clear; does not require mechanical suctioning.
Patient is able to effectively communicate needs and has been referred to speech therapist/center for rehabilitation.
Patient is exhibiting positive coping behaviors and expresses desire to resume usual activities.
Patient cares independently for stoma and discusses measures to protect stoma and ensure adequate humidity.
Patient incorporates surgical outcomes into a revised but positive sense of self.

DISORDERS OF THE LOWER AIRWAY

There are many disorders of the lower airway, but the most significant are those that are chronic. They cause significant impact on life-style and are a frequent cause of permanent disability. The discussion of lower airway disorders in this chapter follows the restrictive and obstructive disorders classification, although the diseases rarely fall into just one category.

A. RESTRICTIVE LUNG DISORDERS

Restrictive disorders are those causing a restriction in lung volume and reduction in lung compliance. They include diseases that restrict lung movement and inhibit proper inspiration.

PNEUMONIA

Pneumonia may be caused by a variety of bacterial and viral organisms. It occurs most commonly in winter and early spring, affects individuals of all ages, and accounts for over 10% of all hospital admissions. It usually results from inhalation of infected material, although its specific communicability is dependent on the infecting organism.

PATHOPHYSIOLOGY

Pneumonia results in inflammation of the lung tissue. The infecting organism causes inflammatory exudate to fill the alveolar air spaces, producing lung consolidation. Gas exchange cannot occur in affected alveoli. Hypoxemia may occur depending on amount of lung tissue affected. Typical symptoms are listed in Table 9-1.

MEDICAL MANAGEMENT

Once sputum smears and cultures have been obtained, antibiotic therapy is instituted for the causative organism. Supportive care is offered for fever, fatigue, and decreased respiratory function. Response to appropriate therapy usually occurs within 24 to 48 hours.

Supplemental oxygen may be needed for patients who are markedly hypoxemic. Supportive measures are offered to assist the patient to open and clear the airway.

Strict isolation is necessary for staphylococcal pneumonia. Staff protection is ensured by good hand washing for most other types.

NURSING MANAGEMENT

Assessment

Subjective

History and duration of symptoms

History of recent upper respiratory tract infection

Location and degree of chest pain or discomfort

Patient's complaints of the following:

Fatigue

Anorexia

Dyspnea

Fever and chills

Objective

Baseline vital signs, tachycardia and tachypnea, elevated temperature

Auscultate lungs—presence of decreased breath sounds, inspiratory rales, cyanosis

Dullness to percussion

Productive cough: greenish, purulent, rusty sputum

Splinting chest during inspiration

Tachypnea; use of accessory muscles, nasal flaring

Presence of expiratory grunt

Nursing Diagnoses

Diagnoses may vary slightly depending on the severity of the disease but commonly include the following:

Activity intolerance related to hypoxemia and overwhelming fatigue

---

TABLE 9-1 Pneumonia

Type	Etiology	Signs and Symptoms
Classical	*Streptococcus pneumoniae* *Haemophilus influenzae* *Staphylococcus aureus* *Klebsiella pneumoniae*	Abrupt onset Fever 39° to 40° C with shaking chills Cough productive of green, purulent or rusty sputum Pleuritic chest pain and restricted chest movement Rapid shallow respirations Inspiratory rales and dullness to percussion; cyanosis may be present
Atypical	*Mycoplasma pneumoniae* Viruses	Gradual onset over 3 to 4 days Malaise, headache, and dry cough
	Legionella pneumophila *Pneumocystis carinii*	Above symptoms plus: Abdominal pain and diarrhea Chills and fever >40° C Renal failure and electrolyte imbalance
Aspiration	Any material entering airway by aspiration	When hospital acquired, staphylococcal or gram-negative organisms may be involved After insidious onset, condition can take a rapid downhill course of bacteremia and septic shock
Hematogenous	Occurs when pathogenic organisms are spread to the lungs via the blood stream; *Staphylococcus aureus* and *Escherichia coli* are among the most common	Pulmonary symptoms are minimal compared with the symptoms of septicemia Nonproductive cough and pleuritic chest pain are common

Ineffective airway clearance related to increased mucus production, inflammation, and alveolar consolidation

Pain related to pleural irritation

Ineffective breathing pattern related to restricted chest movement and splinting

Potential fluid volume deficit related to fever and anorexia

Expected Outcomes

Patient will have sufficient energy to return to normal pattern of activities.

Lungs will become progressively clear to auscultation.

Patient will experience minimal chest pain.

Patient will return to a normal breathing pattern, fully inflating all lung segments.

Patient will receive sufficient fluids orally and intravenously to compensate for losses and maintain a normal fluid balance.

Nursing Interventions

Position patient in semi-Fowler's position to facilitate breathing. Do not position on affected side. Encourage frequent position changes.

Monitor vital signs frequently, especially temperature and respirations.

Assess adequacy of ventilatory effort.

Observe for cyanosis, use of accessory muscles.

Auscultate lungs.

Collect adequate sputum specimens before administration of antibiotics.

Administer medications as prescribed:

Antibiotics

Analgesics

Antipyretics, expectorants, antitussives

Monitor for hypersensitivity

Provide comfort measures: linen, bathing for elevated temperature, mouth care if cough is productive

Administer parenteral fluids as ordered.

Offer fluids orally as tolerated.

Record intake and output accurately.

Ensure adequate fluids.

Offer small frequent meals high in protein and carbohydrates.

Encourage adequate rest.

Assist patient with activities of daily living as needed.

Prevent spread of disease:

Use scrupulous hand-washing procedures.

Teach patient about coughing and tissue disposal.

Use respiratory isolation for staphylococcal pneumonia.

Ensure adequate room humidity. Administer oxygen if prescribed.

Encourage patient to cough and deep breathe effectively.

Administer mild analgesics if chest pain is severe.

Splint chest while coughing.

Utilize chest physical therapy if patient cannot clear airway by coughing.

Encourage patient to restrict activity level until disease resolves to prevent relapse.

Complete full course of antibiotic therapy.

Evaluation

Patient resumes normal activities without reoccurrence of fatigue or dyspnea.

Patient's vital signs are normal, cough is resolving, and lungs are clear to auscultation.

Patient's chest pain has resolved.

Patient's ventilatory movements return to normal—no chest splinting is used.

Patient meets body needs for fluid through ingestion of normal oral diet.

TUBERCULOSIS

Tuberculosis (TB), although considered both preventable and controllable, is still a significant health problem in the United States. Statistics have shown a slight increase in urban regions, and it is a significant health problem among minority populations. The over-65 population is at particular risk. Recent increases in incidence are a reflection of the increase of TB in persons infected with the HIV virus.

PATHOPHYSIOLOGY

Tuberculosis is caused by the *Mycobacterium tuberculosis* bacillus, a gram-positive and acid-fast bacillus. The disease is spread by the inhalation of tubercle-laden droplets. When a person with no previous exposure to TB inhales a sufficient number of tubercle bacilli into the alveoli, a TB infection occurs. Inflammation occurs within the alveoli, and natural body defenses attempt to counteract the infection. The body's reaction depends on the susceptibility of the individual, the size of the dose, and the virulence of the organism. NOTE: Most individuals infected by organism do not develop active disease but demonstrate only positive skin testing and x-ray evidence of calcified nodes or cavities. Active disease may later occur during a period of intense or prolonged physical or emotional stress. If the initial immune response is not adequate, clinical disease will then occur.

MEDICAL MANAGEMENT

The diagnosis is carefully established through a combination of skin testing, x-ray examinations, and culture of the sputum. Most persons with TB do not have positive smears, and a full culture is required. Because the tubercle bacillus grows slowly, the full culture may take 3 to 6 weeks.

The foundation of treatment is drug therapy, with at

least two drugs given together to prevent the development of resistant strains. Drugs commonly prescribed are summarized in Table 9-2. Drugs are administered for 9 to 24 months. Preventive chemotherapy usually involves the daily administration of INH for 6 months, or 1 year if HIV antibodies are present. Preventive therapy is given to individuals who develop positive skin tests without other evidence of active disease. Many positive reactors who take INH for 6 months convert back to a negative skin test.

Adequate rest and optimal nutrition are the other components of basic care. Management is also directed at preventing the spread of the disease. Basic hygiene precautions for coughing and sputum disposal are important, but strict isolation at home is not necessary. Family and social contacts are skin tested, and high-risk individuals may receive preventive drug therapy.

NURSING MANAGEMENT

Assessment

Subjective
History and progression of symptoms
History of TB exposure
Family composition—members at risk
Patient's complaints of the following:
    Fatigue and malaise
    Anorexia and weight loss
    Afternoon or night sweats
Patient's perceptions of or attitudes toward the diagnosis of tuberculosis

Objective
Vital signs; presence of low-grade fever, particularly in the afternoon
Productive cough, character of sputum (may be blood streaked)
Decreasing weight
Positive skin test, chest x-ray

Nursing Diagnoses
Diagnoses may be variable with acuity and stage of the disease but commonly include the following:
    Activity intolerance related to fatigue generated by inflammatory response
    Ineffective airway clearance related to excess mucus production
    Potential for ineffective individual or family coping related to long-term therapy or social stigma associated with tuberculosis
    Knowledge deficit related to tuberculosis, its treatment, and prevention of its spread
    Altered nutrition: less than body requirements, related to the anorexia and nausea associated with both the acute stage of tuberculosis and side effects of medications

Expected Outcomes
Patient will experience increased energy and be able to resume normal activities of daily living.
Patient will experience decreased sputum production and maintain a clear airway.
Patient and family will make positive adaptation to the diagnosis and implications of treatment regimen.
Patient will be knowledgeable about the tuberculosis disease process, need for long-term therapy, and measures to prevent spread of the disease.
Patient's appetite will increase; patient will plan and eat a well-balanced diet and maintain a stable body weight.

Nursing Interventions
Administer medications as prescribed (see Table 9-2).
    Teach patient about expected side effects, especially gastrointestinal disturbances.
Patient should take supplemental vitamin B_6 while taking first-line drugs.

TABLE 9-2 Drugs used to treat tuberculosis

Drug	Dosage	Side Effects
First-Line Drugs		
Isoniazid (INH)	5-10 mg/kg/day	Peripheral neuritis, hepatic toxicity, hypersensitivity (skin rash, fever, arthralgia)
Ethambutol (EMB)	15-25 mg/kg/day	Optic neuritis, peripheral neuritis, skin rash, gastrointestinal (GI) upset
Rifampin	10-20 mg/kg/day	Hepatitis, fever, GI upset, peripheral neuropathy
Streptomycin	15-20 mg/kg/day	Auditory toxicity, nephrotoxicity
Second-Line Drugs		
Para-aminosalicylic acid (PAS)	150 mg/kg/day	GI upset, hypersensitivity, hepatotoxicity
Ethionamide	750-1000 mg/day	GI upset, hepatotoxicity
Kanamycin	0.5-1 g/day	Auditory toxicity, nephrotoxicity
Capreomycin	1 g/day	Auditory toxicity, nephrotoxicity
Pyrazinamide (PZA)	15-30 mg/kg/day	Hyperuricemia, hepatotoxicity
Cycloserine	750 mg/day	Psychosis, personality change, skin rash

Tell patient taking Rifampin that it turns body secretions orangy red.

Teach patient importance of taking all medications for as long as prescribed (may be 9 to 24 months).

Stress importance of routine follow-up to monitor for toxic effects of medications.

Establish degree of respiratory isolation indicated.

Teach patient rationale for restrictions.

Teach patient importance of covering mouth when coughing or sneezing.

Teach patient proper technique for disposal of contaminated tissues and importance of good hand washing.

Follow strict hand-washing precautions.

Employ appropriate nursing measures to increase patient's comfort level: linen changes, tepid baths.

Encourage patient to allow for adequate rest until energy level improves.

Space and limit activities.

Assist patient with activities of daily living as required.

Explore ways to modify food patterns to meet nutritional needs within the constraints of persistent anorexia.

Encourage patient and family to verbalize feelings and concerns about diagnosis of tuberculosis.

Reinforce the importance of completing the full course of therapy to prevent the incidence of resistant organisms.

Teach family importance of ongoing screening for family members exposed to tuberculosis.

Teach patient facts about possibility of future recurrence and importance of being alert to symptoms.

Evaluation

Patient's energy level returns to normal; patient resumes normal occupational, social, and leisure roles.

Patient's mucus production decreases—lungs are clear to auscultation.

Patient and family accept tuberculosis diagnosis and make a positive commitment to compliance with treatment regimen.

Patient is knowledgeable about tuberculosis, its transmission, and the therapy regimen.

Patient's appetite returns; patient eats a balanced diet and maintains a stable body weight.

LUNG CANCER

Lung cancer is the leading cause of death from cancer in both men and women. Over 150,000 new cases are diagnosed each year, and only 13% of these individuals are expected to live 5 or more years after diagnosis. The mortality of the disease is dependent on the specific type of cancer cell involved and the location and size of the tumor at diagnosis. A history of cigarette smoking for 20 or more years is the prime risk factor, although chronic exposure to carcinogens such as asbestos is also important. Most individuals are over 50 years of age at the time of diagnosis.

PATHOPHYSIOLOGY

Most lung tumors arise in the bronchi. The patient may be asymptomatic or simply have a cough. As the tumor grows, hemoptysis, shortness of breath, and unilateral wheezing are common. When tumors grow peripherally, they may perforate the pleural space and create extrapulmonary symptoms such as pleural effusion or pain and friction rub. The incidence of weight loss and debility usually indicates the presence of metastases.

MEDICAL MANAGEMENT

Medical management is complicated by the difficulty in early diagnosis of the disease. Specific treatment is dependent on the tumor histology and disease staging. Treatment options include surgery with either local resection or wide excision, radiation, and chemotherapy, which may be used as primary, adjuvant, or palliative therapy. Table 9-3 describes the basic types of lung surgery.

NURSING MANAGEMENT

Assessment (Preoperative)
Subjective
Patient's complaints of the following:
Cough and dyspnea, pain associated with breathing
Hemoptysis
Fever and chills
Fatigue and weight loss

TABLE 9-3 Types of lung surgery

Procedure	Description
Pneumonectomy	Entire lung is removed. Phrenic nerve is crushed to allow diaphragm to rise and partially fill space. Drainage tubes are not used.
Lobectomy	One lobe of a lung is removed. Remaining tissue must be capable of overexpanding to fill up the space. Two chest tubes are used for postoperative drainage.
Segmental resection	One or more lung segments are removed. Procedure attempts to preserve maximum amount of functional lung tissue. Two chest tubes are used for postoperative drainage. Air leaks may delay reexpansion.
Wedge resection	Well-circumscribed diseased portion is removed without regard for segmental planes. Two chest tubes are used for postoperative drainage.

Smoking history: amount, duration, type

Occupational exposure to carcinogens

Understanding of diagnosis and proposed treatment

Objective

Visible shortness of breath

Unilateral wheezing

Positive chest x-ray and bronchoscopy findings

Cough productive of blood-tinged sputum

Nursing Diagnoses

Diagnoses will vary based on the acuity and stage of the disease. Common diagnoses include the following:

Ineffective airway clearance related to increased mucus production

Pain related to bone infiltration or postoperative incision pain

Potential for ineffective individual or family coping related to the diagnosis and prognosis of lung cancer

Knowledge deficit related to treatment modalities for lung cancer

Expected Outcomes

Patient will maintain a clear airway and optimum oxygen and carbon dioxide exchange.

Patient's pain will be adequately controlled.

Patient and family will be supported as they work through their feelings about both diagnosis and prognosis.

Patient will be knowledgeable about all aspects of the planned treatment protocol.

Nursing Interventions: Preoperative

Teach patient about diagnostic tests and proposed surgical procedure.

Teach patient about equipment to be used in care.

Prepare patient for intensive care unit (ICU) environment.

Teach patient abdominal breathing and proper coughing technique and their importance in the postoperative period.

Teach patient the range of motion exercises to be used for the arm and shoulder in the postoperative period.

Nursing Interventions: Postoperative

Monitor for patency of water seal drainage system (see Figure 9-2 and the box on the next page for basic principles).

Assist patient to a semi-Fowler's position once hemodynamic stability is reestablished.

Provide supplemental oxygen at 4 to 6 liters per minute.

Initiate coughing and deep breathing every hour for first 24 hours.

Assist patient to sit up and manually splint the chest wall.

Record vital signs frequently.

Monitor for signs of excessive bleeding.

Assess for signs of subcutaneous emphysema.

Provide adequate pain relief. *ALERT:* Patient cannot adequately cough and deep breathe without sufficient pain relief.

Keep fluid intake high to liquify secretions.

Ensure adequate room humidity.

Initiate range of motion exercises for arms and shoulders.

Encourage ambulation early in postoperative period.

Position patient on good side with operative side uppermost to promote reexpansion of lung tissue.

ALERT: Patients undergoing pneumonectomy are posi-

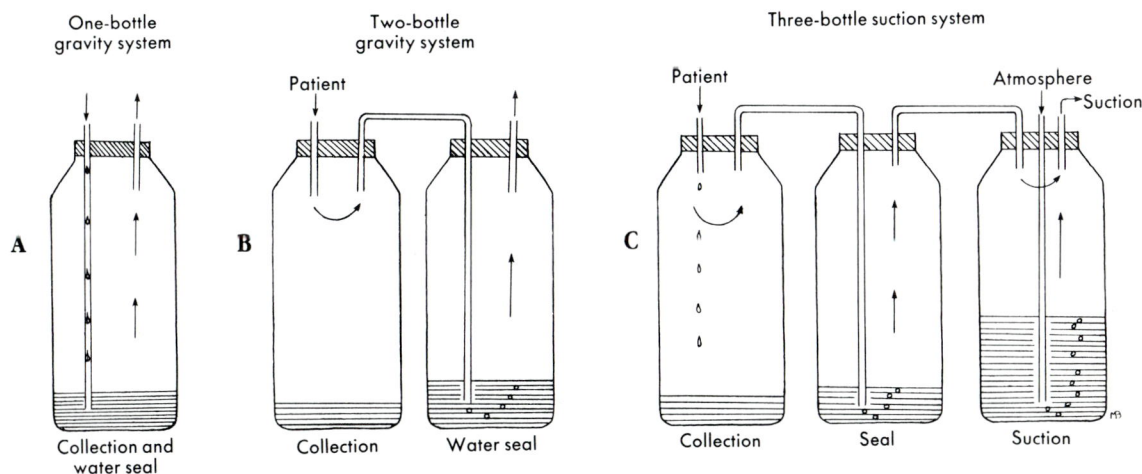

FIGURE 9-2 A, One-bottle drainage system. **B,** Two-bottle drainage system. **C,** three-bottle drainage system. (Illustrations from Hirsch J and Hannock L: Mosby's manual of clinical nursing procedures, St Louis, 1981, The CV Mosby Co.)

PRINCIPLES AND BASIC MANAGEMENT OF WATER SEAL CHEST DRAINAGE

WATER SEAL DRAINAGE

Purpose: to remove fluid and air from the intrapleural space to allow for lung reexpansion

Equipment: one-, two-, or three-bottle chest drainage setups or self-contained disposable units such as Pleurevac (see Figure 9-2)

One-bottle water seal—provides for gravity drainage of the chest; air and fluid are forced out on inspiration

Two-bottle water seal—allows for either the addition of suction to aid in chest reexpansion or a separate bottle for drainage collection

Three-bottle water seal—has separate bottles for water seal, drainage collection, and suction

Pleurevac—provides for three-bottle setup in one unit, but may be used as one- or two-bottle unit also

NURSING INTERVENTIONS

Mark level in drainage bottle regularly—check every hour while drainage is heavy.

Check all connections to ensure that they are taped securely.

Fasten tubing to bed to prevent dependent loops.

Check frequently to be sure water is oscillating in water seal. Tip of chest tube should be 1 to 2 cm below the water level. Water level rises during inspiration and falls on expiration.

If water is not moving, check system for obstruction, such as patient lying on tubes.

Water will cease oscillating when lung is fully reexpanded.

Milk or strip chest tubes only if specifically ordered. This procedure is controversial since it significantly increases negative pressure in the chest.

Keep two hemostats at bedside to clamp chest tube if bottle is accidentally broken. *ALERT:* Clamping is never done except in emergency or with direct order. It can cause tension pneumothorax. If emergency occurs, reconnect tubes with new sterile setup as quickly as possible.

Never lift chest tube bottles above level of the chest, which would allow fluid to be pulled into the chest.

If suction is in use, check regularly to ensure that it is at the prescribed level.

Ensure that side rails and bed will not come down on top of bottle.

Encourage patient to cough and deep breathe.

Ambulation may be encouraged with water seal drainage.

Monitor patient's status regularly—answer all questions about equipment and precautions.

---

tioned *only* on their back or operative side to protect the intact lung from fluid drainage.

Evaluation

Patient's lungs are clear to auscultation; remaining lung tissue provides for adequate oxygen and carbon dioxide exchange.

Patient's pain is controlled and patient ambulates and coughs effectively.

Patient and family openly discuss diagnosis and prognosis and make decisions about additional treatment.

Patient is knowledgeable about treatment regimen and understands the importance of follow-up care.

Patient recovers from surgery without complications.

CHEST TRAUMA

Injuries to the chest range from fractured ribs to major trauma of chest, heart, lungs, and blood vessels. Most patients receive initial treatment in the emergency room and then follow-up surgical repair. Nursing management basically parallels that of the patient with lung cancer treated with thoracic surgery and water seal drainage. The box on the next page describes the common forms of chest trauma.

B. CHRONIC AIRFLOW LIMITATION-OBSTRUCTIVE LUNG DISEASE

The category of diseases traditionally called chronic obstructive pulmonary disease (COPD) has been broadened to include diseases of airflow limitation in which actual obstruction is not the only or even the major pathophysiologic component. Common airflow limitation diseases are listed in the box on the next page. The term COPD remains in common use.

COPD is a major health problem in the United States, and both its morbidity and mortality are continuing to increase. An estimated 10 million persons suffer from COPD, and deaths caused by these diseases are increasing at an annual rate of nearly 9%. The diseases are more common among men, are predominant in middle to late middle age, and are related to cigarette smoking, environmental pollution, chronic infection, and hypersensitivity.

The following discussion is separated into the major categories of bronchitis, emphysema, and asthma for convenience. Most patients exhibit variable mixes of the predominant disease types. The major physiologic components of chronic airflow limitation include the following:

Chronic mucus hypersecretion
Airway hyperactivity
Changes in small airways
Destruction of the pulmonary parenchyma

CHRONIC BRONCHITIS

Chronic bronchitis is defined clinically by its symptoms: hypersecretion of mucus, and recurrent or chronic productive cough for at least 3 months per year for at least 2 years. Physiological signs are hypertrophy and hypersecretion of the bronchial mucus glands. It is caused by inhalation of chemical or physical irritants, or by bacte-

CHEST TRAUMA

BLUNT INJURIES

Trauma involving the chest cage without penetration of chest itself.
1. *Fractured ribs.* The most common type of injury. Damage normally involves fourth to eighth ribs, caused by blows or crushing injury.
   Unless rib fragments penetrate the pleura, treatment is conservative, with tight strapping of the affected side.
2. *Flail chest.* When ribs or the sternum are fractured in more than one place and a portion of the chest wall separates from the chest cage, the chest wall on the affected side becomes unstable. There is insufficient bony support to maintain bellows functions of lungs, and paradoxic breathing results.
   Treatment is by internal stabilization of the flail segment. A tracheostomy is performed and patient is placed on a volume-controlled ventilator to stabilize and control respiration until bone union occurs.

PENETRATING INJURIES

Trauma involving the chest cage and underlying structures.
1. *Pneumothorax.* Air enters the pleural space between the lung and chest wall, usually from an opening that exposes the intrapleural space to atmospheric pressure. Pneumothorax may also occur spontaneously or as the result of blunt injury. Atmospheric pressure builds up in pleural space, and lung on affected side collapses.
   Treatment involves reinflation of the lung with chest tube drainage
   Tension pneumothorax. Positive pressure buildup on the affected side may cause mediastinal shift, compressing the opposite lung and interfering with cardiac action. Becomes a life threatening emergency.
2. *Hemothorax.* Blood leaks into pleural space and collapses the affected lung; this often occurs with pneumothorax.
   Treatment involves drainage and reexpansion with chest tubes.
3. *Cardiac tamponade.* Blood accumulates in the pericardial sac, gradually compressing the heart and interfering with function.
   Treatment involves emergency pericardiocentesis to remove pressure, followed by appropriate surgical repair.

CHRONIC AIRFLOW LIMITATION DISORDERS

Chronic bronchitis	Parenchymal fibrosis or granulo-
Asthma	matosis
Emphysema	Pulmonary lymphangiomyomatosis
Bronchiolitis	Tracheal stenosis
Cystic fibrosis	

From Bates DV: Respiratory function in disease, ed 3, Philadelphia, 1989, WB Saunders.

rial and viral infections. Cigarette smoking is the most common irritant.

PATHOPHYSIOLOGY

Two pathologic changes typify chronic bronchitis: hypertrophy in the mucus-secreting glands and chronic inflammatory changes in the small airways. The excessive mucus and impaired ciliary movement increase susceptibility to infection. Increased airway resistance results from tissue changes in the bronchial walls, and the excessive mucus frequently triggers bronchospasm. As the disease progresses, altered O_2 and CO_2 exchange occurs, typically resulting in progressively severe hypoxemia, hypercapnia, and respiratory acidosis.

EMPHYSEMA

Emphysema is a disorder characterized by increased lung compliance, decreased diffusing capacity, and increased airway resistance. The cause is unknown, but imbalances in proteolytic enzymes and inhibitors have been widely investigated. The pathophysiologic changes apparently begin many years before the onset of overt symptoms. Symptoms typically appear during the fourth decade, with disease disability occurring between 50 and 60 years of age. The typical patient is a male with a long history of cigarette smoking.

PATHOPHYSIOLOGY

The diagnosis of emphysema is made from pulmonary function tests showing a decrease in airflow. Pathologically emphysema is characterized by destructive changes in the alveolar walls and enlargement of the air spaces distal to the terminal bronchioles. The proteolytic enzyme imbalance results in the gradual destruction of the connective tissue of the lungs. Enzyme inhibitor deficiencies may be inherited, and other imbalances are clearly related to the effects of cigarette smoke and other pollutants.

MEDICAL MANAGEMENT

The management of bronchitis and emphysema frequently overlap, and it is not known why some smokers develop predominantly one disease process rather than the other. Therapy is individualized on the basis of the patient's symptoms, blood gases, and pulmonary function study results. General supportive measures include nutrition, avoiding irritants, relaxation and breathing retraining, physical rehabilitation, oxygen therapy, and drug therapy, which may include bronchodilators, antibiotics, corticosteroids, and aerosol therapy.

The box on this page lists major symptoms associated with bronchitis and emphysema.

NURSING MANAGEMENT

Assessment

Subjective

History and severity of disease symptoms
Medications and treatments in use
Smoking history
Family history and occupational exposures
History of upper respiratory infections
Knowledge of disease process
Patient's and family's response to progressive disability
Patient's complaints of the following:
    Shortness of breath
    Sleep disturbances

SIGNS AND SYMPTOMS OF CHRONIC BRONCHITIS AND EMPHYSEMA

CHRONIC BRONCHITIS

Early
    Productive AM cough
Later
    Noticeable shortness of breath and use of accessory muscles
    Cyanosis common
    Bloated appearance, distended neck veins
Advanced disease
    Frequent complications:
        Right-sided congestive heart failure
        Cor pulmonale
        Respiratory failure
Blood gases
    Low resting Po_2
    Elevated Pco_2

EMPHYSEMA

Early
    Dyspnea on exertion
Later
    Severe dyspnea—acute distress, use of accessory muscles
    Increased A-P chest diameter
    Ruddy color—cyanosis uncommon
Advanced disease
    Severe hypercapnia
    Cor pulmonale and respiratory failure
Blood gases
    Resting Po_2 normal—falls with activity
    Normal Pco_2 until disease is advanced

Chronic cough
Anorexia
Fatigue
Perception of general health and fitness

Objective

Pulmonary inspection and auscultation
Forward leaning posture
Use of pursed lip breathing, prolonged exhalation
Dyspnea at rest or with speech or exercise
Use of accessory muscles in respiration
Diminished chest excursion
Increased anteroposterior (A-P) chest diameter
Decreased breath sounds—crackles and rhonchi
Presence and degree of cyanosis
Productive cough—amount and appearance of sputum
Vital signs—presence of tachycardia and tachypnea
Signs of right sided congestive heart failure, edema
Normal or decreased lung volumes
Blood gases—hypoxemia, hypercapnia, respiratory acidosis

Nursing Diagnoses

Diagnoses depend on the stage and severity of the disease. Common diagnoses include the following:

Activity intolerance related to shortness of breath and imbalance between tissue oxygen supply and demand
Ineffective airway clearance related to excessive mucus production and decreased expiratory force
Impaired gas exchange related to destructive changes in the alveolar membrane
Knowledge deficit related to measures to increase general health status and lessen symptoms
Altered nutrition: less than body requirements, related to severe dyspnea and fatigue
Ineffective breathing pattern related to airway changes and fatigue

Expected Outcomes

Patient will have sufficient energy to remain independent in the activities of daily living.
Patient will adequately clear the airway with appropriate use of medications and coughing and deep breathing exercises.
Patient will demonstrate improved ventilation and oxygenation.
Patient will be knowledgeable about disease process, prescribed medications, and measures to delay disease progression.
Patient will maintain an adequate nutritional intake and a stable weight.
Patient will utilize an effective breathing pattern.

Nursing Interventions: General Health

Teach patient about disease progression and home management.

Assist patient and family members to give up smoking.

Discuss modification of life-style and home environment to reduce exposure to pollutants.

OXYGEN THERAPY

GENERAL CONSIDERATIONS

Oxygen therapy is drying and irritating to mucous membranes.

High-dose oxygen must be adequately humidified and nebulized.

Humidification and delivery equipment must be changed frequently to prevent or contain bacterial growth.

No-smoking regulations must be posted and enforced.

Flow rates should be monitored frequently, especially for COPD patients.

METHODS OF ADMINISTRATION

Low-flow systems

Oxygen provided mixes with the room air, which alters the actual percentage received.
1. Nasal prongs or cannula
    Safe, simple, and well tolerated
    Difficult to position properly, easily dislodged
    Can deliver 1 to 6 liters (24% to 45%)
    Concentration depends on patient's breathing pattern
2. Simple face mask
    Delivers oxygen through an entry port
    Concentration varies with breathing pattern
    Efficient for rapid short-term delivery
    Poorly tolerated as tight seal is needed around mouth
3. Partial rebreather mask
    Uses a face mask and reservoir bag
    Mixes expired air from the lung's dead space with oxygen entering the reservoir to increase the overall concentration of oxygen
    Poorly tolerated because of tight fit around mouth
4. Transtracheal catheter
    Catheter is inserted directly into the trachea between the tracheal cartilage
    Does not interfere with eating or talking
    Delivers oxygen throughout the respiratory cycle

High-flow systems

Delivers all of the patient's inspired air. Concentration of oxygen is not affected by changes in respiratory pattern.
1. Nonrebreather mask
    Mask and reservoir are separated by a one-way valve
    Can delivery up to 100% oxygen
    High humidity is not possible
    Mask is tight and uncomfortable
2. Venturi mask
    Oxygen passes through a restricted port that increases the velocity of the gas flow
    High flow rate makes accuracy of oxygen delivery high
    Mask is poorly tolerated

Teach patient measures to avoid infection. Minimize contacts with crowds and young children.

Patient should contact physician promptly if changes occur in the color or amount of the sputum.

Patient should receive an annual flu vaccine and be immunized against pneumonia.

Avoid extremes of hot and cold. Ensure adequate humidity in winter.

Teach patient importance of balanced, nutritious diet and maintaining normal weight.
    Use small, frequent feedings if anorexic.
    Ensure protein adequacy but limit the amount of carbohydrates as they produce CO_2 in the body.

Ensure adequate fluid intake.

Reinforce the importance of maintaining or increasing activity level. Explore the availability of a structured rehabilitation program.

Avoid bed rest at all costs.

Nursing Interventions: Medications

Administer medications as prescribed:
    Methylxanthines—aminophylline or theophylline
    Sympathomimetics—isoproterenol, terbutaline, isoetharine
    Corticosteroids—for short-course acute symptom control

Teach patient about prescribed medications and side effects.

Nursing Interventions: Respiratory Therapy

Administer and teach patient proper use of aerosol therapy.
    Teach use of humidifiers and nebulizers.
    Teach proper use of hand-held inhalators.

Administer oxygen if prescribed (see box on this page).

Encourage patient to use O_2 continuously for best results

ALERT: Only low-flow oxygen is used (1 to 2 L) because chronic carbon dioxide retention causes decreased Po_2 to be the primary respiratory drive and this decreased Po_2 level cannot be removed.

Monitor for signs of hypoxemia and hypercapnea:
    Headache and irritability
    Confusion
    Increasing somnolence

Nursing Interventions: Exercise

Teach patient progressive relaxation exercises.

Assist patient to adjust breathing pattern by doing the following:
    Use pursed lips breathing to prolong exhalation and stabilize airway.
    Practice diaphragmatic or abdominal breathing.
    Exhale with activity.
    Assume leaning forward posture for rest.

Assist patient with muscle reconditioning as tolerated.

Teach patient and family how to do postural drainage and chest physiotherapy (see Figure 9-3 and box on next page).

Reinforce principles of effective deep breathing and coughing. Assist patient to consciously slow breathing rate, inhaling over 5 seconds and exhaling over 10 seconds.

Evaluation

Patient's activity level increases with participation in a pulmonary rehabilitation program.

Patient is able to fully clear airway as needed.

Patient avoids situations that interfere with alveolar gas exchange, and improves alveolar exchange through appropriate exercises.

Patient is knowledgeable about disease and can discuss prescribed medications and correctly demonstrate prescribed treatments.

Patient can discuss safe use of oxygen therapy in the home.

Patient maintains a stable weight and adequate nutrient intake.

Patient demonstrates an effective breathing pattern and uses breathing exercises during activity and exertion.

ASTHMA

Asthma is known to affect 9.6 million people in the United States, two thirds of whom are adults. The disease is characterized by an increased responsiveness of the trachea and bronchi to various stimuli that cause airway narrowing. Asthma has been traditionally classi-

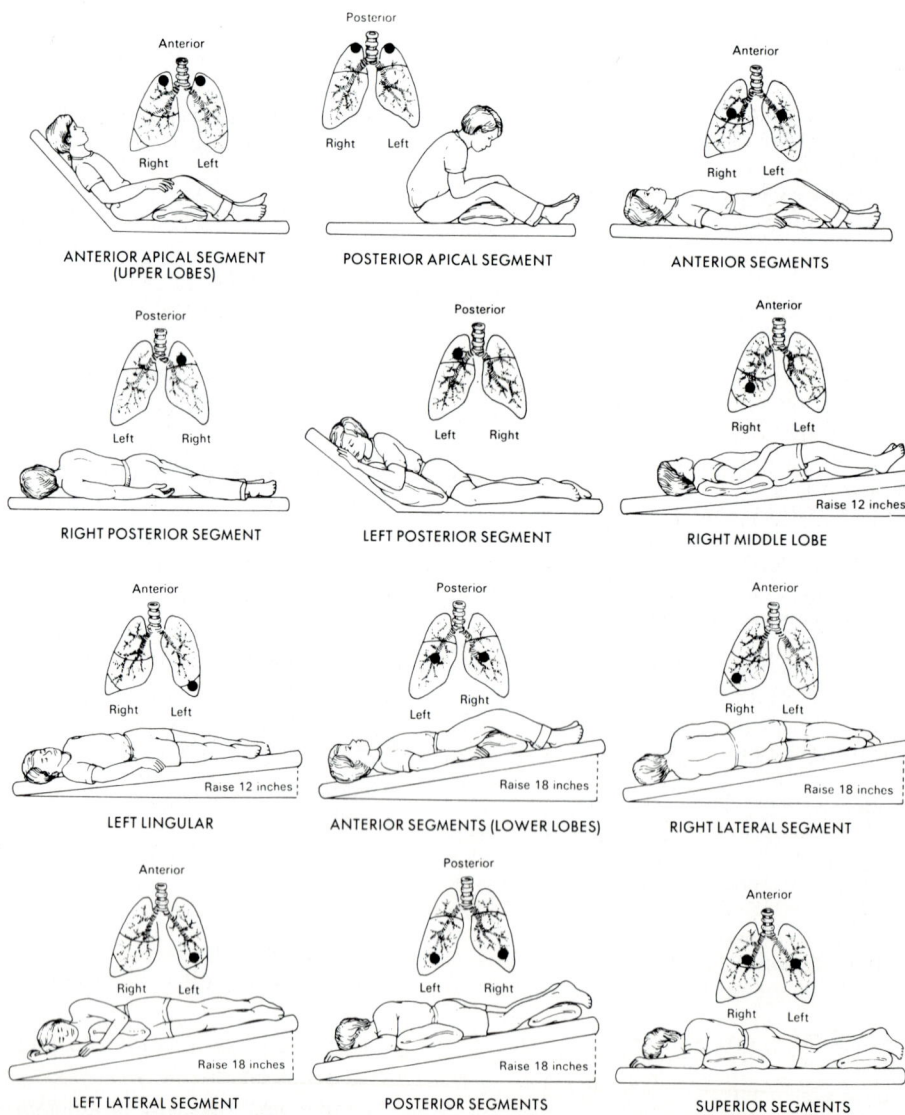

FIGURE 9-3 Correct positions for postural drainage. (From Hirsch J and Hannock L: Mosby's manual of clinical nursing procedures, St Louis, 1981, The CV Mosby Co.)

CHEST PHYSIOTHERAPY—CLAPPING AND VIBRATION

PURPOSE

To combine the force of gravity with natural ciliary activity of the small bronchial airways to move secretions upward toward the main bronchi and the trachea.
Usually combined with postural drainage (see Figure 9-3 for positions).

PROCEDURE

Help patient assume appropriate position for lung segment to be drained.
Clap over area with cupped hands for approximately 1 minute to loosen secretions and stimulate coughing.
At conclusion of clapping, instruct patient to breathe deeply; apply vibrating pressure during the expiratory phase.
Have patient cough effectively to clear the airway.
Repeat as needed and include all appropriate positions.

GENERAL INFORMATION

Modify desired positions as needed to increase patient tolerance.
Clapping is not done over bare skin—provide cloth barrier.
Time treatments for maximal benefit:
   Soon after arising
   At bedtime
   More often as prescribed and tolerated
   Complete procedure at least 1 hour before meals
Provide rest and mouth care after procedures.
Auscultate lungs before and after treatment to assess effectiveness.
Humidity and bronchodilators may be given 15 to 20 minutes before treatment.

fied as immunologic (allergic, extrinsic), nonimmunologic (intrinsic), and mixed. Clinically, however, most people fall into the mixed category, limiting the usefulness of the classification. The current trend is to classify the disorder on the basis of precipitating factors and individual response patterns. Common precipitating factors are listed in the box on this page.

PATHOPHYSIOLOGY

An asthmatic attack is the result of several physiologic alterations. Immunologic asthma is the result of an antigen-antibody reaction in which chemical mediators are released and cause three major reactions:

1. Constriction of large and small airway smooth muscles, resulting in bronchospasm
2. Increased capillary permeability that results in mucosal edema
3. Increased mucus gland secretion and production

The patient then struggles to breathe through a narrowed airway that is in spasm. Increased airway resistance and compliance combined with an impaired mucociliary function can alter the lung's ability to maintain normal oxygen and carbon dioxide exchange. The airway is basically asymptomatic between attacks and exhibits no structural damage.

MEDICAL MANAGEMENT

The treatment plan attempts to provide symptomatic relief from attacks, control specific causative factors, and promote optimum health. The chief aim of drug therapy is to provide the patient immediate and ongoing bronchial relaxation. Oxygen therapy is used as needed during acute attacks. Other medical efforts are aimed at identifying and controlling precipitating factors in the environment.

NURSING MANAGEMENT

Assessment
  Subjective
  History of disease and its treatment
  History of onset of attack
  Factors that precipitate attack
    Allergy history
  Medications in use and patient's knowledge of them and their correct usage
  Other self-care methods used to control symptoms
  Patient's complaints of the following:
    Shortness of breath
    Severe anxiety
    Feeling of suffocation

COMMON PRECIPITATING FACTORS OF ASTHMA

Environmental factors:
  Changes in air temperature or humidity
  Smoke or irritating fumes
  Strong odors
  Pollutants
Aspirin ingestion (prostaglandin inhibitor)
Exercise
Emotional stress
Infection (usually viral)

Objective

Presence of inspiratory wheezing, prolonged expiration, rhonchi

Productive or nonproductive cough

Presence and severity of dyspnea, tachycardia, and tachypnea

Apparent respiratory distress
  Use of accessory muscles to breathe
  Forward positioning to breathe

Transient cyanosis, diaphoresis

Blood gases—early changes are mild hypoxemia and respiratory alkalosis; late effects are severe hypoxemia and acidosis

Nursing Diagnoses

Diagnoses commonly include the following:

  Anxiety related to inability to effectively move air in lungs

  Ineffective airway clearance related to excess mucus production in lungs

  Impaired gas exchange related to bronchospasm and ventilation perfusion imbalance

  Knowledge deficit related to disease mechanism and optimum treatment

Expected Outcomes

Patient's anxiety will decrease as a result of improved disease control.

Patient will successfully employ treatment measures to maintain a clear airway.

Patient will experience improved gas exchange in the lungs.

Patient will be knowledgeable concerning disease and proposed treatment plan.

Nursing Interventions: Acute Attack

Establish calm environment; reassure patient. Do not leave patient alone.

Position patient in high Fowler's position.

Encourage relaxation and controlled breathing.

Monitor vital signs and respiratory status regularly.

Auscultate lungs.
  Observe for cyanosis.

Administer humidified oxygen as ordered.

Administer bronchodilators as ordered.

Monitor IV rates carefully.

Monitor patient for medication's side effects: tachycardia, palpitations, sweating.

Encourage fluids by mouth.

Assist patient to cough effectively. Administer chest physiotherapy if coughing is ineffective.

Promote comfort measures for diaphoretic patient.

Nursing Interventions: Chronic Management

Teach patient to avoid potential allergens and precipitating factors if possible, such as smoking, exertion, cold air, dust.

Teach patient to seek prompt treatment of upper respiratory tract infections.

Teach patient breathing exercises and use of chest physiotherapy if appropriate.

Teach patient to maintain optimum nutrition, adequate rest, and sufficient fluids.

Teach patient about medications and their safe use. Teach patient to use inhaled bronchodilators before planned exercise.

Teach patient relaxation and stress management techniques.

Encourage patient to maintain a symptom diary to identify patterns.

Evaluation

Patient is in knowledgeable control of disease process, experiences infrequent attacks, seeks appropriate care promptly.

Patient is able to cough effectively and maintain a clear airway to auscultation.

Patient has adequate gas exchange in lungs and does not experience hypoxemia or hypercapnia.

Patient is knowledgeable about disease process and can discuss the purpose and side effects of prescribed medications and treatments.

NURSING CARE PLAN

CHRONIC OBSTRUCTIVE PULMONARY DISEASE

Nursing Diagnoses	Expected Patient Outcomes	Nursing Interventions
Ineffective airway clearance related to increased mucus production and decreased expiratory force	Patient is able to clear the airway effectively.	1. Assess breath sounds. 2. Give prescribed bronchodilators; dilute in water if given by aerosol. 3. Teach patient to use aerosol correctly and to use only prescribed number of inhalations (excess use may result in overdosage with side effects). 4. Provide fluid intake of 2000 to 2500 ml/day to thin secretions (unless contraindicated, such as with cor pulmonale). 5. Avoid giving patient fluids that are very hot or cold (may cause bronchospasm or increased secretions). 6. Administer postural drainage and clapping as prescribed. 7. Keep room air humid (30% to 50%) and free of inhalant irritants (such as smoke). 8. Avoid abrupt changes in temperature and use air conditioning as appropriate. Patient should stay indoors when pollution levels are high.
Impaired gas exchange related to a decrease in effective lung surface area	Patient's hypoxemia gradually resolves.	1. Assess respiratory status. 2. Provide prescribed low-flow oxygen. 3. Provide breathing retraining: pursed lip breathing, leaning forward position for exhalation, abdominal breathing techniques, inhalation-exhalation exercises, and exhalation with exertion. 4. Teach relaxation techniques as appropriate (relaxation exercises, meditation).
Activity intolerance related to dyspnea and peripheral tissue hypoxia	Patient will have sufficient energy to maintain independence in the activities of daily living.	1. Provide additional time to carry out the activities of daily living. 2. Provide for rest periods. 3. Teach patient to use controlled breathing techniques and to time activity with exhalation. 4. Encourage the patient to follow a progressive muscle conditioning and exercise program. 5. Teach patient to avoid bed rest and immobility.
Altered nutrition: less than body requirements, related to severe dyspnea and the effort of breathing	Patient ingests required nutrients and maintains a stable body weight.	1. Monitor nutrient intake daily and weigh weekly. 2. Provide meals at intervals that promote increased intake; several small meals may be better tolerated. 3. Give high-protein supplementary feedings. 4. Avoid heavy meals and foods that patient perceives as gas producing. Avoid high carbohydrate intake. 5. Avoid very hot or cold foods. 6. Provide mouth care prior to eating if secretions are excessive. 7. Provide comfortable, pleasant environment and time for eating to decrease fatigue and encourage increased intake. 8. Encourage patient to use supplemental O_2 during meals if ordered.

Continued.

CHRONIC OBSTRUCTIVE PULMONARY DISEASE—cont'd

Nursing Diagnoses	Expected Patient Outcomes	Nursing Interventions
Potential for ineffective individual coping related to the limitations of chronic disease	Patient will make a positive adjustment to disease restrictions.	1. Give patient opportunities to express concerns about limitations imposed by COPD. 2. Provide rationale for necessary activities and information about positive effects. 3. Discuss with family/friends the need for patient to maintain role relationships and to feel worthwhile. 4. Assist patient to identify personal strengths. 5. Provide information about community resources, such as group meetings with other persons with COPD.
Knowledge deficit related to measures to increase general health status and disease management	Patient is knowledgeable about the therapeutic regimen and measures to increase general health.	1. Teach patient the following: a. Nature of COPD and need to follow prescribed therapy and activities. b. Home medication and treatment programs. c. Home exercise program. d. Avoidance of respiratory irritants and infections. e. Signs requiring medical attention. f. Professional and community resources. g. Importance of a "smoke-free" home environment.
Potential for infection related to increased secretions and decreased motility in lungs	Patient does not develop infection.	1. Teach patient the following: a. To avoid large crowds b. To avoid contact with persons with respiratory infections c. To contact physician if quantity or color of sputum changes d. To obtain annual flu shots and be immunized against pneumonia

RESPIRATORY INSUFFICIENCY AND FAILURE

Respiratory *insufficiency* occurs when the exchange of oxygen and carbon dioxide is inadequate to meet body needs during normal activities. It is usually accompanied by dyspnea. *Failure* occurs when the exchange of oxygen and carbon dioxide is inadequate to meet body needs at rest and hypoxemia, hypercapnea, and acidosis exceed predetermined levels.

These conditions may occur as a result of any of the disorders discussed in the chapter as well as a variety of other acute or chronic, surgical, neurologic, and neuromuscular disorders. Diagnosis is made from blood gas results, pulmonary function testing, and the patient's clinical status. The following criteria are used:

Po_2 <50-60 mm Hg on room air
Pco_2 >45-50 mm Hg
pH ≤7.35
　Vital capacity <15 ml/kg
　Respiratory rate >30/min or <8/min

In acute failure there is often a marked decrease in vital capacity. The signs and symptoms of failure often depend more on the rate of change than on absolute values since in patients with COPD the basic imbalances are present chronically.

PATHOPHYSIOLOGY

Regardless of the cause, without adequate ventilation and gas exchange, the arterial Po_2 falls and body cells become hypoxic. Accumulating CO_2 alters the pH and the patient becomes acidotic. Clinical manifestations are related to either the elevated CO_2 or decreasing oxygen levels.

MEDICAL MANAGEMENT

Therapy often begins with identifying the underlying disease state and removing or decreasing the cause if possible. Specific interventions are based on the degree of severity and are aimed at improving oxygenation and ventilation. Supplemental oxygen is given at the lowest effective rate. The airway is kept clear through positioning, suctioning, and physiotherapy. Mechanical ventilation may be necessary to support ventilatory effort.

NURSING MANAGEMENT

Assessment

Subjective
History of respiratory problems or associated disorders
Patient's complaints of the following:
　Recent change in respiratory status
　Severe fatigue
　Increased shortness of breath
　Headache

Objective
Quality of ventilatory effort:
　Respiratory rate and rhythm
　Breath sounds
　Use of accessory muscles
Vital signs—tachycardia and tachypnea
Signs of cyanosis in mucous membranes, lips, ear lobes
Position used for breathing
Diaphoresis; cool, clammy skin
Drowsiness, restlessness, mood fluctuation, general mental status
Visible dyspnea—inability to complete sentences because of shortness of breath

Nursing Diagnoses
Common diagnoses include the following:
　Activity intolerance related to the fatigue of tissue hypoxia
　Ineffective airway clearance related to excess mucus or fluids or neuromuscular weakness
　Impaired gas exchange related to obstructive or restrictive lung disorders
　Altered tissue perfusion related to hypoxemia

Expected Outcomes
Patient's energy level will increase with improved oxygenation of tissues.
Patient will maintain a clear open airway through effective coughing or suctioning.
Patient will experience improved oxygen and carbon dioxide exchange in the lung.
Patient will have improved perfusion to body organs and tissues.

Nursing Interventions
Monitor patient carefully for subtle changes in oxygenation status. Monitor respiratory effort.
Administer humidified oxygen as prescribed. Use lowest concentration of oxygen that will maintain Po_2.
　Monitor COPD patient for carbon dioxide narcosis.
　Help patient tolerate mask delivery systems if needed.
Monitor vital signs, lung sounds, and blood gases.
Keep airway open.
　Suction as necessary.
　Position patient comfortably in upright position.
　Coach patient to slow and control rate of breathing.
　Administer ultrasonic mist if prescribed.
　Perform postural drainage and chest physiotherapy.
　Administer intermittent positive pressure breathing (IPPB) if prescribed.
Manage artificial airway and volume ventilator if in use.
Keep patient calm and at rest to decrease oxygen needs.
Maintain neutral environmental temperature.
Reassure patient and control anxiety.

Explain all procedures and treatments.

Maintain adequate hydration.

Monitor IV fluids.

Keep accurate intake and output records.

Facilitate communication for intubated patient or patient with a tracheostomy.

Keep call bell close—answer promptly.

Provide pad and pencil or magic slate.

Evaluation

Patient progressively resumes responsibility for self-care.

Patient's airway is clear to auscultation.

Patient's respirations are unlabored; blood gases are within normal limits.

Patient exhibits no signs of cyanosis and is mentally alert and aware.

ADULT RESPIRATORY DISTRESS SYNDROME

Adult respiratory distress syndrome (ARDS) is an often fatal syndrome associated with shock, trauma, overdose of drugs, inhaled substances, and pulmonary infections. It is characterized by severe dyspnea, hypoxemia, and

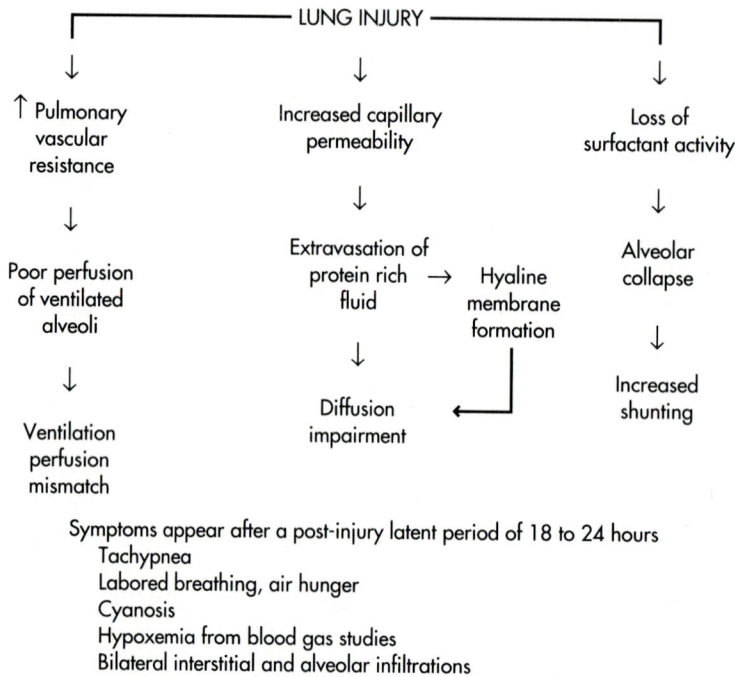

FIGURE 9-4 Pathophysiology of adult respiratory distress syndrome.

TABLE 9-4 Types of mechanical ventilators

Types		Basic Function Mode
Positive pressure ventilator		Types of positive pressure ventilators are based on how inspiratory phase is ended.
Pressure-cycled ventilator	(Require intubation)	Inspiration ends at a preset pressure limit; time and volume are variable.
Time-cycled ventilator		Inspiration is preset for a given time interval; volume and pressure are variable.
Volume-cycled ventilator		Preset volume of air is delivered. Time and pressure are variable. However, volume-cycled ventilators often have pressure- and time-cycled capacities.
Negative pressure ventilator (intubation not required)		Thorax, at least, is encapsulated. When ventilator expands, it creates negative pressure by pulling the thorax outward. Air rushes into the airways because of the pressure gradient created.
High-frequency ventilation (requires intubation)		System is still under clinical investigation. There are several variants of this system. All high-frequency ventilators use high respiratory rates to deliver small tidal volumes at low pressures.

From Phipps WJ, Long BC, and Woods NF: Medical-surgical nursing: concepts and clinical practice, ed 4, St Louis, 1990, Mosby–Year Book, Inc.

diffuse bilateral pulmonary infiltrations. Figure 9-4 describes the pathophysiologic process of ARDS.

Patients with ARDS are critically ill. They are treated with mechanical ventilatory support (see Table 9-4) and frequently require the addition of positive end expiratory pressure (PEEP) to support ventilation. Other interventions are similar to those used for the patient in respiratory failure.

BIBLIOGRAPHY

Barry MA and others: Tuberculosis infection in urban adolescents: results of a school based testing program, Am J Public Health **80:**439-441, 1990.

Bradley RB: Adult respiratory distress syndrome, Focus Crit Care **14:**48-59, 1989.

Carroll PL: Lowering the risks of endotracheal suctioning, Nursing 88 **18**(15):46-50, 1988.

Caruthers DD: Infectious pneumonia in the elderly, Am J Nurs **90:**56-60, 1990.

Chisholm S and others: Duck bill prosthesis: words of hope for the laryngectomy patient, Nursing 86 **16**(3):29-31, 1986.

Cornell C: Tuberculosis in hospital employees, Am J Nurs **88:**484-486, 1988.

Engelking C: Lung cancer, Am J Nurs **87:**1434-1440, 1987.

Feinstein D: What to teach the patient who's had a total laryngectomy, RN **50**(4):53-57, 1987.

Fuchs CP: Caring for ventilator patients, Nursing 86 **16**(6):34-39, 1986.

Griffin CW and others: Learning to swallow again, Am J Nurs 87:314-315, 1987.

Hanley MV and Tyler ML: Ineffective airway clearance related to airway infection, Nurs Clin North Am **22:**135-149, 1987.

Harris LL and Kraege J: After T-E puncture: relearning to speak, Am J Nurs **86:**55-58, 1986.

Hoffman LA and Maskiewicz RC: The specifics of suctioning, Am J Nurs **87:**44-53, 1987.

Johnson A: The elderly and COPD, J Gerontol Nurs **14:**20-24, 1988.

Larson J and Kim MJ: Ineffective breathing pattern related to respiratory muscle fatigue, Nurs Clin North Am **22:**207-224, 1987.

Madsen LA: Tuberculosis today, RN **53**(3):44-51, 1990.

McNaull FW: Lung cancer: What are the odds?, Am J Nurs **87:**1430-1432, 1987.

Shekelton ME: Coping with chronic respiratory difficulty, Nurs Clin North Am **22:**569-581, 1987.

Vasbinder-Dillon D: Understanding mechanical ventilation, Crit Care Nurse **8**(7):42-56, 1988.

Witta K and others: Myths and facts about mechanical ventilation, Nursing **18:**25, 1988.

CHAPTER 10

Disorders of the Gastrointestinal System

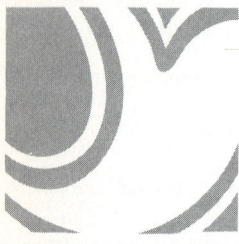

Problems involving the gastrointestinal (GI) system include a wide variety of common and uncommon, acute and chronic disorders. Ingestion and digestion are essential to health and survival and are closely linked to enjoyment of life. Because they are also closely linked with cultural habits and values, disorders involving the GI tract present challenging situations for medical and nursing management.

Disorders presented in this chapter include problems of both the upper and lower gastrointestinal tract, and encompass infections, obstructions, and tumors, as well as structural alterations. Figure 10-1 shows the anatomical structure of the digestive system.

DISORDERS OF THE UPPER GASTROINTESTINAL TRACT

ORAL CANCER

Cancers involving the lips, oral cavity, and the tongue represent 4% of all cancers in men and 2% of all cancers in women. The incidence is higher among older individuals with a history of both heavy smoking and alcohol consumption. The mortality rate for cancer of the tongue and floor of the mouth is high because of the vascularity and extensive lymph drainage of the area.

PATHOPHYSIOLOGY

Most forms of oral cancer are basically asymptomatic. Premalignant lesions such as leukoplakia (white patches on the tongue or mucosa) may become cancerous, but a small ulcer or growth is often the only sign. Parotid tumors often present as painless lumps that can be easily palpated. They cause minimal interference, if any, with function in early stages.

MEDICAL MANAGEMENT

Treatment depends on the location and staging of the tumor. Most oral cancers are treated initially with surgery, external radiation, or the implant of radioactive seeds or needles. The treatment for advanced disease is basically palliative. Surgery usually includes wide excision that significantly interferes with major oral functions such as eating and speaking. Prosthetic reconstruction to gradually restore appearance and function is a common adjunct to this type of surgery.

NURSING MANAGEMENT

Assessment

Subjective

History of symptoms and knowledge of disease process

History of smoking and alcohol use

Patient's understanding of proposed surgery or treatment plan, including the following:

　Extent of tissue destruction

　Degree of interference with communication

　Loss of or interference with eating function

　Planned method for nutrition postoperatively

Patient's stage of grief, attitude about altered body image

Objective

Condition of mouth

Presence of leukoplakia, ulcerated lesion, or palpable lump

General health and nutritional status

Nursing Diagnoses

Diagnoses will depend on the nature and extent of proposed treatment but commonly include:

Impaired verbal communication related to destruction of structures essential for speech

Potential for ineffective individual coping related to alterations in eating, swallowing, and speaking functions

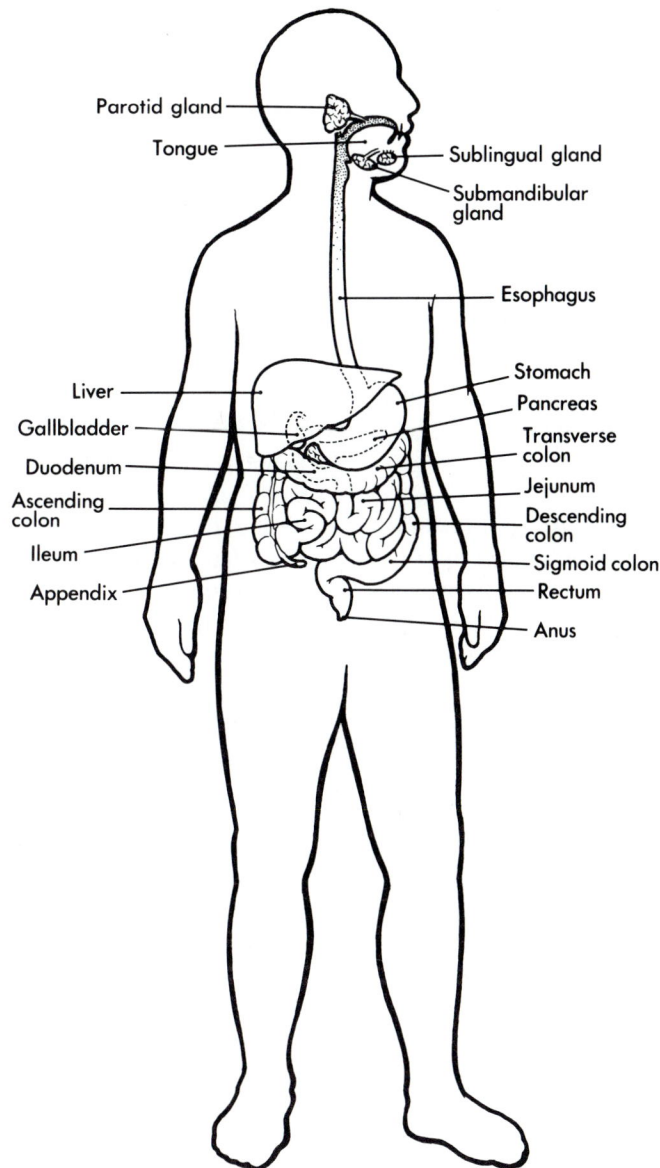

FIGURE 10-1 Digestive system.

Altered nutrition: less than body requirements, related to structural alterations in mouth

Body image disturbance related to visible structural changes in mouth and throat

Altered oral mucous membranes related to surgical wounds or effects of radiation and chemotherapy

Knowledge deficit related to techniques of mouth care and feeding techniques after surgery

Expected Outcomes

Patient will successfully communicate with staff and family and begin vocal therapy as healing progresses.

Patient will cope effectively with diagnosis and treatment and demonstrate an optimistic attitude toward the future.

Patient will ingest all needed fluid and nutrients and maintain a stable weight.

Patient will incorporate body changes into an altered but positive body image.

Patient's mouth and neck will heal without complications or infection.

Patient will be knowledgeable about self-care skills necessary to accomplish feeding and mouth care.

Nursing Interventions: Preoperative

Teach patient about proposed surgery and its outcomes. Be specific and honest about the resulting changes in appearance and function.

Clarify misconceptions.

Ensure that patient's perceptions are accurate.

Encourage patient and family to verbalize their feelings and concerns about body changes. Support appropriate grieving.

Explain expected postoperative measures such as suctioning, nasogastric tube, drains.

Begin prescribed preoperative mouth preparation.

Nursing Interventions: Postoperative

Position patient to maintain airway and promote drainage of secretions from the mouth—usually in side-lying and then semi-Fowler's position when reactive.

Assist patient to remove saliva from mouth with suction, gauze wick, or emesis basin. Provide constant monitoring if patient cannot swallow.

Maintain patency of drainage tubes.

Assess for facial nerve damage or return of function—ask patient to raise eyebrows, frown, pucker lips.

Provide frequent oral hygiene care with mouth irrigations. Avoid use of toothbrush.

Use saline, water, or dilute hydrogen peroxide and sterile equipment.

Teach patient technique for oral hygiene. Encourage patient participation as able.

Provide nutrition through a liquid diet administered with a catheter, tube, or syringe.

Teach patient technique for feeding. Place syringe or spoon on back of tongue to facilitate swallowing. Avoid use of fork.

Advance patient to soft foods as healing progresses.

Provide privacy during feeding if patient prefers.

Teach patient to rinse mouth carefully after meals.

Establish effective communication with patient.

Use magic slate or pad and pencil.

Use yes or no questions initially.

Initiate speech retraining when healing occurs.

Teach patient to use throat and not lips for speech clarity.

Encourage patient to speak slowly.

Reassure patient that speech is possible as long as vocal cords are intact.

Listen carefully and validate messages.

Refer to speech therapy for retraining.

See Chapter 2 for appropriate interventions for patients receiving external or internal radiotherapy.

ALERT: Oral irradiation causes inflammation and tissue sloughing of mucous membranes, bad odor, and dry mouth. Meticulous oral hygiene and diet modifications are mandatory.

Put patient and family in contact with community agencies that can provide assistance.

Encourage patient to express feelings about surgery in order to reach grief resolution.

Encourage family to include patient in family gatherings and social events to foster acceptance of changed appearance.

Evaluation

Patient is able to communicate needs accurately and maintains social interaction with family and friends.

Patient's surgical incisions heal without complications.

Patient demonstrates correct technique for mouth and incisional care and feeds self independently.

Patient ingests balanced nutrients and maintains a stable weight.

Patient demonstrates active coping and resumes familial roles.

Patient communicates gradual acceptance of body changes and resumes social and occupational roles.

ESOPHAGEAL DISORDERS

Esophageal disorders are relatively uncommon but include problems involving acid reflux, difficulty in swallowing, tumors, and structural disorders. Esophageal reflux occurs fairly commonly but is usually referred to by the patient as simple heartburn. Table 10-1 summarizes some of the basic esophageal disorders and their treatment.

PEPTIC ULCER DISEASE

Peptic ulcer is a common disorder affecting 5 to 10% of the adult population, men more often than women. It is frequently a chronic disease characterized by periodic reoccurrences. Duodenal ulcers occur about four times more frequently than gastric ulcers.

The risk and precipitating factors for peptic ulcers remain unclear despite significant research. Smoking and hereditary factors are clearly linked, as are ulcerogenic drugs such as aspirin, nonsteroidal antiinflammatory drugs (NSAIDs), and corticosteroids. The role of life stress remains unclear.

PATHOPHYSIOLOGY

A peptic ulcer is an ulceration involving the mucosa and deeper structures of the distal esophagus, stomach, or duodenum. Duodenal ulcers are related to an increase in acid secretion, particularly between meals. Patients also demonstrate a markedly increased rate of gastric emptying that results in an increased amount of acid content entering the duodenum.

Gastric ulcers are not directly related to acid secretion or rate of gastric emptying. Ulceration appears to occur from decreased resistance of mucosa to acid. Infection by *Campylobacter pylori* bacteria is also being carefully investigated as a potential cause of the mucosal breakdown.

MEDICAL MANAGEMENT

Drug therapy is the basis of medical intervention. Commonly used drugs are summarized in Table 10-2. Anticholinergics used to be a basic component of drug therapy but are rarely used anymore. There is no evidence that modifying the diet accelerates the healing of un-

TABLE 10-1 Esophageal disorders

Disorder	Description	Treatment
Achalasia (cardiospasm)	Absence of peristalsis in esophagus Failure of esophageal sphincter to relax after swallowing Esophagus dilates above the constriction Dysphagia is major symptom	Forceful dilation of the constricted sphincter Peristalsis is not restored
Esophageal diverticula	Bulging of esophageal mucosa through weakened portion of muscular layer Portions of ingested food may enter diverticula Causes regurgitation of food from diverticula	Surgical excision if symptoms are severe
Esophageal tumors	Incidence higher in persons who have other esophageal problems and those with history of excessive alcohol intake Causes progressive dysphagia to solid food	Radiation therapy Surgical excision
Diaphragmatic hernia	Protrusion of part of the stomach through the diaphragm and into the thoracic cavity Precipitated by any condition increasing intraabdominal pressure Causes heartburn and reflux of gastric contents, especially when patient is in recumbent position	Minor problems treated with antacids, small frequent feedings, bland diet, and avoiding lifting Surgery to repair hernia via thoracic or abdominal route
Gastroesophageal reflux disease	Condition in which acidic gastric contents reflux back into the lower esophagus. May be related to hiatal hernia, increased abdominal pressure, or reduced esophageal sphincter pressure	Small frequent meals—high protein, low fat Remain upright for 1 to 2 hours after meals Sleep with head of bed elevated 6 to 10 inches Avoid smoking and heavy lifting Take antacids as needed

complicated ulcers, but the patient should avoid all irritating substances.

Rest, with cessation of normal activities, has been shown to be very effective in healing uncomplicated ulcers.

Surgery may be necessary if ulcers perforate, if they recur frequently, or if risk of cancer is high. Table 10-3 describes common types of ulcer surgery.

NURSING MANAGEMENT

Assessment

Subjective

History of pain and home treatment attempted
Patient's description of pain: presence, location, character, time of occurrence in relation to eating and sleeping. NOTE: Ulcer pain typically occurs 1 to 3 hours after eating, often at night, and is usually relieved by food or antacid. It is located in the epigastric area and may radiate to the back.
Patient's complaints of nausea or bloating
Smoking and alcohol history
Intake of potentially ulcerogenic drugs: aspirin, steroids, antiinflammatory drugs
Family history of peptic ulcer
Personal and career stress levels
Knowledge of peptic ulcers and therapy

TABLE 10-2 Drug therapy in peptic ulcer disease

Drug	Action	Comments
Antacids: Maalox, Gelusil, Mylanta, Riopan, Amphogel	Neutralize gastric acid	Generally heal ulcers in 4 to 6 weeks Side effects of constipation and diarrhea are common Lack of adherence to regimen by many patients
Histamine H_2 receptor antagonists: Cimetidine, ranitidine, famotidine	Inhibit acid secretion	Generally heal ulcers in 4 to 6 weeks Side effects of confusion, dizziness, weakness, diarrhea, and cramps may interfere with adherence to regimen
Sucralfate	Coats ulcer; prevents action of acid and pepsin on ulcer	Generally heals ulcers in 4 to 6 weeks Longer time span before reoccurrence Large capsule—difficult to swallow Constipation

TABLE 10-3 Surgery used to treat ulcers

Procedure	Description	Procedure	Description
Vagotomy	Removes acid secreting stimulation and reduces responsiveness of stomach parietal cells; usually included in duodenal ulcer management. Types include: truncal **(A)**; selective **(B)**; proximal or parietal cell **(C)**.	Subtotal gastrectomy	
		Billroth I	Removal of one half to two thirds of lower part of stomach and anastomosis of remaining segment to the duodenum (see **A** below).
		Billroth II	Same procedure as Billroth I with anastomosis of remaining segment to the side of the proximal jejunum (see **B** below).
		Gastrectomy	Removal of the entire stomach with anastomosis to duodenum or jejunum; presents many problems to patients and is usually done only for gastric cancer (see **C** below).
Pyloroplasty	Procedure to alter the pyloric outlet, usually to widen it to prevent gastric stasis after vagotomy. A longitudinal incision across pylorus is pulled apart and closed in a transverse position to widen pyloric outlet.		

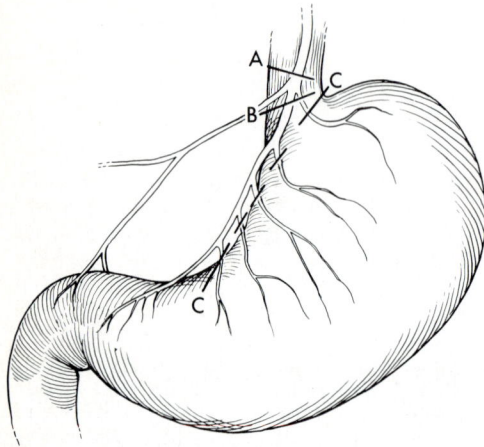

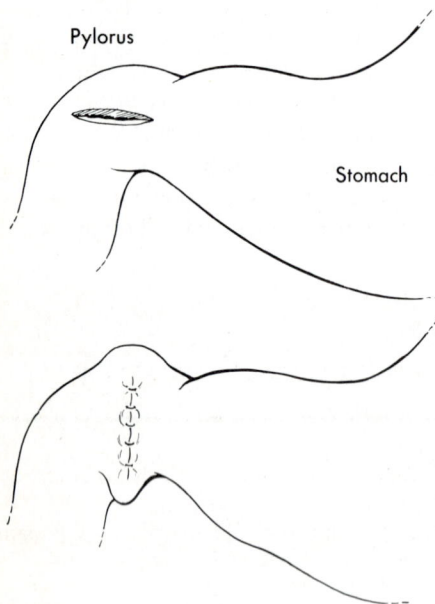

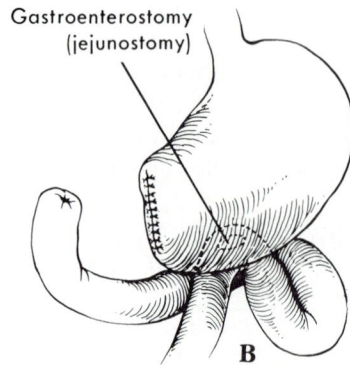

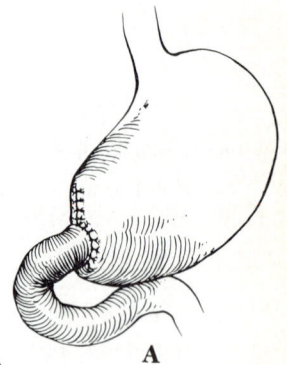

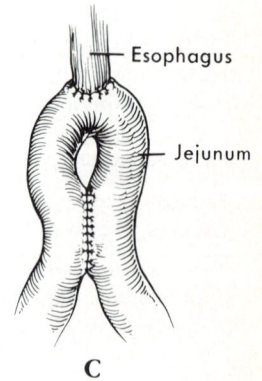

Illustrations from Phipps WJ, Long BC, and Woods NF: Medical-surgical nursing: concepts and clinical practice, ed 4, St Louis, 1990, Mosby–Year Book, Inc.

Objective
Guaiac-positive stools
Iron deficiency anemia
Hematemesis—frank GI bleeding
Signs of ulcer perforation:
   Rigid boardlike abdomen
   Decreased bowel sounds
   Signs of shock or sepsis
Positive results from upper GI series, gastroscopy, or
   gastric analysis

Nursing Diagnoses
Diagnoses will depend on the severity of the ulcer but
commonly include:
   Pain related to action of gastric secretions on the in-
      flamed mucosa
   Knowledge deficit related to treatment regimen nec-
      essary to promote healing
   Sleep pattern disturbance related to the occurrence
      of ulcer pain at night

Expected Outcomes
Patient's discomfort will gradually decrease.
Patient will be knowledgeable concerning medications
   prescribed and life-style modifications to promote
   healing.
Patient will enjoy restful, uninterrupted sleep.

Nursing Interventions: Conservative Treatment
Administer medications as prescribed.
   Teach patient about side effects of antacids and their
      management.
   Assess effectiveness of medications.
   Monitor pattern of bowel elimination.
Teach patient proper timing of medications.
   Give histamine receptor antagonists 30 to 60 minutes
      before meals or as a single nighttime dose (60% of
      gastric acid is secreted at night).
   Give antacids 1 to 3 hours after meals and as needed.
Teach patient to avoid medications known or suspected
   to be ulcerogenic, such as aspirin, steroids, antiin-
   flammatory drugs.
Teach patient to avoid foods that cause discomfort. Pa-
   tient should do the following:
   Avoid substances high in caffeine.
   Modify meal pattern to six small meals if it helps to
      control symptoms.
   Avoid gastric overdistention, which triggers reflux.
Teach patient importance of decreasing or eliminating
   cigarette smoking and alcohol intake.
Help patient to rest during ulcer attack. Explore with
   patient life-style modification to reduce or better han-
   dle stress.
Encourage a regular pattern of planned exercise.

Nursing Interventions: Preoperative
Provide appropriate patient teaching about proposed
   surgery and routines to be followed after the operation, including IVs and nasogastric tube. Respiratory
   care will be particularly important

Nursing Interventions: Postoperative
Initiate frequent position changes; use mid-Fowler's to
   high Fowler's position to facilitate chest excursion.
Encourage patient to cough and deep breathe. Ensure
   adequate analgesia. Splint the incision.
Measure and observe nasogastric drainage frequently.
   Provide good mouth care.
ALERT: Nastrogastric tubes are not routinely irrigated
   after stomach surgery. Clarify order before irrigating.
   Drainage should contain no fresh blood after first 12
   hours.
Monitor for signs of leakage (peritonitis).
Monitor patient for signs of fluid and electrolyte imbal-
   ance or anastomosis leakage.
Record intake and output accurately.
Introduce liquid and small amounts of bland food after
   nasogastric tube is removed—about 7 days after sur-
   gery—usually as three to six small meals daily.
Monitor for signs of early satiety and dumping syndrome (see box on this page). Avoid stress after
   meals; rest after eating.

DUMPING SYNDROME

Dumping syndrome is likely to occur following gastric resection but may occur with vagotomy, antrectomy, and
gastroenterostomy procedures.

EARLY DUMPING SYNDROME
Occurs within first hour after eating
Entrance of hyperosmolar food mixture into jejunum
   causes fluid to be drawn from the bloodstream to the
   jejunum
Symptoms: weakness, faintness, diaphoresis, palpitations,
   nausea, discomfort; diarrhea may follow

LATE DUMPING SYNDROME
Occurs between meals, 2 to 4 hours after eating
Sudden rise in blood sugar from hyperosmolar food mix-
   ture stimulates the release of insulin from the pancreas,
   followed by hypoglycemia
Symptoms: weakness, fatigue, diaphoresis, severe anxiety

SYMPTOM MANAGEMENT
Teach patient to eat meals low in carbohydrates, high in
   fats and proteins.
Teach patient to take fluids only between meals.
Teach patient to eat small, frequent meals.
Teach patient to lie down on left side after eating.
Anticholinergic drugs may be used to control symptoms.

Teach patient means of controlling symptoms.

Teach patient to monitor weight carefully and report signs of malabsorption and steatorrhea.

Teach patient to keep head elevated when lying down if reflux heartburn occurs.

Teach patient the importance of follow-up monitoring for malabsorption or pernicious anemia.

Evaluation

Patient is free of ulcer pain.

Patient is knowledgeable about prescribed medications and has adjusted diet to eliminate substances that trigger ulcer pain.

Patient maintains a stable weight, shows no signs of malabsorption, and is able to control any symptoms of dumping syndrome.

Patient is able to enjoy uninterrupted sleep.

COMPLICATIONS OF PEPTIC ULCER

A peptic ulcer may perforate the stomach wall, obstruct the pyloric outlet of the stomach, or perforate a major blood vessel causing hemorrhage. Perforation and obstruction are usually treated surgically. Postoperative management for perforation involves supportive care for patient in severe shock. The mortality rate is quite high.

Peptic ulcers cause bleeding in about 15% to 20% of all cases. Management of this commonly occurring emergency is dealt with in the box on this page.

STRESS ULCERS

Acute ulcers are a common result of life-threatening events such as trauma, burns, sepsis, and shock. They are believed to be the result of decreased mucosal resistance, and two thirds occur in the stomach. Pain is rarely present so their presence may go unnoticed until complications develop. Prevention is the key. All at-risk patients should receive histamine receptor antagonists and antacids to keep the stomach pH greater than 4.

CANCER OF THE STOMACH

The incidence of stomach cancer has decreased significantly over the last 50 years, but it remains a problem with a high mortality rate. It is a disease of later middle age, affecting more men than women. The early symptoms are vague or nonexistent and usually do not appear until the tumor has spread to other structures. The risk factors are unknown. Surgery remains the primary therapy, with subtotal or total gastrectomy followed by chemotherapy. Care is similar to that described for peptic ulcer disease.

MANAGEMENT OF ULCER HEMORRHAGE (GI BLEEDING)

SYMPTOMS

Vomiting of bright red or coffee ground blood (usually occurs with gastric ulcers)

Tarry stools (more common with duodenal ulcers)

Signs of early and progressive hypovolemic shock
Faint feeling, dizziness, thirst
Feelings of apprehension, restlessness
Dyspnea, pallor, rising pulse, falling blood pressure

INTERVENTIONS

Place patient on bed rest.

Patient should receive nothing by mouth.

Administer sedative to control restlessness if prescribed.

Monitor vital signs frequently (every 15 minutes).

Administer IV fluids and blood transfusions as prescribed.
Record accurate intake and output; assess response to treatment.
If bleeding is minor, administer antacids hourly.
If bleeding is acute, insert nasogastric tube and irrigate with tap water or saline until clear.
Provide mouth care after patient vomits—a weak solution of hydrogen peroxide helps remove blood from oral mucous membranes.

Monitor stools for increasing blood content after episode.

Prepare patient for endoscopy procedure if indicated.

Explain all procedures, keep calm, and reassure patient as much as possible.

DISORDERS OF THE LOWER GASTROINTESTINAL TRACT

INFLAMMATORY DISORDERS: APPENDICITIS

Acute inflammation of the appendix occurs most commonly in people between 10 and 30 years, more often in males than females. No specific causes of the disease have been identified. Classic symptoms include the following:

Pain in right lower quadrant of the abdomen, which may localize at McBurney's point

Anorexia, nausea and vomiting

Fever of 38° to 38.5° C.

White blood cell count >10,000

Some patients may have less defined symptoms and require a more careful diagnostic workup.

PATHOPHYSIOLOGY

Occlusion of the lumen of the appendix by feces or kinking may impair the circulation and lower resistance to colon organisms. Mucosa becomes reddened, edematous, and often infected. Abscess, necrosis, or rupture can occur. The most serious risk is rupture, which results in acute peritonitis.

PEPTIC ULCER

Nursing Diagnoses	Expected Patient Outcomes	Nursing Interventions

Pain related to the action of gastric secretions on the inflamed mucosa	Patient's pain decreases or resolves.	1. Give prescribed medications:
		  a. Antacids: 1 and 3 hr after meals and at bedtime for best effect; may be given as often as every 30 min for severe pain
		  b. Histamine H_2 blockers with meals and at bedtime or single large bedtime dose
		  c. Sucralfate: 1 hr before meals and at bedtime
		  d. Do not give antacids concurrently with cimetidine or sucralfate.
		2. Avoid substances high in caffeine.
		3. Eliminate foods that trigger gastric pain.
		4. Use a five to six meal pattern if it reduces incidence of ulcer pain.
		5. Assist patient to rest.

Potential for injury related to ulcer perforation or hemorrhage	Patient does not experience bleeding.	1. Monitor patient for signs of complications:
		  a. Signs of overt bleeding: hematemesis, tarry stools
		  b. Signs of shock
		  c. Signs of perforation: severe sharp abdominal pain
		2. If signs of complications occur, give patient nothing by mouth and prepare to insert nasogastric tube for lavage.
		3. Eliminate ulcerogenic medications if possible, particularly aspirin, antiinflammatories, steroids

Ineffective individual coping related to life stresses	Patient is able to understand and identify stressors and effectively problem solve to reduce them.	1. Assist patient to identify:
		  a. Any present stressors in daily life
		  b. Feelings and responses to identified stressors
		  c. Usual coping mechanisms
		  d. Individuals who can serve as support persons when new stressors occur
		2. Assist patient to explore alternative ways of coping.
		3. Teach patient stress management techniques, such as relaxation response, as appropriate.
		4. Encourage activities that promote relaxation (recreation, hobbies).
		5. Assist patient to do the following:
		  a. Identify specific health-risking behaviors that may aggravate the ulcer (such as smoking, caffeine, alcohol, stressful situations)
		  b. Explore ways of modifying the behaviors, such as ways to stop smoking or drinking, or to avoid certain stressful situations

Knowledge deficit related to peptic ulcer treatment regimen	Patient is knowledgeable concerning prescribed medications and life-style modifications necessary to promote healing.	1. Teach patient the following:
		  a. Nature of peptic ulcers
		  b. Factors that contribute to healing and decreased occurrence of ulcers
		  c. Medication regimens
		  d. Methods to reduce stress and promote relaxation
		  e. Need to report symptoms of bleeding, perforation, and pyloric obstruction to physician immediately

MEDICAL AND NURSING MANAGEMENT

The appendix is removed through a small incision, and healing is usually prompt. Drains may be inserted if an abscess is found. Bowel function returns promptly after surgery, and the convalescence is short.

Nursing management involves monitoring and supportive care while the diagnosis is being established and general postoperative surgical care. The hospitalization is usually brief.

CHRONIC INFLAMMATORY BOWEL DISORDERS

Crohn's disease and ulcerative colitis are two major inflammatory disorders of the large bowel, ulcerative colitis being twice as common. Specific causes have not been identified, but both disorders tend to affect primarily young white adults in Western society. They follow recurrent patterns of exacerbation and remission and cause significant disruption to an individual's normal activity pattern. Table 10-4 compares some major aspects of the two disorders.

PATHOPHYSIOLOGY

Crohn's disease is characterized by cobblestone granulomas along the mucosa, thickening of the intestinal wall, and scar tissue formation. Lesions commonly perforate and form fissures with the intestinal wall or other hollow organ. Scar tissue interferes with normal bowel absorption. Lesions may occur in an ascending pattern throughout the bowel, often separated by patches of normal tissue.

Ulcerative colitis consists primarily of mucosal ulcerations that begin in the rectosigmoid colon and spread upward through the colon. The ulcers may bleed or perforate. The bowel mucosa becomes edematous and thickened. The formation of scar tissue thickens the colon and causes loss of elasticity.

MEDICAL MANAGEMENT

There is no specific treatment for inflammatory bowel disease. The patient is offered symptomatic supportive care through diet modification and medications to provide comfort, decrease bowel motility, and prevent or treat local infection. During exacerbations care is primarily supportive, with rest and nutritional support. Commonly prescribed medications include the following:

Sulfasalazine (Azulfidine)—used for its antiinflammatory effects; most patients receive this drug, and it may sustain long-term remissions

Corticosteroids—suppress inflammation and may induce remission but cannot effect a cure

Antibiotics—administered during acute exacerbations in patients with fistulas or signs of peritoneal irritation

Bulk hydrophilic agents such as psyllium (Metamucil)—given in preference to antimotility drugs for diarrhea.

Surgery is indicated when the patient does not respond to medical management. Surgery is performed in Crohn's disease for obstruction, fistula, or abscess drainage. It usually consists of bowel resection and anastomosis. Most procedures for ulcerative colitis are curative in nature and remove most or all of the colon. Options include total proctocolectomy with ileostomy or continent ileostomy, and total colectomy with ileorectal or ileoanal anastomosis.

TABLE 10-4 Comparison of Crohn's disease and ulcerative colitis

	Crohn's Disease	Ulcerative Colitis
Age occurring	20-30 years 40-50 years	Young adults
Area affected	Mainly terminal ileum, cecum, and ascending colon	Colon and rectum only, primarily the descending portion
Extent of involvement	Segmental areas of involvement	Continuous, diffuse areas of involvement
Character of stools	No blood; may contain fat; three to five semisoft stools per day	Blood present; frequent liquid stools; no fat content
Abdominal pain	Colicky cramping pain in right lower quadrant, which may be severe	May occur, usually prior to defecation
Complications	Fistulas; perianal disease; strictures; vitamin and iron deficiencies	Pseudopolyps; hemorrhage; cachexia; infrequently perforation
Reasons for surgery	Fistulas; obstruction	Poor response to medical therapy; hemorrhage; perforation
Type of surgery	Colon resection with anastomosis	Total proctocolectomy with permanent ileostomy; continent ileostomy

NURSING MANAGEMENT

Assessment

Subjective

History of the disease and treatment

Patient's response to chronic disease

Patient's understanding of disease process, treatment plan, and precipitating factors if any

Diet pattern followed at home; food intolerances

Medications in use; patient's knowledge of action and side effects

Report of or signs of stress and anxiety in daily life

Patient's report of bowel pattern: frequency, consistency, incontinence

Patient's report of pain or cramping

Patient's complaints of fatigue, anorexia, nausea

Effects of disease on social and sexual relationships

Objective

Body weight and recent changes

General appearance and nutritional status

Presence of perianal excoriation

Stool assessment—presence of blood, pus, or fat

Assessment of skin and mucous membranes for dehydration

Intake and output

Vital signs; presence of fever

Positive results from stool analysis, sigmoidoscopy or colonoscopy, barium enema

Nursing Diagnoses

Diagnoses depend on stage and severity of the disorder but commonly include the following:

Activity intolerance related to extreme fatigue and debilitating effects of the disease

Diarrhea related to inflammation and ulceration of the bowel

Pain and cramping related to bowel ulceration and inflammation

Potential for ineffective individual coping related to chronic disabling effects of the disease

Actual or potential fluid volume deficit related to excessive GI losses through diarrhea

Altered nutrition: less than body requirements, related to inadequate intake and GI losses through diarrhea

Actual or potential impairment of skin integrity in perianal area related to excoriation from frequent diarrhea

Knowledge deficit related to treatment regimen

Expected Outcomes

Patient's energy level will increase; patient will gradually resume normal activity pattern.

Patient will have less diarrhea and return to a nearly normal pattern of bowel elimination.

Patient will be relieved of discomfort of chronic diarrhea.

Patient will make a positive adjustment to chronic disease and maintain normal occupational and social activities.

Patient will reestablish a normal fluid and electrolyte balance.

Patient will gain weight to an appropriate level and select meals appropriate to dietary restrictions.

Patient will regain and maintain an intact skin.

Nursing Interventions

Provide sufficient uninterrupted rest. Encourage rest after meals.

Help patient to meet physical needs as indicated.

Discuss appropriate relaxation and stress management. Assist patient with positive coping efforts.

Space activities to avoid fatigue.

Avoid complications of bed rest.

Provide regular skin care for cachectic patient.

Protect bony prominences with sheepskin or pads.

Provide perianal care when diarrhea is severe. Apply zinc oxide or other protective barrier.

Encourage regular use of sitz baths.

Apply analgesic ointment (Nupercainal) to painful tissue.

Administer prescribed medications.

Teach patient about action and side effects of medications. (See Chapter 12 for teaching concerning corticosteroids.)

Monitor stools accurately: number, amount, and character.

Maintain accurate intake and output records, assess for dehydration.

Give patient nothing by mouth during exacerbations.

Teach patient principles of diet modification if prescribed.

Encourage patient to take oral nutrition or elemental diet when permitted.

Encourage patient to explore use of high protein, high-calorie, high-vitamin, low-residue diet if food tolerances permit. Avoid milk and milk products.

Eliminate foods that irritate the bowel. Use alcohol, caffeine, and raw fruits and vegetables cautiously.

Provide adequate fluids, at least 2500 ml/day.

Weigh patient daily.

Make environment as pleasant as possible.

Offer ongoing emotional support to patient.

Encourage patient to express feelings about disorder.

Keep room as clean and odor free as possible.

Empty bedpan promptly.

Provide appropriate care for patients undergoing total colectomy and ileostomy (see box on p. 154).

NURSING CARE PLAN

ULCERATIVE COLITIS

Nursing Diagnoses	Expected Patient Outcomes	Nursing Interventions
Altered nutrition: less than body requirements, related to inadequate intake and losses through diarrhea	Patient's weight stabilizes at an appropriate level. Patient selects meals appropriate to dietary restrictions.	1. Give nothing by mouth or only prescribed feedings during acute episode. 2. If elemental feedings are required, chill the fluids and offer a variety of flavors, as taste is poor. 3. Provide a high-protein, low-residue, high-carbohydrate diet after acute episode subsides. Offer supplemental vitamins. 4. Identify foods, such as those high in fats or fiber, spicy foods, or milk products, that are poorly tolerated by patient and eliminate these foods from the diet. 5. Use measures to encourage increased food intake (pleasant environment, reduction of stress at mealtime, between-meal snacks). 6. Give prescribed vitamins. 7. Monitor weight two to three times a week.
Actual or potential fluid volume deficit related to excessive GI losses	Patient maintains a balance of intake and output.	1. Monitor intake and output daily. 2. Encourage fluids to 2500 ml/day if patient is on oral diet. 3. Assess skin turgor and status of mucous membranes daily. 4. Give mouth care as needed to keep membranes moist and encourage eating.
Diarrhea related to inflammation and ulceration of the bowel	Patient passes soft, formed stools without cramping or urgency.	1. Monitor stools for characteristics and frequency. 2. Give prescribed antiinflammatory medications (sulfasalazine, corticosteroids) and monitor for side effects. 3. Give prescribed bulk hydrophilic agents (Metamucil). 4. Give prescribed antidiarrheals or antibiotics as ordered. 5. Encourage patient to lie quietly after meals to reduce peristalsis.
Pain and abdominal cramping related to bowel inflammation and perianal irritation	Patient is relieved of abdominal discomfort.	1. Facilitate easy access to toilet, commode, or bedpan (abdominal cramping is relieved by bowel movements). Empty promptly. 2. Provide soft toilet tissue or medicated wipes (Tucks). 3. Keep anal area clean with mild soap and water and dry well. Apply zinc oxide or other protective ointments after cleaning. 4. Provide sitz baths for rectal comfort, as necessary. 5. Use analgesic ointments (Nupercaine) as needed. 6. Protect and massage pressure areas developing from prolonged toilet/bedpan sitting. Keep sheepskin or eggcrate mattress on bed. 7. Use room deodorizers, as needed. 8. Examine anus at intervals for signs of perianal fissures.

NURSING CARE PLAN

ULCERATIVE COLITIS—cont'd

Nursing Diagnoses	Expected Patient Outcomes	Nursing Interventions

Potential for ineffective individual coping related to chronic disabling effects of disease	Patient makes a positive adjustment to chronicity of disease and maintains usual occupational and social roles.	1. Assess patient's knowledge of disorder and provide information as needed.
		2. Schedule regular time periods to interact with patient and begin to develop a trust relationship.
		3. Give patient opportunities to express feelings about condition (frustration, depression, anger) and identify content related to these feelings.
		4. Help patient identify the following:
		  a. Life stressors and usual response to the stressors
		  b. Usual coping mechanisms and alternative methods of coping
		5. Encourage patient to participate in planning activities and assuming self-care.
		6. Discuss effects of stress on disease exacerbations.

Activity intolerance related to extreme fatigue and debilitating effects of the disease	Patient will experience an increasing energy level and gradually resume a normal activity pattern.	1. Encourage rest during exacerbations. 2. Space activities to conserve energy. 3. Provide privacy and quiet for uninterrupted rest. 4. Assist with activities of daily living as needed. 5. Encourage patient to gradually resume responsibility for self-care as condition improves. 6. Discuss need for independence with family. 7. Explore need for vitamin or iron therapy to reverse anemia. 8. Teach patient to monitor pulse for improvement in activity tolerance.

CARE OF THE PATIENT WITH AN ILEOSTOMY

PREOPERATIVE CARE

Teach patient in detail about the proposed surgery:
 Size and appearance of stoma
 Amount and consistency of drainage
 Appliances used and their basic care, if any
Encourage patient to ask questions and express feelings
 about major alteration in body appearance and function.
Provide emotional support for stage of grief or acceptance
 patient exhibits.
Provide for initiation of teaching and visits by en-
 terostomal therapist. Therapist usually does stoma site
 selection.
Assist with complete bowel preparation as ordered.

POSTOPERATIVE CARE

Monitor fluid and electrolyte balance carefully:
 Measure all output accurately.
 Maintain patency of IV lines and nasogastric drainage
 system.
 Observe for early signs of shock.
Monitor stoma and suture line carefully:
 Stoma should be pink–bright red; dark blue–red indi-
 cates impaired circulation and should be reported im-
 mediately.
 Note amount and type of drainage
 Mucus and serosanguineous discharge occurs for first
 24 to 48 hours.
 Liquid drainage occurs with returning peristalsis—
 may initially be as much as 1500 ml per day. Ter-
 minal ileum will begin absorption in about 2 weeks
 and drainage will then thicken.
Teach patient the symptoms of dehydration.
Protect skin around stoma from fecal drainage:
 Cleanse skin carefully and dry.
 Apply skin barrier.
 Change pouch as needed if leaking occurs—never sim-
 ply add tape.

Reassure patient and support all efforts at self-care.
Encourage patient to look at stoma and observe care.
Teach patient stoma management:
 Teach technique for pouch application and skin care.
 Teach emptying and disposal or cleansing of pouch.
Advance diet and fluids as prescribed:
 Begin with bland low-residue diet.
 Avoid foods that cause increased gas or odor, such as
 corn, celery, cabbage, onions, and spiced foods.
Teach patient that some foods and substances (seeds, ker-
 nels, enteric or slow-release medications) will pass
 through stoma unchanged. Use liquid or chewable med-
 ications when available.
Encourage patient to maintain an adequate fluid intake.
Discuss with patient the following modifications in life-
 style necessitated by ileostomy:
 Modify clothing.
 Adjust recreational pursuits—contact sports should be
 avoided, but most other activities may be resumed.
 Make adaptations for traveling.
 Hand carry all necessary ostomy supplies.
 Use disposable equipment and take extra supplies.
 Eat moderately—use restraint with new foods and
 water.
Put patient in touch with local ostomy associations.
Encourage patient to discuss concerns regarding resump-
 tion of sexual activity.
Teach patient importance of reporting any early signs of
 complications. Patient should be alert to the following:
 Changes in color, consistency, or odor of stool
 Bleeding from stoma
 Persistent diarrhea or lack of stool
 Changes in stoma contour (prolapse or inversion) or
 signs of infection
 Skin irritation that doesn't respond to basic treatment

Evaluation

Patient has sufficient energy to perform all self-care activities and resume normal life-style.

Patient has normal pattern of bowel elimination or stabilizes colon output through ileostomy stoma.

Patient is free of cramping and discomfort.

Patient learns self-care management of ileostomy, establishes control over disease process, and resumes normal life-style.

Patient maintains a normal fluid and electrolyte balance.

Patient tolerates a normal diet and maintains desired
weight.

Patient maintains an intact skin.

INFLAMMATORY DISORDERS: DIVERTICULITIS

Diverticula are small outpouchings of mucosa through
defects in the muscular wall of the colon. This disorder
occurs in late middle age and appears to be related to

low intake of dietary fiber. Symptoms occur when diverticula become inflamed, causing painful spasms, or
when complications develop such as perforation, obstruction, or hemorrhage.

 Basic treatment consists of a diet high in fiber. Psyllium (Metamucil) may also be prescribed to increase
stool bulk. Antispasmodics (Pro-Banthine, Bentyl) may
be prescribed during attacks of inflammation, along
with analgesics, antibiotics, and bowel rest. Colon resection surgery may be indicated for the patient who experiences complications.

BOWEL OBSTRUCTION

Intestinal obstruction refers to blockage of the movement of intestinal contents through the small or large
intestine. Mechanical obstructions occur from physical
blockage of the passage. Common causes are identified
in the box on the next page. Paralytic obstruction occurs when peristalsis is inhibited as a result of the ef-

CAUSES OF MECHANICAL BOWEL OBSTRUCTION

Obstruction from causes that physically impede passage of intestinal contents:

  Adhesions
  Neoplasms
  Inflammatory bowel disease
  Foreign bodies, gallstones
  Fecal impaction
  Congenital strictures
  Radiation strictures
  Intussusception (telescoping of segment of bowel within itself)
  Volvulus (twisting of the bowel)

---

fects of trauma or toxins on the autonomic control of intestinal motility in the presence of an open passageway. The bowel manipulation associated with abdominal surgery is one of the most common causes.

PATHOPHYSIOLOGY

An increase in peristalsis occurs near the obstruction in an effort to move intestinal contents. As intraluminal pressure increases, the proximal intestine dilates, smooth muscle becomes atonic, and peristalsis ceases. Large amounts of isotonic fluid then move from the plasma into the distended bowel, and normal reabsorption of intestinal gas and fluid is impeded. The tissue becomes edematous, and mucosal blood flow is decreased. Large amounts of gas collect from air swallowing and the action of intestinal bacteria.

The end result may be severe dehydration and electrolyte imbalance with possible perforation or strangulation of the colon. The severity of the symptoms will depend on the site and degree of obstruction, and the amount of time that elapses before the patient seeks help.

MEDICAL MANAGEMENT

Treatment of intestinal obstruction may include nasogastric or intestinal intubation and decompression, fluid and electrolyte replacement, and surgical relief of the source of obstruction if necessary. The operative procedure will vary with the cause and location but may include release of adhesions, bowel resection, and temporary or permanent colostomy.

NURSING MANAGEMENT

Assessment

Subjective

  History and course of the symptoms
  Location and severity of pain, cramping, tenderness
  Patient's complaints of bloating or distention, nausea
  Timing and consistency of latest bowel movement
  Passage of flatus

Objective

  Auscultation of the abdomen for:
    Loud high-pitched sounds early in obstruction
    Diminished or absent sounds late in obstruction
  Vomiting
    Profuse, nonfecal if proximal small bowel
    Infrequent fecal type if distal bowel
  Abdominal distention and girth
  Signs of dehydration
  Changes in vital signs
  Abdominal x-ray studies showing air and fluid in the bowel and a gradually worsening electrolyte profile

Nursing Diagnoses

Diagnoses may vary with cause and severity of obstruction but frequently include the following:

  Pain related to pressure and accumulation of fluid and gas in the bowel
  Fluid volume deficit related to accumulation of excess fluid in the bowel
  Altered nutrition: less than body requirements, related to bowel obstruction and prolonged NPO period during treatment

Expected Outcomes

Patient will experience relief of pain and distention.
Patient will return to a normal fluid and electrolyte balance; intravascular volume will be restored.
Patient will return to a normal diet that meets daily nutritional requirements.

Nursing Interventions

Begin to prepare patient for any needed surgery.
Maintain accurate intake and output records.
Assess for fluid and electrolyte imbalance.
Monitor IV fluids carefully.
Monitor vital signs for indications of shock, fluid overload, or peritonitis.
Provide good supportive care.
  Position patient comfortably and change positions frequently.
  Use Fowler's position to support ventilation.
  Assist patient as needed with activities of daily living.
  Provide regular skin care.
  Offer frequent, scrupulous mouth care, especially if patient is vomiting.
  Ensure adequate pulmonary ventilation; encourage deep breathing.
  Patient should avoid mouth breathing and air swallowing.
Auscultate for bowel sounds, passage of flatus.
Measure and record abdominal girth.
Maintain patency of nasogastric or intestinal tubes (see Table 10-5).

TABLE 10-5 Use of intestinal tubes

Purpose	Types	Tube Use and Patient Care
To drain fluids and gas that accumulate above a mechanical obstruction and to decompress the bowel	Miller-Abbot (double-lumen tube). One lumen leads to the balloon and the other has openings for drainage or irrigation. Mercury is inserted into the balloon after placement. Cantor (single-lumen tube). Cantor tube has only one opening used for drainage; balloon must be injected with mercury before insertion. Both tubes have balloons that, when inflated, act like a bolus of food, stimulating peristalsis and advancing along the intestinal tract. If peristalsis is absent, the weight of mercury in the balloon carries it forward.	Special care is taken during insertion, as the presence of the balloon makes passage through the nose quite difficult. After tube passes into the stomach, its progression is aided by positioning the patient. Encourage patient to lie on right side for 2 hours. Patient switches to lying on back for 2 hours with head elevated. Patient lies on left side for 2 hours. Walking about stimulates further movement by increasing peristalsis. Advance tube 2 to 10 cm (1 to 4 inches) at specified intervals to provide slack for peristaltic action. Never tape tube in place until it reaches desired position. Pin excess tubing to clothing. Provide comfort measures for nose and throat. Irrigate tube for patency if ordered— return aspiration is often not feasible. If tube is well advanced in bowel, light food and fluid may be permitted. Monitor patient for return of bowel sounds, passage of flatus, or spontaneous bowel movement.

Evaluation

Patient has normal and regular patterns of bowel elimination.

Abdominal girth returns to normal.

Patient experiences no pain in the abdomen.

Patient has a normal fluid and electrolyte balance as evidenced by laboratory reports and intake and output balance.

Patient returns to a normal nutritional intake, regains lost weight, and meets body's basic nutritional needs.

HERNIA

A hernia is a protrusion of an organ or structure (usually the bowel) from its normal cavity through a congenital or acquired defect.

A reducible hernia can be returned to its own cavity by manipulation, whereas an irreducible hernia cannot. If the blood supply becomes occluded, the hernia is said to be strangulated.

Hernias typically occur in the umbilical or inguinal area, particularly in men.

PATHOPHYSIOLOGY

Hernias produce a distinct local swelling that usually disappears when the person lies down. They typically produce no symptoms beyond the palpable physical defect. Pain is usually the result of local irritation of the peritoneum. Severe pain is usually associated with strangulation, which may produce all of the problems of intestinal obstruction and necessitate emergency surgery.

MEDICAL MANAGEMENT

Initial treatment may consist of local support and restrictions on lifting. The only cure for a hernia is surgical repair of the defect, which is often performed today in an outpatient surgical center.

NURSING MANAGEMENT

Assessment

Subjective

History of the hernia: onset, reducibility, change in size

Presence of pain or tenderness

Occupation and leisure activities, particularly those that that involve heavy lifting

Presence of factors that cause chronic coughing— smoking habit, allergies, upper respiratory tract infection

Knowledge of planned surgery

Objective
Appearance, size, and tenderness of hernia
Lung sounds; presence of chronic cough

Nursing Diagnoses
Pain related to tenderness of the hernia or postoperative incisional pain
Activity intolerance related to postoperative pain and edema at incisional site

Expected Outcomes
Patient will have a decrease in pain and tenderness at hernia site.
Patient will gradually resume normal activity pattern and use good body mechanics when performing heavy lifting.

Nursing Interventions
Report to physician presence of any respiratory disorder that may place extra strain on repair sutures.
Teach patient importance of frequent ambulation and deep breathing since minimal postoperative coughing is preferred.
  Splint incisional area firmly if patient is coughing.
  Assist patient to gradually assume an upright posture.
Patient should avoid any abdominal straining. Provide stool softeners or cathartics as needed.
Monitor postoperative voiding carefully. Assist patient out of bed to promote voiding.
Provide sufficient analgesia to enable patient to ambulate.
Provide icebags and scrotal support for inguinal hernias.
Monitor integrity and healing of the incision carefully.
Teach patient to refrain from driving and heavy lifting after discharge. Clarify the physician's specific restrictions.
Reinforce and teach importance of using good body mechanics.

Evaluation
Patient experiences no residual pain or tenderness at hernia site.
Patient resumes prior activities and utilizes good principles of body mechanics in moving and lifting.

CANCER OF THE BOWEL

Malignant tumors of the colon and rectum are among the most common cancers affecting adults of both sexes. These cancers represent a serious health problem, affecting over 140,000 persons per year. Their cause remains unknown, but both environmental and genetic factors are implicated. Dietary factors are under intense investigation. The incidence of bowel cancer increases with age, with a peak in the seventh decade. It occurs primarily in developed countries.

PATHOPHYSIOLOGY

Colon cancer may develop as a polyplike lesion or as an annular lesion that encircles the lumen of the colon. Polyps may ulcerate but rarely obstruct. In the descending and rectosigmoid portion of the colon, the constricting tumor may present with symptoms of bowel obstruction. Specific symptoms vary with position and type of tumor growth pattern. The tumor may alter bowel elimination patterns, trigger nausea or vomiting, or produce blood in the stool. Diagnosis is confirmed by proctoscopy or biopsy. Lesions eventually penetrate the colon wall and extend into adjacent tissue.

MEDICAL MANAGEMENT

The treatment of colon cancer is surgical removal of the tumor, surrounding colon, and lymph nodes. If possible, the remaining portions of the bowel are anastomosed. Since greater than 70% of the tumors occur in the sigmoid and descending colon, however, permanent colostomy is almost always necessary. Preoperative work-up includes a thorough bowel prep with laxatives, antibiotics, and enemas to empty and cleanse the bowel.

NURSING MANAGEMENT

The nursing management associated with bowel cancer is very similar to that described for intestinal obstruction in general. Preoperative and postoperative care for a patient with a colostomy also closely follows that outlined for the ileostomy patient. Problems with altered body image are often more severe for bowel cancer patients, who are often older individuals and have little time to comprehend and internalize the implications of the diagnosis and treatment. Depending on the location of the colostomy, the patient may choose irrigation to facilitate management. The procedure for colostomy irrigation and the general principles of care for a patient with bowel surgery are outlined in the boxes on the next page.

ANORECTAL LESIONS

Common anorectal lesions are described in Table 10-6. Of these, hemorrhoids are the most frequently occurring and cause a great deal of pain and discomfort. Causes that have been identified include heredity, prolonged sitting or standing, chronic constipation, and any situation that increases intraabdominal pressure such as pregnancy, cirrhosis, or congestive heart failure.

PATHOPHYSIOLOGY

Congestion in the hemorrhoidal plexus leads to varicosities in the lower rectum or the anus. Internal hemorrhoids (above the internal sphincter) often bleed on defecation. External hemorrhoids (outside the anal sphinc-

COLOSTOMY IRRIGATION

Position patient on toilet, or on padded chair next to toilet if perineal wound has not healed.

Remove old pouch.

Clean skin and stoma with water.

Apply irrigating sleeve and belt.

Fill bag with desired amount of tepid water (250 to 1000 ml).

Hang bag so bottom of bag is at shoulder height.

Remove air from tubing.

Gently insert irrigating cone snugly into stoma, holding it parallel to floor.

Let water run in slowly until patient identifies need to expel stool.

Remove cone and allow solution to drain into container.

When most of stool is expelled (about 15 minutes), rinse sleeve with water and close up bottom end.

Encourage activity to complete bowel emptying (about 30-45 minutes).

Remove sleeve and apply clean pouch:

1. Trace pattern ⅛ inch larger than the stoma on paper side of the skin barrier (Stomadhesive, Hollihesive, Reliaseal, Colly Seal).
2. Cut hole on pattern line and round the edges.
3. Trace pattern on pattern side of the pouch, making it slightly larger than hole for the skin barrier.
4. Cut hole on pattern line and round the edges.
5. Remove paper backing from pouch and apply to shiny side of the skin barrier.
6. Warm skin barrier slightly, remove paper backing, and press and seal to dry clean skin around the stoma.

CARE OF THE PATIENT HAVING BOWEL SURGERY

PREOPERATIVE CARE

Give patient low-residue diet during workup period.

Give patient clear liquids for day prior to surgery.

Administer prescribed laxatives and enemas.

Administer prescribed bowel-cleansing antibiotics.

Provide adequate perianal cleansing and ointments.

Reinforce teaching about proposed surgery and postoperative routines and equipment.

POSTOPERATIVE CARE

Encourage maximum possible activity, coughing, and deep breathing.

Maintain patency of IV and drainage apparatus.

Monitor intake and output accurately; assess for signs of fluid imbalance.

Monitor for signs of returning peristalsis—bowel sounds, flatus.

Provide good oral hygiene; keep nose and mouth well lubricated.

MEASURES SPECIFIC TO ABDOMINAL PERINEAL RESECTION

Monitor perineal dressings; initial drainage is profuse.

Reinforce or change dressings as ordered; wound is often open.

Encourage leg exercises; risk of thrombophlebitis is high.

Maintain patency of drainage tubes, and suction if in use.

Initiate normal saline perineal irrigations as prescribed. Hold dressings in place with T-binders.

Substitute sitz baths for irrigations when patient is fully ambulatory.

Help patient to find comfortable positions for rest and sleep—usually side-lying position is best tolerated.

---

ter) bleed relatively rarely and seldom cause pain unless a vein ruptures and causes a thrombosis.

MEDICAL MANAGEMENT

A variety of treatments are available for hemorrhoids. Conservative management involves diet and exercise, stool softeners, and the local application of ice and analgesic ointments. Internal hemorrhoids may be treated through the injection of sclerosing substances or rubber band ligation. Standard surgical ligation may be performed for either type.

TABLE 10-6 Common anorectal lesions

Lesion	Description	Signs and Symptoms	Medical Treatment
Anal fissure	Slitlike ulceration in epithelium of anal canal	Pain with defecation; bleeding; constipation	Stool softeners; analgesic ointments; sitz baths; surgical removal of fissure if medical therapy is ineffective
Anal abscess	Abscess in tissue around anus	Persistent throbbing anal pain with walking, sitting, defecation; systemic signs of infection	Incision and drainage of abscess
Anal fistula	Hollow track leading through anal tissue from anorectal canal through skin near anus	Purulent discharge near anus	Fistulectomy or fistulotomy
Hemorrhoids	Varicosities of lower rectum and anus	Bleeding with defecation; pain if thrombosed	Analgesic ointments for mild discomfort; injection, ligation, or hemorrhoidectomy for severe discomfort

From Phipps WJ, Long BC, and Woods NF: Medical-surgical nursing: concepts and clinical practice, ed 4, St Louis, 1990, Mosby–Year Book, Inc.

NURSING MANAGEMENT

Assessment

Subjective

History of condition
Self-treatment methods used
Medications in use
Normal diet and exercise pattern
Amount and severity of pain and bleeding
Normal defecation pattern

Objective

Appearance of stool
Presence of blood in stool

Nursing Diagnoses

Constipation related to fear and pain associated with defecation

Pain related to defecation or postsurgical incisional discomfort

Knowledge deficit related to the effects of diet and exercise on normal bowel patterns

Expected Outcomes

Patient will reestablish a regular pattern of bowel elimination without pain or bleeding.

Patient will not have pain or discomfort with defecation.

Patient will be knowledgeable about diet and exercise effects on patterns of bowel elimination and modify patterns to enhance regular elimination.

Nursing Interventions: Preoperative

Administer bowel preparation as prescribed.

Encourage normal intake of food or low-residue diet.

Teach use of sitz bath for postoperative period.

Teach patient about surgical procedure and management of pain and elimination in the postoperative period.

Nursing Interventions: Postoperative

Administer pain medication liberally as prescribed.

Assist patient to position of comfort, usually side lying. Patient should avoid sitting and supine position.

Monitor rectal area for signs of bleeding. Carefully inspect dressings if in use.

Monitor for adequate urinary elimination. Encourage patient to be out of bed to void.

Administer ice packs, warm compresses, or ointments as prescribed.

Initiate use of sitz baths three or four times daily. Monitor patient for hypotension during first sitz bath.

Administer stool softeners, mineral oil, or bulk formers to assist in stool passage.

Provide analgesia before and monitor patient for fainting during first bowel movement.

Encourage use of sitz bath after defecation.

Cleanse rectal area carefully after each defecation until healing is complete.

Provide discharge teaching about the following measures to promote proper bowel function:

Ingest high-fiber diet.
Keep fluid intake high.
Engage in regular moderate exercise.
Respond promptly to defecation stimulus.
Continue use of stool softeners if indicated.

Evaluation

Patient establishes pattern of regular bowel elimination, passes soft formed stool without straining.

Patient passes stool without pain or bleeding.

Patient eats a diet with adequate fiber, maintains a liberal fluid intake, and exercises regularly.

BIBLIOGRAPHY

Alterescu KV: Colostomy, Nurs Clin North Am **22**:281-290, 1987.

Anderson BJ: Tube feeding: is diarrhea inevitable?, Am J Nurs **86**:705-706, 1986.

Atkins JM and Oakley CW: A nurse's guide to TPN, RN **49**(6):20-24, 1986.

Benedict P and Haddad A: Post op teaching for the colostomy patient, RN **52**(3):85-90, 1989.

Dobkin KA and Broadwell DC: Nursing considerations for the patient undergoing colostomy surgery, Semin Oncol Nurs **2**:249-255, 1986.

Erickson P: Ostomies: the art of pouching, Nurs Clin North Am **22**:311-320, 1987.

Feickert DM: Gastric surgery: your crucial pre and post op role, RN **50**(1):24-35, 1987.

Foltz AT: Nutritional factors in the prevention of gastrointestinal cancer, Semin Oncol Nurs **4**:239-245, 1988.

Joachim G and others: Inflammatory bowel disease: effects on lifestyle, J Adv Nurs **12**:483-487, 1987.

Kinash RG: Inflammatory bowel disease: implications for patients, challenges for nurses, Rehabil Nurs **12**:82-89, 1987.

Konopad E and Noseworthy T: Stress ulceration: a serious complication in critically ill patients, Heart Lung **17**(4):339-348, 1988.

McConnell EA: Meeting the challenge of intestinal obstruction, Nursing 87, **17**(7):34-41, 1987.

Medvec BR: Esophageal cancer: treatment and nursing intervention, Semin Oncol Nurs **4**:246-256, 1988.

Neufeldt J: Helping the inflammatory bowel disease patient cope with the unpredictable, Nursing 87, **17**(8):47-49, 1987.

Schulmeister L: Join the fight against oral cancer, Nursing 87 **17**(5):66-67, 1987.

Shipes E: Psychosocial issues: the person with an ostomy, Nurs Clin North Am **22**:291-302, 1987.

Smith CE: Assessing bowel sounds, Nursing 88 **18**(2):42-44, 1988.

CHAPTER 11

Disorders of the Liver, Biliary System, and Pancreas

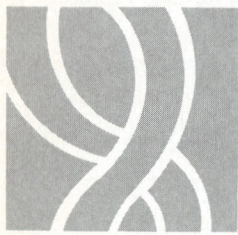

The liver, biliary system, and pancreas are affected by a variety of pathologic processes, many of which are chronic in nature and require significant adjustments in life-style. They include disorders caused by infectious organisms as well as those that result from changes in structure or function.

LIVER DISORDERS

The liver is subject to a wide variety of disorders ranging from trauma and abscess through infection and cancer. The two most common disorders, hepatitis and cirrhosis, are the focus of discussion in this chapter. Figure 11-1 illustrates the portal circulation.

HEPATITIS

The term hepatitis is used to refer to several clinically similar but etiologically distinct infections involving acute liver inflammation. It can be caused by viruses, bacteria, or toxic injury to the liver. There are some pathologic differences, but the management of the different types of hepatitis is very similar. Viral hepatitis represents a significant health problem both in the United States and worldwide.

Type A viral hepatitis primarily affects older children and young adults. The route of infection is primarily oral-fecal through contaminated food or water. It has an abrupt, often febrile onset and usually resolves without complications.

Type B viral hepatitis affects all age groups but primarily younger adults. The route of infection is primarily parenteral through contaminated blood or blood products, but direct and sexual transmission can occur. It typically has an insidious onset, runs a more protracted course, and may lead to chronic disease.

Non-A–non-B viral hepatitis affects all age groups but primarily adults. The route of infection is primarily parenteral through needles or other blood-contaminated equipment, sexual contact, and close household contacts. It has an insidious onset and frequently results in chronic disease.

Delta hepatitis, the most recently recognized form, affects the same age groups and is transmitted via the same routes as hepatitis B. It can occur as a superinfection in hepatitis B and causes a high incidence of chronic disease. Table 11-1 details the major differences among the four forms.

PATHOPHYSIOLOGY

Viral hepatitis causes diffuse inflammatory infiltration of hepatic tissue with local necrosis. The pathologic process is evenly distributed throughout the liver. Inflammatory destruction and regeneration occur almost simultaneously. The liver cells become very swollen, bile flow is interrupted, antigen-antibody complexes activate the complement system, and bilirubin diffuses into the tissues and is excreted by the kidney. Bile salts accumulate under the skin, and both hepatomegaly and splenomegaly frequently occur.

MEDICAL MANAGEMENT

There is no specific medical therapy for hepatitis. Once an accurate diagnosis has been made, treatment is aimed at providing sufficient rest and nutrition to allow the liver to heal itself. Although the disease usually persists for 2 to 4 months, recovery is usually complete. Corticosteroids may be prescribed to control inflammation in acute fulminant forms of the disease.

Another major focus of disease management is the prevention of its spread. Recommendations for the prevention of hepatitis are summarized in the box on the next page.

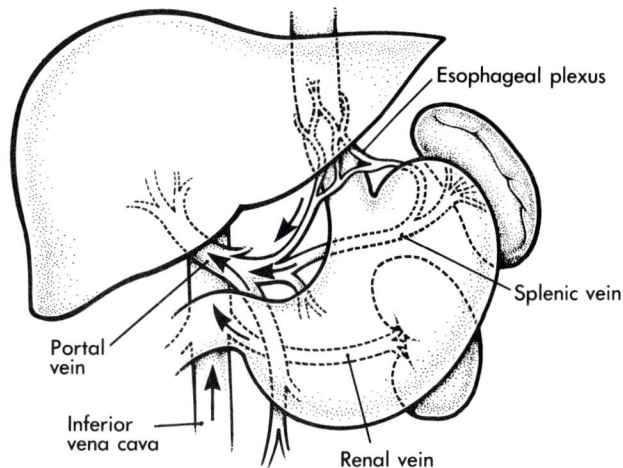

FIGURE 11-1 Portal circulation.

NURSING MANAGEMENT

Assessment
Subjective
History of symptoms

History of exposure to hepatotoxic agents, infected persons, injections, or blood transfusions

Knowledge of the disease and its treatment
Preicteric stage
Patient's complaints of the following:

Headache

Fever

Chills

Severe anorexia, nausea, and vomiting

Severe fatigue and malaise

Tenderness or aching in the right upper quadrant of the abdomen

Pruritus (itching)

Objective
Icteric phase
Elevated temperature

Yellow sclera and jaundiced skin

Dark amber urine

Clay-colored stools

Hepatomegaly and acute tenderness in right upper quadrant of the abdomen

Nutritional and fluid intake

Skin rashes, lesions from scratching

Abnormal liver function tests—SGOT (serum glutamic oxidase transaminase), SGPT (serum glutamic pyruvate transaminase), direct and indirect bilirubin

Nursing Diagnoses
Diagnoses will vary depending on the severity and stage of the disease but commonly include the following:

PREVENTION OF HEPATITIS

GENERAL PREVENTIVE MEASURES
Practice good hand washing—particularly with type A hepatitis.

Treat all body fluids and excretions as potentially infectious.

Handle all contaminated needles and syringes with great care—do not attempt to recap needles.
Type A
Place patient on enteric precautions during period of infectivity.

Wear gown and gloves when handling feces or contaminated items.

Disposable eating dishes and utensils are recommended.

Instruct patient not to donate blood.
Type B, non-A–non-B, and delta hepatitis
Place patient on blood/body fluid precautions.

Wear gown and gloves when in contact with blood or body fluids. Protect open areas on skin.

Avoid sexual contact during period of infectivity.

Instruct patient not to donate blood.
HEPATITIS PROPHYLAXIS
Hepatitis A
Postexposure—For close household and sexual contacts, administer immune globulin.
Hepatitis B
Preexposure—For health care workers, hemodialysis patients, sexually active homosexual men, IV drug abusers, and blood product recipients, hepatitis B vaccine is recommended.

Postexposure—For close household and sexual contacts, administer either hepatitis B vaccine or anti-HB immune globulin.
Non-A–non-B hepatitis
Prophylaxis has shown limited effectiveness.
Delta hepatitis
No prophylactic measures presently exist.

Activity intolerance related to extreme fatigue

Pain related to liver tenderness, pruritus, and arthralgia

Diversional activity deficit related to bed rest and the protracted course of the disease

Altered nutrition: less than body requirements, related to pronounced anorexia and nausea

Potential impairment of skin integrity related to severe pruritus

Fatigue related to imbalance in body energy production

Expected Outcomes
Patient will gradually resume a normal activity level as energy increases.

Patient will not experience pruritus or abdominal discomfort.

Patient will receive appropriate meaningful stimulation and not experience boredom or depression.

_____

TABLE 11-1 Characteristics of different types of hepatitis

Characteristic	Hepatitis A	Hepatitis B	Non A–Non B Hepatitis	Delta Hepatitis
Onset	Abrupt, febrile	Insidious, seldom febrile	Insidious, often nonicteric	Insidious
Incubation period	15-50 days	45-180 days	14-150 days	Unknown
Transmission	Primarily person to person through oral-fecal contamination; rare by blood; *not* transmitted by kissing or sharing utensils	Infected blood or body fluids; introduced by contaminated needles and sexual contact; spread by direct household contact is possible; *not* transmitted by oral-fecal route or contaminated water	Infected blood transfusion or parenteral drug abuse	Same routes as hepatitis B
Mortality	Less than 0.5%	1%-5%	Unknown	Unknown
Age groups	Older children, young adults, particularly custodial or day care situations	Young adults, particularly immigrants and refugees from endemic areas, drug abusers and hemodialysis patients and personnel	All ages, particularly those receiving frequent blood transfusions	Same as hepatitis B
Incidence of chronic disease	Virtually absent	About 10%	20%-70%	Frequent with superinfections
Carrier state	Does not occur	6%-10%	8%	80% with superinfections

Adapted from Phipps WJ, Long BC, and Woods NF: Medical-surgical nursing: concepts and clinical practice, ed 4, St Louis, 1990, Mosby–Year Book, Inc.

_____

Patient will resume a normal nutritional intake that meets all basic body needs.

Patient will maintain an intact skin.

Patient will experience a return of energy and vigor.

Nursing Interventions

Maintain patient on bed rest during acute phase.

Caution patient to resume activity very gradually.

ALERT: Relapses are believed to be frequently related to too rapid increases in activity.

Promote patient comfort while on bed rest.

Provide frequent position changes.

Keep environment cool and quiet with low levels of stimuli.

Encourage the restriction of visitors during acute phase.

Group care activities and assist patient with activities of daily living as needed. Provide for periods of uninterrupted rest.

Encourage oral fluid intake (to 3000 ml/day). Use IV route if nausea or vomiting is severe.

Maintain accurate intake and output records.

Discuss food preferences with patient.

Fruit juices, carbonated beverages, and hard candy are usually well tolerated.

Diet high in protein and carbohydrates but low in fats is optimal.

Provide frequent mouth care—keep environment pleasant and odor free.

Provide or encourage good skin care.

Implement measures to treat pruritus.

Give tepid water baths; avoid use of heat and rubbing as they increase vasodilation and itching sensation. Use lotions and creams for dry skin.

Avoid use of wool or any constricting clothing.

Encourage patient to keep nails trimmed short.

Administer medications if prescribed—antiemetics, antihistamines, vitamins.

Maintain precautions appropriate to the source of the virus.

Provide separate toilet facilities if feasible.

Use disposable dishes and utensils.

Take special precautions with excreta, blood, and blood-drawing equipment.

Avoid direct contact.

Provide diversionary activities to prevent boredom.

Teach patient importance of continuing to restrict activity during home convalescence, and provide follow-up care to monitor blood values.

Teach family measures for continuing care at home.

Describe symptoms indicative of relapse—increasing fatigue, return of nausea and vomiting, incidence of bleeding or easy bruising.

Encourage patient to avoid alcohol during the recovery period.

Evaluation

Patient maintains limited activity until liver enzymes return to normal and then gradually resumes all preillness activities.

Patient experiences minimal discomfort or pruritus.
Patient maintains social interactions and avoids boredom and depression.
Patient eats a normal diet and meets all basic nutritional needs.
Patient's skin is intact and without abrasions.
Patient's energy level and vigor return to preillness levels.

CIRRHOSIS

Cirrhosis is a term applied to several diseases that are characterized by diffuse liver inflammation and fibrosis leading to severe structural changes and significant loss of liver function. Table 11-2 describes the common forms of cirrhosis. Laënnec's cirrhosis, the most common variety, can occur at any age but is most common in 45- to 65-year-old white males and nonwhites of both sexes.

PATHOPHYSIOLOGY

Fatty infiltration of the liver is the first change seen. Acute inflammation leads to liver cell death, scar tissue formation, and cell regeneration that result in nodules of liver parenchyma surrounded by fibrous tissue. These changes distort the structure and obstruct the hepatic blood flow of the portal vein. As much as three fourths of the liver is destroyed before physiologic functioning is altered. The body attempts to circumvent the obstruction by establishing collateral circulation. Early degenerative changes produce general gastrointestinal symptoms. Later symptoms include jaundice, ascites, and edema.

MEDICAL MANAGEMENT

There is no specific treatment for cirrhosis. The emphasis is on removing or treating causative factors, provid-ing supportive care, and preventing further damage to the liver. Therapy includes diet modification, balance of rest and exercise, supplemental vitamins, and treatment of specific complications. Liver biopsy may be used to confirm the diagnosis. The box on the next page outlines the care associated with a liver biopsy.

NURSING MANAGEMENT

Assessment: Subjective

Early phase

Patient's complaints of the following:
  Weight loss
  Anorexia, nausea, and indigestion
  Intestinal dysfunction
  Pain, particularly in right upper quadrant
  Weakness and fatigue
History and severity of symptoms
History of other health problems
Normal dietary pattern
History of alcohol or drug intake

Later phase

Patient's complaint of the following:
  Easy bruising
  Hair loss—axilla, pubic area
  Menstrual irregularities or impotence

Assessment: Objective

Later phase

Jaundice
Ascites—increased abdominal girth
Muscle wasting, decreased muscle strength
Emotional behavior, orientation
Peripheral edema
Changes in amount and color of urine and stool
Presence of dilated visible abdominal veins (caput medusae)

TABLE 11-2 Types of cirrhosis

Type	Etiology	Description
Laënnec's cirrhosis (nutritional, portal, or alcoholic cirrhosis)	Alcoholism, malnutrition	Massive collagen formation; liver in early fatty stage is large and firm; in late state is small and nodular
Postnecrotic cirrhosis	Massive necrosis from hepatotoxins, usually viral hepatitis	Liver is decreased in size, with nodules and fibrous tissue
Biliary cirrhosis	Biliary obstruction in liver and common bile duct	Chronic impairment of bile drainage; liver is first large and then becomes firm and nodular; jaundice is a major symptom
Cardiac cirrhosis	Right side congestive heart failure (CHF)	Liver is swollen and changes are reversible if CHF is treated effectively; some fibrosis with long-standing CHF
Nonspecific, metabolic cirrhosis	Metabolic problems, infectious diseases, infiltrative diseases, gastrointestinal diseases	Portal and liver fibrosis may develop; liver is enlarged and firm

From Phipps WJ, Long BC, and Woods NF: Medical-surgical nursing: concepts and clinical practice, ed 4, 1990, Mosby–Year Book, Inc.

CARE OF THE PATIENT HAVING A LIVER BIOPSY

PROCEDURE
A specially designed needle is inserted through the chest or abdominal wall into the liver, and a small piece of tissue is removed for study.

PREPROCEDURE CARE
Be sure that patient understands the nature and risks of the test; informed consent is frequently required.

Explain the need to hold breath during the procedure to stabilize the liver.

Check prothrombin levels; administer supplemental vitamin K as ordered.

POSTPROCEDURE CARE
Maintain patient on bed rest for 8 to 24 hours.

Turn patient on right side for first few hours with pillows or sandbags against the abdomen to provide pressure.

Monitor patient carefully for signs of hemorrhage.

Check vital signs and do site inspection every 15 minutes for 1 hour.

Continue checking vital signs and site every 30 minutes and then hourly for remaining 24 hours.

Hemorrhoids

Palmar erythema (red palms)

Spider angiomas (tiny, red, pulsating arterioles)

Gynecomastia (breast development in males)

Decreasing level of consciousness

Abnormal liver function tests

Anemia, leukopenia, and thrombocytopenia

Nursing Diagnoses
Diagnoses depend on stage and severity of the disorder but commonly include the following:

Activity intolerance related to chronic fatigue, anemia, weight of ascites, and peripheral edema

Fluid volume excess related to increased intraabdominal pressure and decreased osmotic gradient

Potential for injury related to thrombocytopenia and leukopenia

Noncompliance with diet modification and alcohol restrictions

Altered nutrition: less than body requirements, related to fatigue and anorexia

Body image disturbance related to jaundice and ascites

Potential impairment of skin integrity related to decreased activity, ascites, and peripheral edema

Knowledge deficit related to the regimen for disease management

Expected Outcomes
Patient will have sufficient energy to maintain independence in self-care activities.

Patient will not have bleeding or infection related to depressed blood values of white cells and platelets.

Patient will make a positive adjustment to disease and express desire to comply with treatment regimen.

Patient will reestablish a normal fluid and electrolyte balance.

Patient will eat sufficient nutrients to meet the body's basic needs.

Patient will adapt to changes in appearance.

Patient will maintain an intact skin.

Patient will be knowledgeable about diet and life-style changes required by treatment regimen.

Nursing Interventions
Encourage patient to balance rest and activity.

Encourage moderate planned exercise within patient's tolerance.

Encourage patient to remain independent in activities of daily living.

Patient should maintain good hygiene and avoid exposure to infections and toxins. Alcohol is contraindicated. Patient should not take any drug not prescribed by physician.

Work with patient to modify diet yet include food preferences. Diet should include the following:

Sufficient protein to meet body repair needs (approximately 40 g of high biologic value)

Carbohydrates for energy

Low fat

Restricted sodium, adequate potassium

Make environment pleasant to encourage patient to eat. Try frequent small feedings.

Incorporate food preferences where possible.

Administer vitamins as prescribed.

Discuss measures to increase compliance with treatment regimen. Remind patient that controlling disease will be a lifelong process.

Implement measures to control pruritus.

Provide or encourage good skin care. Use antipressure foam mattresses if on bed rest.

Use high Fowler's position to support gas exchange. Encourage frequent position changes and regular deep breathing.

Encourage patient to verbalize concerns over changes in body image and function.

Teach patient the following bleeding precautions to be observed if patient is thrombocytopenic:

Use gentle mouth care and soft toothbrush.

Avoid use of straight razor.

Avoid trauma. Avoid intramuscular and subcutaneous injections.

Report presence of blood in stools or urine.

Check for bruises and petechiae daily.

Maintain pressure over venipuncture sites for several minutes.

NURSING CARE PLAN

CIRRHOSIS

Nursing Diagnoses	Expected Patient Outcomes	Nursing Interventions
Activity intolerance related to chronic fatigue, anemia, and weight of ascites	Patient has sufficient energy to remain independent in self care activities.	1. Encourage bed rest during acute phase. 2. Encourage increasing activity but space activity to allow for uninterrupted rest. 3. Intervene if patient shows fatigue after prolonged visits by family and/or friends. 4. Encourage patient to remain independent in activities of daily living.
Altered nutrition: less than body requirements, related to fatigue and anorexia	Patient ingests sufficient balanced nutrients to meet the body's basic needs.	1. Assess nutrient intake. 2. Teach patient how to plan and implement a well-balanced, high-carbohydrate diet that limits fat and total protein. 3. Focus on complete amino acids, high biologic value proteins. 4. Restrict sodium intake and explore use of alternate seasonings or salt substitutes. 5. Give antiemetics and mouth care if nausea is present. Make environment pleasant. 6. Suggest small frequent meals. 7. Administer vitamins as prescribed.
Fluid volume excess related to increased intraabdominal pressure and impaired aldosterone metabolism	Patient's fluid and electrolyte values return to normal. Patient maintains a stable weight without evidence of edema. Abdominal girth decreases.	1. Monitor for signs of peripheral edema; measure abdominal girth and weigh daily. 2. Monitor intake and output until excess fluid is excreted. 3. Teach patient rationale for sodium restriction. 4. Encourage bed rest when ascites is severe. 5. Give prescribed medications (diuretics, salt-free albumin infusions). 6. Restrict fluids if prescribed; provide fluids that are best tolerated and space these fluids throughout the day.
Potential impairment of skin integrity related to decreased activity, ascites, and poor nutrition	Patient's skin remains intact.	1. Use preventive measures to reduce effects of pressure. 2. Assess skin daily for signs of pressure or breakdown. 3. Prevent skin breakdown during bedrest. Keep skin clean and moisturized. 4. Avoid heat and heavy clothing or linens; provide a cool environment. 5. Apply antipruritic lotion to skin after bathing. 6. Keep fingernails cut short. 7. If patient must scratch, provide a soft cloth to prevent excoriations. 8. Support abdomen when positioned on side.

Continued.

NURSING CARE PLAN

CIRRHOSIS—cont'd

Nursing Diagnoses	Expected Patient Outcomes	Nursing Interventions

• Potential for injury related to thrombocytopenia and leukopenia	Patient will not experience bleeding or infection from depressed blood values.	1. Monitor for signs of infection. Auscultate lungs every 4 hours.
		2. Encourage pulmonary hygiene.
		3. Use sterile technique for all intrusive procedures.
		4. Restrict patient exposure to persons with infections.
		5. Monitor for bleeding:
		  a. Check urine and stool for blood.
		  b. Check skin and mucous membranes for signs of bleeding.
		  c. Assess regularly for petechiae and easy bruising.
		6. Avoid injections, if possible; apply pressure at all puncture sites for several minutes.
		7. Give prescribed vitamin K.
		8. Teach patient to use soft toothbrush and to avoid use of straight razor.
		9. Provide frequent gentle mouth care.

Body image disturbance related to jaundice and ascites	Patient will adapt to changes in appearance and maintain positive sense of self.	1. Encourage patient to participate in goal setting and decision making. 2. Help patient identify personal strengths and give positive feedback. 3. Assist family to understand patient's need for a positive body image and how they can help. 4. Encourage patient to verbalize concerns over body image changes. 5. Assist patient to explore ways to diminish overt signs of jaundice and ascites and thus help body image.

Knowledge deficit related to treatment regimen and needed lifestyle modifications	Patient is knowledgeable about the disease and expresses the desire to comply with the treatment regimen.	1. Teach patient:
		  a. Basis of symptoms and therapeutic regimen
		  b. Dietary and fluid restrictions
		  c. Medication therapy
		  d. Avoidance of infection and substances toxic to liver
		  e. Importance of avoiding alcohol use
		  f. Signs requiring immediate medical follow-up
		  g. Importance of regimen adherence as disease requires lifelong management.

Keep accurate intake and output records. Check weight and abdominal girth daily.

Evaluation

Patient maintains independence in the activities of daily living and resumes some preillness social activities.

Patient is free of fluid overload; electrolyte values are within normal limits.

Patient is free of infection and does not experience bleeding.

Patient is knowledgeable about treatment regimen and can discuss diet and activity modifications.

Patient maintains a stable weight and is able to eat a healthy diet within prescribed restrictions.

Patient integrates body changes and continues normal pattern of social interactions.

Patient maintains an intact skin.

COMPLICATIONS OF CIRRHOSIS

Complications tend to appear in patients with long-standing chronic liver disease. Common serious complications include ascites, portal hypertension–esophageal varices, and hepatic encephalopathy.

ASCITES

Ascites is one of the most common complications of cirrhosis and is associated with portal hypertension. The mechanisms of ascites are poorly understood but seem to be related to the following:

Decreased hepatic synthesis of albumin necessary for adequate colloid osmotic pressure

Increased portal vein pressure, which moves fluid into the peritoneal space

Obstructed hepatic lymph flow

Increased serum aldosterone level

A vicious cycle is established as escaped albumin further aggravates the osmotic balance. Fluid is retained in the abdomen and throughout the body. The abdominal fluid accumulation may be profound.

Medical Management

Restriction of sodium significantly limits the formation of ascitic fluid. Sodium is usually restricted to 1 g daily. Fluid restrictions may be required if there is evidence of dilutional hyponatremia. Bed rest facilitates reabsorption of fluid.

If conservative measures fail, then diuretics may be administered. Spironolactone (Aldactone) may be used to inhibit the reabsorption of sodium. Furosemide (Lasix) may also be used with careful monitoring of the serum potassium. Albumin may be administered to retain adequate vascular volume. If other measures fail, a peritoneovenous shunt may be placed to allow for continuous reinfusion of ascitic fluid back into the venous circulation. Special attention must be paid to position-ing, skin care, and pulmonary ventilation for patients with massive edema.

PORTAL HYPERTENSION–ESOPHAGEAL VARICES

Portal hypertension occurs when peripheral resistance is increased as distorted hepatic structures obstruct the portal blood flow. As pressure increases in the portal veins, a back flow of blood occurs into the veins that empty the spleen, stomach, and esophagus. These collateral channels become distended and varicosed as they are not anatomically equipped to handle large volumes of blood. Bleeding may occur spontaneously or be precipitated by straining, coughing, or sneezing. Severe hematemesis and resultant shock are not uncommon. The mortality rate associated with hemorrhage is 50%.

Medical Management

Treatment for bleeding varices begins with establishing the source of the bleeding. Esophagoscopy is frequently used. Measures are instituted to restore blood volume and control the bleeding. Gastric lavage may be accompanied by the injection of vasopressin (Pitressin) to reduce portal pressure and blood flow. Injection sclerotherapy may be attempted by introducing an endoscopic tube and injecting a sclerosing substance into the bleeding varicosities. Esophagogastric tamponade with a Sengstaken-Blakemore tube may also be used in cases of massive bleeding (see box on the next page and Figure 11-2). Portacaval shunting may be attempted as a last effort to control bleeding, but the mortality associated with this procedure is very high.

PORTAL SYSTEMIC ENCEPHALOPATHY

Hepatic coma is a form of metabolic encephalopathy of the brain associated with liver failure. It is believed to be precipitated by factors that increase the ammonia level or depress liver function. In liver failure, ammonia (a waste product of the breakdown of protein in the intestine) is not converted to urea and accumulates in the blood. It adversely affects the brain, and the patient exhibits changes in level of consciousness:

Impaired attention span

Irritability and restlessness

Apathy, loss of interest, lethargy, somnolence

Coma

The serum ammonia may or may not be significantly elevated. The diagnosis is made on the basis of clinical signs.

Medical Management

Treatment centers around identifying and reversing the precipitating cause. Strain on the liver is reduced by severely restricting protein in the diet temporarily, administering antibiotics to reduce ammonia-forming bacteria in the bowel, and administering enemas or cathartics to

CARE OF THE PATIENT WITH A SENGSTAKEN-BLAKEMORE TUBE

DESCRIPTION OF TUBE

The esophagogastric tube has three lumens and two balloons:

Nasogastric suction lumen
Lumen to inflate gastric balloon
Lumen to inflate esophageal balloon
Gastric balloon
Esophageal balloon

PATIENT CARE

Monitor output from tube. Correct balloon inflation will exceed portal pressure and cause esophageal bleeding to stop.

Stomach may be lavaged with ice water to provide vasoconstriction as well as pressure.

All blood must be removed from stomach to prevent its breakdown to ammonia in intestine, which can lead to hepatic coma.

Monitor patient carefully for respiratory problems.

Any shift in the tube can cause obstruction of the airway.

Patient cannot swallow around the tube and may aspirate secretions.

Measure and record balloon pressures every hour.

Provide emesis basin and tissues to handle saliva.

Use suction if needed.

Provide mouth and nasal care frequently, every 1 to 2 hours.

Administer blood or IV fluids to counter shock. Monitor vital signs frequently.

Administer medications as prescribed.

Magnesium sulfate is used to hasten excretion of blood in gastrointestinal (GI) tract.

Antibiotics lessen bacterial action on blood in GI tract.

Antacids reduce acidity and prevent esophageal reflux.

Administer enemas as prescribed to cleanse GI tract of blood.

Provide comfort measures and support to patient. Carefully explain all interventions.

Esophageal balloon is left inflated for a maximum of 48 hours.

Gastric balloon must be deflated regularly to prevent erosion and ulceration.

Instill saline cathartics or lactulose through the tube as ordered.

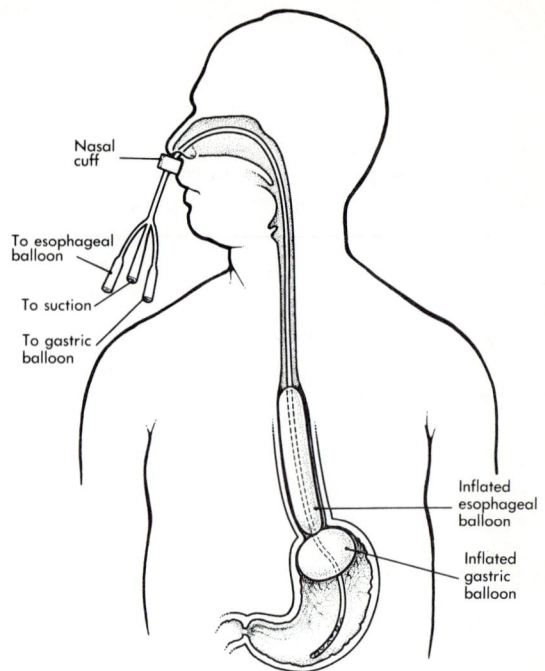

FIGURE 11-2 Sengstaken-Blakemore tube.

empty the bowel and prevent ammonia formation. Lactulose may also be given to decrease ammonia formation. General supportive care and monitoring are maintained with special attention to the prevention of infection.

BILIARY DISORDERS

The biliary system consists of the gallbladder and its associated ductal system. The principal disorders are cholecystitis (inflammation of the gallbladder) and cholelithiasis (presence of stones in the biliary tract).

These are very common disorders affecting about 20 million adults of both sexes in the United States.

CHOLECYSTITIS/CHOLELITHIASIS

Cholecystitis and cholelithiasis are frequently encountered together. Stone formation may be preceded by inflammation or follow it in a chronic form. These disorders tend to occur in middle age and afflict women more frequently than men. Other identified risk factors include a sedentary life style, multiparity, obesity, use of oral contraceptives, and the presence of associated GI diseases.

PATHOPHYSIOLOGY

Acute cholecystitis results from a blockage of the cystic duct with edema, plus spasms of the ducts and gallbladder itself. The gallbladder becomes very enlarged, thickened, and edematous. A reaction is triggered by retained bile that may impair circulation and produce ischemia. In an acute attack the patient is extremely ill, with nausea, vomiting, and severe abdominal pain. The disease may also follow a chronic pattern, causing permanent scarring and thickening over time.

Three specific factors contribute to the development of gallstones: metabolic factors, stasis, and inflammation. An increase in bile salts, bile pigment, or cholesterol may cause precipitation of the substance. About 75% of gallstones are cholesterol stones. Stasis leads to water absorption and increases the risk of precipitation.

Inflammation alters the bile constituents and may reduce the solubility of cholesterol.

Stones may lodge anywhere in the system. Biliary colic is caused by spasm of the bile ducts as they attempt to move the stone. Diagnosis is usually confirmed by cholecystogram or cholangiogram. Figure 11-3 shows common sites for gallstones.

MEDICAL MANAGEMENT

Medical management has traditionally involved surgery, although extracorporeal shock wave lithotripsy and stone dissolution therapy are now viable options for increasing numbers of patients. Medical therapy during an acute attack of inflammation involves antibiotics, nothing by mouth, analgesics, and IV fluids. A nasogastric tube is used if vomiting persists.

Chenodeoxycholic acid and ursodeoxycholic acid have been shown to be effective in dissolving small cholesterol stones, and lithotripsy is often effective when relatively small numbers of stones are present. Surgery is usually performed after the patient's condition has been stabilized. Cholecystectomy and choledocholithotomy (incision into the common bile duct) are the most common procedures.

NURSING MANAGEMENT

Assessment

Subjective
History of the problem and symptoms
History of fat intolerance, heartburn, dyspepsia
Patient's complaints of mild to severe pain and right upper quadrant tenderness, nausea and vomiting, and fever
Normal dietary pattern

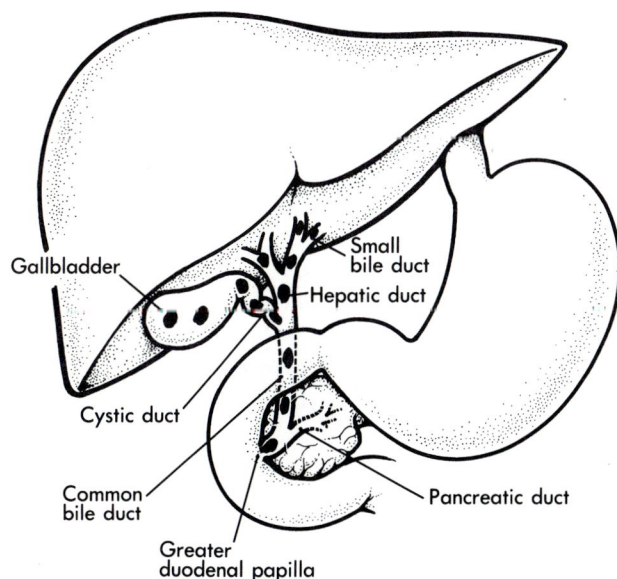

FIGURE 11-3 Common sites for gallstones.

Objective
Fever
Presence and degree of jaundice
Leukocytosis
Tenderness and rigidity in right upper quadrant, distention
Color of urine or stool (dark urine and clay-colored stools indicate obstruction)

Nursing Diagnoses
Diagnoses will depend on the severity of the disorder and approach used to manage it. Diagnoses may include the following:
Pain related to inflammation or obstruction within the gallbladder
Altered nutrition: more or less than body requirements, related to pain and vomiting
Potential impairment of skin integrity related to severe pruritus or postoperative wound drainage
Knowledge deficit related to medical disease regimen or planned surgery

Expected Outcomes
Patient will experience decreasing levels of pain and tenderness.
Patient will reestablish an adequate nutrient intake within the framework of suggested restrictions.
Patient will maintain an intact skin.
Patient will be knowledgeable about diet modifications to be followed after discharge.
Patient who is treated surgically will recover without complications.

Nursing Interventions: Acute Phase
Administer medications as prescribed for pain. Assess for effectiveness.
ALERT: Demerol is usually administered rather than morphine because it does not cause spasm in sphincter of Oddi.
Offer comfort measures. Provide position changes, skin care, fresh linen.
Give patient nothing by mouth.
Keep accurate intake and output records and monitor IV infusion.
Assess hydration status.
Provide oral care.
Maintain patency of nasogastric tube if used.
Administer antiemetics if ordered.
Offer measures to relieve itching.
Monitor stools and urine for signs of bile obstruction.
Assess patient for jaundice.
Monitor for signs of infection.
Administer antibiotics as ordered.
Teach patient principles of low fat diet.

CARE OF THE PATIENT WITH A T-TUBE

PURPOSE

To ensure patency of the common bile duct after surgical exploration. Edema produced by surgical probing can produce obstruction.

ASSOCIATED NURSING INTERVENTIONS

Attach tube to closed gravity drainage.

Never irrigate or clamp tube without direct order.

Avoid pulling or kinking tube; teach patient not to lie on it.

Monitor and record amount and color of drainage each shift.

    Initial output will be 500 to 1000 ml/day and gradually taper off as bile begins to flow again into the duodenum.

    Report presence of blood in drainage.

Change dressings as needed. Cleanse surrounding skin of bile to avoid irritation.

Assess patient's response to on and off clamping regimen if ordered.

Assess stools and urine for indications of returning bile flow.

    Suggest use of smaller, more frequent meals.

    Plan diet for patient to reduce weight if needed.

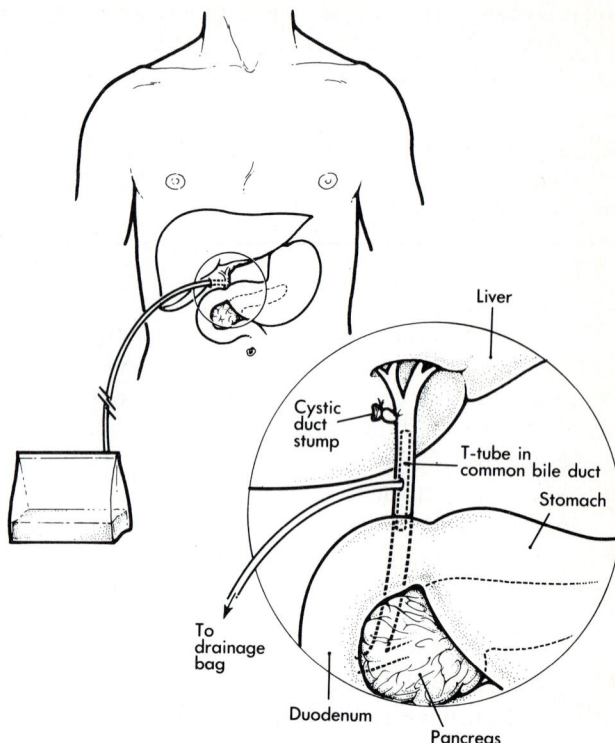

FIGURE 11-4 T-tube insertion into common bile duct.

Nursing Interventions: Preoperative

Teach patient deep breathing and coughing.

NOTE: High abdominal incision makes respiratory hygiene difficult in postoperative period.

Prepare patient for postoperative routine. Explain use of nasogastric tube or T-tube if planned.

NOTE: A T-tube will be placed for bile drainage if the surgery has involved exploration of the common bile duct for stones. Basic care is outlined in the box on this page.

Nursing Interventions: Postoperative

Administer routine postoperative care.

Provide adequate pain relief to enable good ventilation.

    Patient should cough and deep breathe every 1 to 2 hours.

    Change patient's position frequently.

    Keep patient in low Fowler's position to reduce pressure on diaphragm.

Give nothing by mouth until peristalsis resumes.

    Progress to soft, low-fat diet as tolerated.

Maintain patency of nasogastric tube if used.

Encourage ambulation.

Advance diet from clear liquids to regular or low fat.

    Assess patient's response and tolerance.

    Teach patient to avoid excessive fat intake, but no special diet is required.

Change dressing as needed. Keep skin protected from irritating bile.

Maintain patency of T-tube if used (see Figure 11-4).

Evaluation

Patient experiences no gallbladder-related pain or tenderness.

Patient maintains an adequate nutrient intake, chooses foods appropriate to well-balanced, regular or low-fat diet, and reduces to or maintains weight at desired level.

Patient is able to discuss food groups to be reduced or eliminated to maintain a low-fat diet.

Patient's incision and drainage tube sites heal without complications; pruritus is relieved.

Postsurgical patient heals without complications and returns to normal life-style.

NURSING CARE PLAN

CHOLECYSTECTOMY WITH EXPLORATION OF COMMON BILE DUCT

Nursing Diagnoses	Expected Patient Outcomes	Nursing Interventions
Ineffective breathing patterns related to pain and splinting of high abdominal incision	Patient's lungs are clear to auscultation, and chest movements are symmetrical.	1. Monitor respirations and breath sounds (especially right lower lobe) every 2 to 4 hours for 24 hours, then every 4 hours while awake until patient is ambulating well. 2. Place patient in low Fowler's position and encourage patient to change position frequently. 3. Encourage deep breathing and coughing exercises at least every 1 to 2 hours for 24 hours, then every 2 to 4 hours while awake until patient is ambulating well. 4. Provide liberal narcotic analgesia during first 72 hours, especially prior to ambulation. 5. Splint incision to encourage deep coughing. 6. Encourage use of incentive spirometer. 7. Encourage ambulation as permitted.

Potential for injury related to accidental obstruction of bile drainage	Patient does not experience obstruction or dislodgement of T-tube drainage.	1. Maintain patency of T-tube:
		  a. Connect tube to closed gravity drainage.
		  b. Provide sufficient tubing to facilitate patient mobility.
		  c. Explain to patient importance of avoiding kinks, clamping, or pulling of tube.
		2. Monitor amount and color of drainage from T-tube.
		3. Monitor color of urine and stool.
		4. Report signs of peritonitis (abdominal pain or rigidity, fever) immediately.
		5. If clamping of T-tube is prescribed before removal, monitor patient for signs of distress; if this occurs, unclamp tube and notify physician.

Pain related to incisional discomfort	Patient experiences decreasing levels of pain.	1. Assess type and quality of pain. 2. Give analgesics liberally for 48 to 72 hours after surgery. Demerol is the drug of choice. 3. If nasogastric tube is present, give mouth and nose care as needed. 4. Encourage activity. 5. Use other pain-relieving measures, as appropriate. 6. Employ measures to control itching.

Potential impairment of skin integrity related to wound drainage	Skin remains intact—incision heals without complications.	1. Assess skin around incision and stab wound with each dressing change.
		2. Change dressings as needed to maintain a dry dressing as bile is highly irritating to skin.
		  a. Use Montgomery straps if frequent changes are necessary.
		  b. Use soap and water to remove bile drainage from skin.

Knowledge deficit related to necessary diet modifications and care after discharge	Patient is knowledgeable about diet and self-care requirements after discharge.	1. Teach patient the following:
		  a. Techniques of dressing change if drainage is still occurring at time of discharge.
		  b. Any prescribed dietary changes such as low fat or low calories.
		  c. Signs to report to physician (excessive drainage, jaundice, light-colored stools).
		  d. Resumption of normal activities by 4 weeks, but avoidance of heavy activity until 6 weeks.

EXOCRINE PANCREATIC DISORDERS

PANCREATITIS

Pancreatitis is a serious inflammatory disorder of the pancreas that may be either acute or chronic. It is a relatively rare condition that usually resolves without complications but carries a 10% mortality rate. A patient may experience a single episode or recurrent attacks. The disease has been linked to alcoholism, gastrointestinal disorders, biliary tract disease, infections, and trauma. Many forms are idiopathic.

PATHOPHYSIOLOGY

Pancreatitis is theorized to develop from the activation of proteolytic enzymes within the pancreas itself. A process of autodigestion is triggered, creating severe edema, interstitial hemorrhage, coagulation, and fat necrosis. Release of histamine and bradykinin increase vascular permeability and vasodilation. A critical situation involving hypotension, shock, and desseminated intravascular coagulation may result. These processes combine to create the classic symptoms of intense pain, nausea and vomiting, and peritonitis. Serum amylase and lipase levels are significantly elevated.

In chronic pancreatitis there is permanent and progressive destruction of the pancreas, with fibrous tissue replacing the normal. It can lead to chronic insufficiency of the pancreatic hormones, producing diabetes, malabsorption, and malnutrition.

MEDICAL MANAGEMENT

The medical care for both acute and chronic forms of the disease is similar and depends on the nature and severity of the symptoms. Treatment is aimed at resting the injured pancreas while treating the major symptoms and preventing or reversing shock. Management of pain is a primary consideration. The patient is given nothing by mouth until inflammation resolves and may receive TPN (total parenteral nutrition). A nasogastric tube is placed to reduce gastrin release. Careful attention is paid to preventing or treating developing infection.

Long-term management is aimed at preventing future attacks through use of a bland, low-fat diet and frequent small meals. The patient should avoid alcohol and may receive vitamin supplements and antacids to decrease pancreatic stimulation. Lifelong administration of pancreatic extract may eventually be necessary.

NURSING MANAGEMENT

Assessment

Subjective

History of biliary disease
Pattern of alcohol use
Patient's complaints of the following:
Sudden-onset pain (acute, constant, widespread in abdomen, radiating to back, flanks, and substernal area)
Nausea and vomiting
Difficulty in breathing

Objective

Fever
Jaundice
Cyanosis
Signs of incipient shock:
Altered level of consciousness, restlessness
Tachycardia, hypotension
Poor skin turgor, clammy or dry mucous membranes
Abdominal tenderness and rigidity
Decreased bowel sounds
Decreased breath sounds
Presence of elevated amylase and lipase levels; elevated white blood cells, serum bilirubin, and glucose; decreased calcium

Nursing Diagnoses

Diagnoses may vary depending on the severity of the disorder but will commonly include the following:
Severe pain related to inflammation and obstruction within the pancreas
Actual or potential fluid volume deficit related to vomiting and hemorrhage
Altered nutrition: less than body requirements, related to nausea, vomiting, or malabsorption
Knowledge deficit related to diet and life-style modifications appropriate to decrease pancreatic activity
Potential for infection related to decreased respiratory excursion or necrotic tissue in pancreas

Expected Outcomes

Patient will experience decreasing pain.
Patient's fluid and electrolyte balance will be restored to normal limits.
Patient will have basic nutritional needs met and gradually resume oral intake.
Patient will be assisted to maintain adequate ventilation and gas exchange.
Patient will be knowledgeable about diet and life-style modifications appropriate to preventing recurrent attacks of pancreatitis.
Patient is free of preventable infection.

Nursing Interventions

Administer prescribed pain medication liberally. Demerol is usually used because it is not spasmogenic.
Position patient to achieve greatest comfort.
Suggest sitting with trunk flexed.
Suggest side-lying position with knees to chest.
Use noninvasive measures to increase comfort and relaxation.

Monitor intake and output accurately.

Administer IV fluids as ordered.

Assess patient for dehydration and incipient shock.

Monitor vital signs frequently.

Give patient nothing by mouth.

Offer frequent mouth care.

Maintain patency of nasogastric tube.

Assist patient to deep breathe and cough every 2 hours.

Auscultate breath sounds.

Assess for signs of infection.

Check urine or blood for glucose every 4 to 6 hours.

Observe for signs of hypocalcemia. Administer calcium as ordered.

Assess patient for response to oral feedings when initiated. Advance to low-fat, bland diet with five to six meals daily.

Teach patient principles of low-fat and bland diet.

Teach patient to avoid alcohol and rich foods after discharge.

Teach patient signs and symptoms to be reported:

Recurrence of pain, nausea, or vomiting

Change in bowel pattern, weight loss

Teach patient about medications ordered for chronic disease:

Pancreatic extracts given with meals

Bile salts

Oral hypoglycemics or insulin

Evaluation

Patient is free of pain.

Patient's fluid and electrolyte balance is stable as demonstrated by intake and output measures and laboratory reports.

Patient's baseline nutritional needs were met during acute phase; patient is able to ingest low-fat, bland diet without pain or nausea and maintains optimum weight.

Patient's lungs are clear to auscultation; patient is free of infection or atelectasis.

Patient modifies diet and life-style to meet needs of therapy regimen and can state rationale for restrictions.

Patient is free of infection or abscess; pancreatitis resolves.

BIBLIOGRAPHY

Adinaro D: Liver failure and pancreatitis: fluid and electrolyte concerns, Nurs Clin North Am **22**:843-852, 1987.

Anderson FP: Portal systemic encephalopathy in the chronic alcoholic, Crit Care Q **8**(4):40-52, 1989.

Birdsall C and Fiore-Lopez N: How do you manage pancreatic sump tubes?, Am J Nurs **87**:770-771, 1987.

Blake RL: Acute pancreatitis, Primary Care **15**:187-199, 1988.

Brown M: Gastroesophageal varices, Primary Care **15**:175-186, 1988.

Dobberstein K: The liver: to know it is to love it, Am J Nurs **87**:74, 1987.

Dodd RP: Ascites: when the liver can't cope, RN **47**(10):26-30, 1984.

Fain JA and Amato-Vealey E: Acute pancreatitis: a gastrointestinal emergency, Crit Care Nurse **8**(5):47-63, 1988.

Hoofnagle JH: Type D (Delta) hepatitis, JAMA **261**:1321-1325, 1989.

Jeffries C: Complications of acute pancreatitis, Crit Care Nurse **9**(4):38-46, 1989.

Keith JS: Hepatic failure: etiologies, manifestation and management, Crit Care Nurse **5**(1):60-86, 1985.

Lancaster S and Biaro-Marshall D: Gallstone lithotripsy, Am J Nurs **88**:1629-1630, 1988.

Munn NE: When the bile duct is blocked, RN **52**(2):50-57, 1989.

Rowland GA, Marks DA, and Torres W: The new gallstone destroyers and dissolvers, Am J Nurs **89**:1473-1478, 1989.

Schreeder M: Viral hepatitis, Primary Care **15**(1):157-173, 1988.

Taylor EL and Harrington TM: Cholecystitis and cholelithiasis, Primary Care **15**(1):147-157, 1988.

CHAPTER 12

Endocrine Disorders

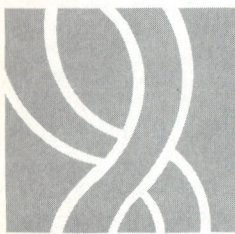

An alteration in the function of the endocrine glands may result in a wide variety of signs and symptoms because of the diversity of physiologic functions that are under hormonal control. Disorders may be primary or secondary to disorders present elsewhere in the body or system. Some of the disorders occur frequently; others are relatively rare. This chapter discusses the major disorders of hyperfunctioning or hypofunctioning of the endocrine glands. Figure 12-1 shows the anatomical structure of the endocrine system.

ANTERIOR PITUITARY DISORDERS

The largest section of the pituitary is the anterior portion, which plays a major role in regulating the functioning of the individual endocrine glands. Table 12-1 lists the major hormones of the anterior pituitary and their functions. Dysfunctions may be related to individual hormones or combinations of them. Table 12-2 presents various anterior pituitary disorders and their distinguishing characteristics.

HYPERPITUITARISM

Hyperpituitarism may result from a primary problem in the pituitary gland or occur secondary to a dysfunction of the hypothalamus. The most common cause of hyperpituitarism is pituitary adenoma. The adenomas are frequently classified according to the type of hormone they secrete. Prolactin-secreting tumors account for 60 to 80% of the total. Adenomas cause symptoms related to the hypersecretion of hormones or pressure on surrounding neurologic tissue. Pituitary hyperfunctioning may also result from hyperplasia of pituitary tissue, usually as a failure of feedback mechanisms.

PATHOPHYSIOLOGY

Hypersecretion of the pituitary hormones—adrenocorticotropic hormone (ACTH), growth hormone (GH), prolactin, and thyroid stimulating hormone (TSH)—is commonly identified during a workup for adrenal, menstrual, or thyroid dysfunction. Depending on which hormone is being oversecreted, a wide variety of effects may be seen (see Table 12-2). Patients frequently wait to seek help until symptoms of rising intracranial pressure occur. The growing tumor may put pressure on surrounding brain structures including the optic chiasm, cranial nerves III, IV, and VI, and the frontal or temporal lobes.

TABLE 12-1 Hormones of the anterior pituitary gland

Hormone	Functions
Thyroid stimulating hormone (TSH)	Stimulates thyroid to secrete thyroxin
Adrenocorticotropic hormone (ACTH)	Stimulates adrenal cortex to secrete cortisol
Gonadotropic hormones	
Luteinizing hormone (LH)	Induces ovulation and stimulates formation of corpus luteum and progesterone secretion in female
Follicle-stimulating hormone (FSH)	Stimulates follicle growth in ovary and secretion of estrogen in female
Interstitial cell–stimulating hormone (ICSH)	Stimulates secretion of testosterone in male
Growth hormone (GH) (somatotropin [STH])	Stimulates body growth; influences protein, carbohydrate, and fat metabolism
Prolactin	Stimulates mammary gland development

Adapted from Long BC and Phipps WJ: Essentials of medical-surgical nursing: a nursing process approach, ed 2, St Louis, 1989, The CV Mosby Co.

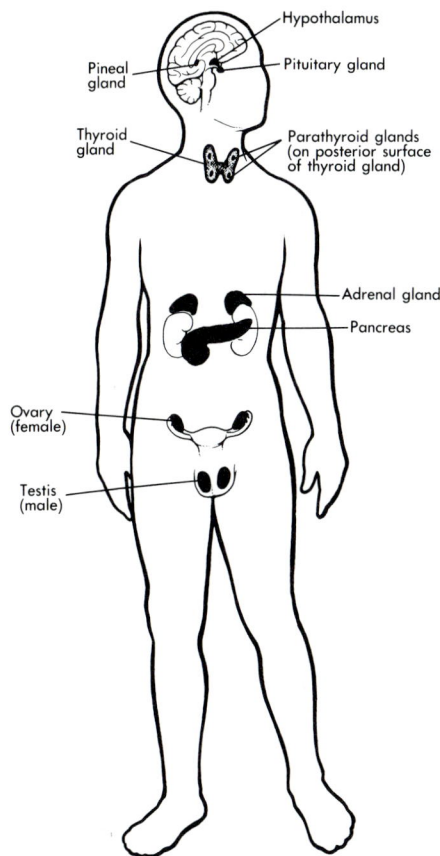

FIGURE 12-1 Endocrine system.

Serum and urine tests reveal elevated hormone levels and CT scans may be used to confirm the presence and size of the adenoma.

MEDICAL MANAGEMENT

Treatment is aimed at decreasing abnormal hormone levels and removing the adenoma. Bromocriptine (Parlodel) may be used with prolactin-secreting tumors to restore hormone levels to normal, restore fertility, and reduce tumor size. GH- and ACTH-secreting tumors are usually treated surgically via transsphenoidal hypophysectomy in which the sella turcica is entered from below through the sphenoid sinus. The patient will require either temporary or long-term replacement of anterior pituitary hormones after surgery.

Radiation therapy may be used as an adjunct or alternative to surgery, but the response rate is slow and the incidence of posttreatment hypopituitarism is high.

NURSING MANAGEMENT

Assessment

Subjective
History of symptoms: progression, severity
Menstrual changes in females
Impotence or changes in libido in males
Patient's understanding of diagnosis and treatment plan
Patient's complaints of the following:
    Visual changes or deficits
    Changes in hat, shoe, or glove size
    Muscle weakness, changes in energy level
    Peripheral sensory changes
    Frontal or temporal headache
    Changes in facial appearance
    Persistent sweating, increased oiliness of skin

Objective
Coarse facial features, enlarged tongue, abnormal body proportions
Husky voice
Warm, moist, coarse skin
Elevated blood pressure
Early signs of increasing intracranial pressure
Changes in cranial nerve functioning
Height and weight changes

Nursing Diagnoses
Diagnoses depend on the severity of the disorder but commonly include the following:
    Knowledge deficit related to etiology and management of endocrine disorders
    Body image disturbance related to effects of excess growth hormone
    Sensory/perceptual alteration (visual) related to pressure of tumor on the optic nerve
    Potential fluid volume deficit related to failure of ADH secretion in postoperative period

Expected Outcomes
Patient will be knowledgeable about the disorder and be able to describe the treatment plan and potential for reversibility of current symptoms.
Patient will be assisted in resolving feelings about changed body appearance into a positive body image.
Patient will learn how to compensate for any permanent changes in visual perception to maintain a safe environment
Patient with diabetes insipidus will reestablish a normal intake and output balance.

Nursing Interventions: Preoperative
Assist patient to control headache—mild analgesics, darkened room, relaxation strategies.
Teach patient about proposed surgical procedure.
    Explain that there is no external incision with transsphenoidal approach. Incision is made through space between upper gums and lip.
    Explain that a graft is taken from leg to pack sella turcica and reconstruct its floor.
Explain that soft tissue changes will gradually decrease but most of the bony changes are irreversible.

TABLE 12-2 Anterior pituitary dysfunction

Alteration in Secretion	Etiology	Signs and Symptoms
GH excess	Pituitary tumors Pituitary hyperplasia	Gigantism in children Acromegaly in adults: growth of soft tissues, cartilages, bones Enlargement and coarsening of facial features Enlarged tongue Visceral enlargement (liver, spleen, heart, kidneys) Warm, moist, coarse skin; increased sweating Husky voice Hypertension
GH deficit	Infection Granuloma Trauma Congenital tumor	Dwarfism in children Immature voice and facial features Sensitivity to insulin Hypoglycemia No symptoms in adults
ACTH excess	Pituitary tumors or hyperplasia Nonpituitary secreting tumor Iatrogenic from chronic steroid use	Similar to Cushing's syndrome (adrenocortical excess)
ACTH deficit	Same as GH deficit Iatrogenic suppression of hypothalamic-pituitary axis by exogenous corticosteroids	Similar to Addison's disease (adrenocortical deficiency) Asthenia (weakness) Nausea, vomiting Hypotension, hypoglycemia Hyponatremia, hyperkalemia
TSH excess	Pituitary tumor or hyperplasia	Same as hyperthyroidism (thyroid hormone excess)
TSH deficit	Same as GH deficit	Same as hypothyroidism (thyroid hormone deficit) Cretinism in newborn Myxedema in adult
Prolactin excess	Pituitary tumor Idiopathic Side effect of certain drugs that interfere with secretion	Amenorrhea, galactorrhea, depressed libido, infertility, impotency, change in secondary sex characteristics
Prolactin deficit	Same as GH deficit	Usually no clinical symptoms in adults
Gonadotropic hormone excess	Same as GH deficit	Hirsutism in female

Gonadotropic hormone deficit	Same as GH deficit	Delayed sexual development in children
		In adults:
		  Amenorrhea, infertility in female
		  Impotence in male
		  Changes in secondary sex characteristics in both males and females

Adapted from Long BC and Phipps WJ: Essentials of medical-surgical nursing: a nursing process approach, ed 2, St Louis, 1989, The CV Mosby Co.

Teach patient rationale for temporary or long-term hormone replacement.

Nursing Interventions: Postoperative—

Transsphenoidal Approach

NOTE: See Chapter 3 for discussion of care of the craniotomy patient.

Assess for cerebrospinal fluid (CSF) leakage—should seal within a few days.

Check patient's complaint of postnasal drip or frequent swallowing.

If leak occurs, patient is maintained on bed rest with head of bed elevated.

Test drainage for halo ring formation on gauze pad or positive glucose test. Send specimen to laboratory.

Instruct patient not to do the following:

Cough, sneeze, or blow nose

Bend over

Strain at isometric exercise or stool

Monitor patient for signs of infection. Administer antibiotics as prescribed.

Encourage frequent oral hygiene. Patient should rinse

mouth with saline or mild mouthwash and clean teeth with toothettes.

ALERT: Patient should not brush teeth at first as this may disrupt the suture line.

Provide oxygen or humidity if prescribed. Encourage deep breathing.

Advance to diet as tolerated but avoid rough foods.

Monitor for signs of diabetes insipidus.

Weigh daily.

Observe for polydipsia and polyuria (>200 ml/hr)

Watch for dilute urine with 1.000 to 1.005 specific gravity.

Keep accurate intake and output records every 2 to 4 hours.

Maintain adequate fluid at bedside.

Teach patient correct use of vasopressin (Pitressin) if diabetes insipidus is not self-limiting or if there is inadequate fluid replacement.

Teach patient about medications prescribed for temporary or long-term replacement: cortisol, gonadotropins, or thyroid replacement.

Explain to patient importance of long-term follow-up and regular checkups.

Evaluation

Patient is knowledgeable about residual hormone deficits and can discuss purpose, schedule, and side effects of prescribed medications.

Patient resolves feelings about altered body image and speaks positively about self and body; patient resumes former social activity pattern.

Patient has adequate visual perception and maintains a safe environment.

Patient compensates for diabetes insipidus by increasing fluid intake; patient maintains normal fluid and electrolyte balance.

HYPOPITUITARISM

Hypopituitarism may result from vascular lesions, developmental disorders, trauma or surgery, and tumors. It may involve only one or all of the hormones of the anterior pituitary. Deficits in growth hormone and gonadotropins appear first. The clinical picture will vary with specific hormones, severity of the deficits, and the age of the patient. Treatment involves identifying the deficiency and replacing the deficient hormones, with careful long-term follow-up.

POSTERIOR PITUITARY DISORDERS

The posterior pituitary secretes two hormones: oxytocin and antidiuretic hormone (ADH). The primary disorders of the posterior pituitary involve excesses and deficits of ADH secretion.

ADH EXCESS: SYNDROME OF INAPPROPRIATE ADH

The syndrome of inappropriate ADH (SIADH) involves a continual release of hormone that is unrelated to serum osmolality. Water is retained, extracellular fluid volume expands, and dilutional hyponatremia occurs. The syndrome is associated with diseases, trauma, and surgery of the nervous system, extreme stressors, and, most commonly, oat cell carcinoma of the lung, where the cells actually secrete ADH.

The patient retains water and exhibits the weakness, lethargy, and central nervous system changes characteristic of hyponatremia (see Chapter 1). Treatment is directed at restoring the plasma sodium levels. Water retention is managed by water restriction of 800 to 1000 ml per day, combined with the administration of hypertonic (3%) saline and diuretics if the patient's condition worsens. The syndrome is usually self-limiting, and responds promptly to treatment.

ADH DEFICIT: DIABETES INSIPIDUS

True diabetes insipidus in which the posterior pituitary fails to secrete ADH is quite rare, but the symptoms are seen fairly commonly after trauma, with pituitary tumor, or after hypophysectomy. Without ADH to stimulate reabsorption from the renal tubules, as much as 15 L of fluid may be excreted daily, with the potential for serious fluid and electrolyte imbalance. If fluid is not replaced. dehydration and vascular collapse occur rapidly.

Treatment is aimed at correcting the underlying condition if possible and providing adequate hormone replacement. Initial therapy will begin with subcutaneous administration of aqueous vasopressin (Pitressin). If long-term management is needed, a synthetic solution of vasopressin is administered by nasal spray or drops. Associated nursing interventions are included in the discussion of anterior hyperpituitarism.

THYROID GLAND DISORDERS
HYPERTHYROIDISM

Hyperthyroidism is a condition that results from excessive secretion of thyroxine (T_4) and/or triiodothyronine (T_3). It is a common disorder that primarily affects women aged 20 to 40. Hyperthyroidism occurs in several forms, all of which share similar clinical symptoms. The two most common forms are Graves' disease and toxic nodular goiter.

PATHOPHYSIOLOGY

Although the exact etiology of Graves' disease is unknown, it appears to involve an autoimmune glandular stimulation by immunoglobulins that may have a genetic or familial component. It follows the classic pattern of exacerbation and remission. Hyperthyroidism from toxic nodular goiter is a generally milder form of the disease that is characterized by the presence of nodules within the thyroid that oversecrete thyroxin.

In the hyperthyroid state the normal regulatory control of thyroid function is lost. The excess thyroid hormone produces increased metabolic rate, increased cardiac and respiratory stimulation, and increased sympathetic adrenergic activity (see Table 12-3 for thyroid hormone functions).

Graves' disease is characterized by a triad of goiter, hyperthyroidism, and exophthalmos. The mechanism behind exophthalmos is poorly understood, but increased deposits of fats and fluids in the tissues behind the eye lead to protrusion of the eye and even incomplete eye closure, which can cause serious damage. Exophthalmos is rarely present in other forms of hyperthyroidism.

MEDICAL MANAGEMENT

Therapy is aimed at reducing thyroid hormone levels and controlling other signs and symptoms. This may be done by using antithyroid drugs, removing thyroid tissue through surgery, or destroying thyroid tissue by radioactive iodine. The choice of treatment approach is based on the patient's age and sex and the size of the goiter. Radioactive iodine is the treatment of choice for most adults with Graves' disease. Drug therapy is usually the initial form of treatment since patients must be in a euthyroid state before definitive treatment is undertaken. Table 12-4 lists drugs frequently used to treat hyperthyroidism.

NURSING MANAGEMENT

Assessment

Subjective

History of symptoms and severity

Family history of thyroid disease

Patient's complaints of the following:

Nervousness and irritability

Exaggerated emotions and mood swings

Heat intolerance

Palpitations, anginal pain

Fatigue and muscle weakness

Increased hunger plus weight loss

Menstrual irregularities, decreased libido and fertility

Abdominal discomfort, frequent soft stools

Objective

Body weight and proportions

Skin appearance and texture:

Dermopathy

TABLE 12-3 Functions of the thyroid gland hormones

Hormone	Functions
Thyroxine (T_4) and triiodothyronine (T_3)	Regulates protein, fat, and carbohydrate catabolism in all cells
	Regulates metabolic rate of all cells
	Regulates body heat production
	Insulin antagonist
	Necessary for muscle tone and vigor
	Maintains cardiac rate, force, and output
	Affects central nervous system development
	Maintains secretion of gastrointestinal tract
	Affects respiratory rate and oxygen utilization
	Maintains calcium mobilization
	Affects red blood cell production
	Stimulates lipid turnover, free fatty acid release, and cholesterol synthesis
Thyrocalcitonin	Lowers serum calcium and phosphorus levels by inhibiting osteoclastic activity
	Decreases calcium and phosphorus absorption in gastrointestinal tract

From Long BC, and Phipps WJ: Essentials of medical-surgical nursing: a nursing process approach, ed 2, St Louis, 1989, The CV Mosby Co.

TABLE 12-4 Drugs used in the treatment of hyperthyroidism

Drug	Actions
Antithyroid Drugs	
Propylthiouracil (PTU) Methimazole (Tapazole)	Block thyroid hormone synthesis; slow-acting drugs that may take 2 to 4 weeks to produce noticeable improvement; approximately 50% achieve remission
Iodine Preparations	
Lugol's solution	Block the synthesis and release of thyroid hormone, producing rapid reduction in metabolic rate; do not have a sustained effect, but reduce gland vascularity and are frequently given preoperatively
Beta-Adrenergic Blockers	
Propranolol (Inderal)	Used to treat tachycardia, arrhythmia, and angina symptoms that may accompany hyperthyroidism; used for all patients in thyroid storm

　　Presence of sweating or reddening
　　Fine thin hair
　Tachycardia; signs of congestive heart failure
　Elevated systolic blood pressure
　Fine tremors
　Exophthalmos;
　Goiter

Nursing Diagnoses

Diagnoses will depend on the severity of the disease and its treatment but commonly include the following:

　Activity intolerance related to easy fatigability of muscles

　Altered nutrition: less than body requirements, related to excess metabolic rate

　Sleep pattern disturbance related to irritability and hyperactivity

　Body image disturbance related to the occurrence of goiter or exophthalmos

　Anxiety and nervousness related to excess nervous system activity

Expected Outcomes

Patient will regain muscle strength and endurance and resume preillness activity pattern.

Patient will ingest sufficient nutrients to meet body needs and maintain desired weight.

Patient will sleep uninterrupted at night for at least 6 hours.

Patient will incorporate body changes into an altered but positive self-concept.

Patient will feel in control of body and environment.

Nursing Interventions

Establish a calm, quiet environment.
　Keep temperature cool.
　Assign patient to room away from major activities.
Assist patient to plan activities to foster rest.
Patient should avoid activities needing fine coordination.
Assist patient to understand physiologic basis for nervousness and moods.
Provide high-calorie, high-protein diet.
　Keep snacks at bedside.
　Maintain adequate fluid intake.
　Patient should avoid caffeinated substances.
Chart daily weights.
Provide care for exophthalmos.
　Restrict dietary sodium.
　Keep head of bed elevated.
　Protect cornea from ulceration and infection; patch eye if lid closure is incomplete.

CARE OF THE PATIENT RECEIVING RADIOACTIVE IODINE THERAPY

Treatment is given on an outpatient basis and involves a one-time oral liquid treatment with ^{131}I. Symptoms decrease slowly, and a euthyroid state is achieved in about 6 months. Patient should be monitored for the development of hypothyroidism in the future.

CARE AND TEACHING

Radiation precautions are not usually needed. Isotope has a short half-life and is quickly bound in the gland.

Small levels of isotope will be excreted in body secretions during first 48 hours:
　Flush toilet two or three times after use.
　Increase intake of oral fluids.
　Avoid prolonged physical contact with infants and young children.

Teach patient to anticipate some soreness and discomfort in the throat after treatment.

Medical follow-up is essential as the treatment may induce hypothyroidism.

　Administer methylcellulose eye drops for comfort.
　Teach patient to use wrap-around sunglasses outdoors for protection from wind, sun, and dust.
　Encourage patient to verbalize feelings about altered appearance.

Teach patient about radioactive iodine treatment if prescribed (see box on this page).

Administer and teach patient about prescribed medications (see Table 12-4).

Provide preoperative teaching if surgery is scheduled.
　Teach patient importance of supporting head with hands after operation to prevent stress on sutures.
　Explain to patient that talking may be difficult initially. (The box on p. 181 presents postoperative care associated with thyroidectomy.)
　Teach patient importance of ongoing medical supervision.

Evaluation

Patient's muscle strength and endurance return to preillness levels.

Patient establishes and maintains desired weight; adjusts intake to meet decreased metabolic needs.

Patient enjoys restful sleep pattern.

Patient incorporates permanent changes into a revised body image and speaks positively of self.

Patient no longer experiences anxiety and feels in control of body and environment.

NURSING CARE PLAN

HYPERTHYROIDISM

Nursing Diagnoses	Expected Patient Outcomes	Nursing Interventions
Anxiety related to excess nervous system activity	Patient understands reason for change in behavior. Emotional lability is minimized. Patient feels in control of environment.	1. Discuss reasons for emotional lability. 2. Maintain calm, relaxed environment. Teach and reinforce relaxation strategies. 3. Encourage visitors who promote relaxation. 4. Provide privacy (such as single room). 5. Explain all interventions. 6. Avoid stimulants such as coffee, tea, cola, alcohol. 7. Help patient identify previous successful coping mechanism or explore new mechanisms. 8. Avoid activities requiring fine motor coordination. 9. Decrease known stressors, explain planned interventions, and listen to patient's concerns. Administer prescribed drugs and document therapeutic response.
Altered nutrition: less than body requirements, related to excess metabolic rate	Patient will ingest sufficient nutrients to meet body needs and maintain desired weight.	1. Monitor weight every other day or weekly. 2. Help patient plan for high-calorie, high-protein, high-carbohydrate diet, selecting foods from all food groups. Assess for abdominal discomfort and frequency of stools. 3. Suggest six small meals per day or between meal snacks. Keep snacks at bedside. 4. Use supplements such as Ensure if necessary. 5. Encourage adequate fluid intake to replace losses.

Potential for sensory/perceptual alterations (visual) related to eye changes of exophthalmos	Patient will employ measures to prevent eye damage.	1. Assess visual acuity, ability to close eyes, photophobia.
		2. Protect eyes from irritants:
		  a. Use patches or glasses for excess light or wind or if eyes cannot completely close.
		  b. Use artificial tears if prescribed to keep eyes moist.
		  c. Elevate head of bed at night.
		3. Encourage patient to restrict dietary sodium.

Potential for hypothermia related to excess heat production	Patient will maintain a stable body temperature and is comfortable in the environment.	1. Control environmental temperature for comfort (fans may be helpful). Monitor vital signs. 2. Suggest patient take frequent showers. 3. Encourage adequate fluid intake to replace losses.
Activity intolerance related to easily fatigued muscles	Patient will regain muscle strength and endurance and resume preillness activity pattern.	1. Assess activity schedule. 2. Suggest ways to modify fatiguing activities. 3. Identify activities that can be done by others until condition is controlled. 4. Balance periods of activity with rest. 5. Encourage activities that promote sleep at night.
Body image disturbance related to the occurrence of goiter or exophthalmos	Patient will incorporate body changes into an altered but positive body image.	1. Encourage patient to verbalize feelings about altered appearance. 2. Provide patient with factual information about the degree of reversibility of symptoms. 3. Support positive coping efforts. 4. Teach patient about self-care.

CARE OF THE PATIENT AFTER THYROIDECTOMY

MONITORING FOR COMPLICATIONS

Check for signs of the following:
　Hemorrhage
　　Bleeding on dressings behind neck and on pillow
　　Increased difficulty in swallowing
　　Choking sensation
　　Sensation of dressing tightness
　Vocal cord edema
　　Hoarseness
　　Dyspnea
　Laryngeal nerve damage
　　Difficulty in speaking, hoarseness
　　Persistent or worsening respiratory distress; obstruction; crowing sound
　Injury to parathyroid glands (hypocalcemia)
　　Positive Chvostek's and Trousseau's signs; tetany
　　Numbness and tingling in fingertips and around lips
ALERT: It is imperative to have a tracheostomy set and calcium gluconate available at the bedside in case of complications.

GENERAL CARE

Introduce fluids and soft diet with caution; supervise swallowing. Advance diet as tolerated.
Maintain patient in semi-Fowler's position to avoid stress on sutures.
Use a humidifier if indicated.
Encourage activity. After 5 to 7 days, initiate range of motion exercises for the neck.
Teach patient about any drugs required after discharge.

HYPOTHYROIDISM

Hypothyroidism is a metabolic state resulting from deficient thyroid hormone, which may occur at any age. It may be idiopathic or result from a congenital deficiency, iodine deficiency, or drugs. The most common cause is surgical or radioactive destruction of the gland. Congenital hypothyroidism produces a condition called cretinism. Myxedema is a severe adult form of hypothyroidism that has a significant mortality.

Hypothyroidism is theorized to occur frequently in the elderly and is frequently undiagnosed. Early signs of hypothyroidism are vague, with cold intolerance, constipation, weakness, and lethargy occurring commonly. Sluggishness, weight gain, and sleepiness are also common. As the disease progresses, the patient exhibits slowed intellectual functioning, dry skin, and diminished reflexes. The patient with advanced myxedema may lapse into coma.

Treatment involves lifelong replacement of deficient thyroid hormone. Synthroid, Cytomel, Trionine, and Euthroid are among the drugs in use. Relief of symptoms begins within 2 to 3 days of therapy.

PARATHYROID DYSFUNCTION

The parathyroid glands secrete parathyroid hormone (PTH), which maintains serum calcium and phosphorus levels by controlling bone resorption, gastrointestinal absorption, and urinary excretion of these minerals. Disorders of the parathyroid glands are extremely rare but are being diagnosed more often as a result of the increased frequency of routine calcium measurement.

HYPERPARATHYROIDISM

The most common cause of primary hyperparathyroidism is benign adenoma. It may also result from the chronic hypocalcemia associated with renal disease or malabsorption. It tends to occur in adults aged 30 to 60, more commonly in females.

PATHOPHYSIOLOGY

Hypersecretion of parathyroid hormone produces an elevated serum calcium level and a decreased phosphorus level. The increased calcium can increase bone resorption, leading to pathologic fracture. The renal calcium reabsorption can predispose the patient to kidney stones and causes gastrointestinal symptoms and mental changes varying from confusion and depression to outright psychosis. Relatively small elevations in calcium may cause impaired mentation and memory, particularly in the elderly. Calcium imbalance is discussed in Chapter 1.

MEDICAL MANAGEMENT

Surgery, usually the removal of three glands and a portion of the fourth, is the treatment of choice for most patients with primary hyperparathyroidism. The electrolyte imbalance must be corrected prior to surgery, however. This is usually accomplished by rehydration and physiologic flushing with isotonic sodium chloride, combined with dietary restriction and a diuretic to enhance calcium excretion. Mithramycin may be used to lower serum calcium in patients whose renal or cardiovascular function is inadequate to handle high-volume sodium chloride flushing. Severe hypocalcemia is common in the immediate postoperative period while calcium is taken up by the bones.

NURSING MANAGEMENT

Assessment
　Subjective
　History and severity of presenting symptoms
　History of renal or cardiovascular disease
　History of renal stones
　Normal dietary pattern
　Patient's complaints of the following:
　　Anorexia, nausea, or vomiting
　　Fatigue and muscle weakness

Bone or joint pain

Polyuria, polydipsia, and constipation

Alteration in mental status or personality, such as depression, stupor, behavior changes

Objective

Intake and output balance

Depressed reflexes and muscle strength

Elevated serum calcium levels, decreased phosphorus levels

Mental status evaluation

Nursing Diagnoses

Diagnoses may vary with the severity of the disorder but commonly include the following:

Constipation related to decreased gastrointestinal functioning

Bone pain related to demineralization

Altered nutrition: less than body requirements, related to anorexia and nausea

Alteration in thought processes related to effects of calcium on cerebral tissue

Potential fluid volume deficit related to excess urination and nausea

Potential for injury related to muscle weakness and bone demineralization

Expected Outcomes

Patient will return to a normal bowel elimination pattern.

Patient will experience decreasing bone pain.

Patient will resume a normal dietary pattern adequate to meet basic body needs.

Patient will return to preillness level of mental functioning and exhibit no ongoing depression or behavioral changes.

Patient will be restored to a normal fluid volume balance.

Patient will not experience injury or fracture.

Nursing Interventions

Monitor vital signs for cardiac problems.

Monitor intake and output accurately.

Maintain IV fluids as ordered.

Assess for signs of renal stones.

Help patient balance rest and activity to preserve energy.

Ensure weight-bearing activity each day to preserve bone structure.

Assist patient with activities of daily living as needed.

Teach patient rationale for low-calcium diet.

Encourage use of acid ash diet or ascorbic acid supplements in diet to acidify urine.

Encourage patient to drink large amounts of fluid.

Encourage frequent mouth care.

Offer small frequent feedings if anorexia is present.

Teach patient importance of fiber and bulk in diet and adequate fluids to prevent constipation. Administer prescribed medications, such as stool softeners or cathartics.

Maintain environmental safety.

Keep side rails up; supervise ambulation.

Assess patient's mental status regularly.

Provide encouragement and stimulation.

Position patient for comfort; handle extremities gently.

Teach patient about proposed surgery and postoperative routine.

Provide standard postoperative care for parathyroidectomy, which is very similar to that for thyroidectomy patients.

ALERT: The serum calcium level will decrease within 24 hours, and patients are monitored closely for tetany as their serum calcium levels fall. Calcium replacement will be given until function normalizes.

Evaluation

Patient has a normal bowel elimination pattern and passes soft stool regularly without need for laxatives or stool softeners.

Patient experiences no further bone pain and is able to resume former activities.

Patient is free of nausea and eats a normal diet; patient modifies diet appropriately if indicated to enrich or restrict calcium content.

Patient's mental status is at preillness levels; patient returns to normal social activities without ongoing depression or behavior changes.

Patient has a normal fluid balance and experiences no inappropriate thirst or urination.

Patient is knowledgeable about any prescribed medications and recognizes the importance of ongoing medical supervision.

Patient does not experience injury during the acute period.

HYPOPARATHYROIDISM

Hypoparathyroidism is a metabolic disorder that results in hypocalcemia. It commonly occurs after thyroid or parathyroid surgery, but may be idiopathic. It can produce serious effects as decreased calcium levels lead to neuromuscular irritability, tetany, laryngeal stridor, and cardiac arrhythmias.

Treatment involves the early identification of symptoms so prompt intervention is possible. Calcium gluconate is given intravenously for immediate replacement. Vitamin D and supplemental dietary and elemental calcium are prescribed, and the patient is taught to follow a vitamin D–rich diet and to recognize the early signs of calcium deficiency.

ADRENAL GLAND DISORDERS

Dysfunction of the adrenal gland may result from hypersecretion or hyposecretion by either the cortex or the medulla. Table 12-5 lists the hormones secreted by the adrenal gland and their functions.

HYPERSECRETION OF THE ADRENAL CORTEX: CORTISOL EXCESS

Excessive levels of glucocorticoids from whatever cause produce a classic group of symptoms called Cushing's syndrome. Primary Cushing's syndrome is seen most frequently in females in the second to fourth decade. Major causes of cortisol excess include the following:

Increased release of ACTH from the pituitary

Excess cortisol secretion from adenoma or carcinoma of the cortex (primary Cushing's syndrome)

Increased release of ACTH from an ectopic source such as bronchogenic or pancreatic cancer

Iatrogenic Cushing's syndrome as a complication of chronic corticosteroid therapy, which is the most frequent cause seen in clinical practice; the end result is cortisol excess with a loss of normal diurnal secretory patterns

PATHOPHYSIOLOGY

The effects of cortisol excess produce widespread changes in body appearance and function. These changes are presented in Table 12-6. The metabolic dysfunctions result from an exaggeration of all known hormone actions affecting all aspects of metabolism, the immune response, and emotional stability. They place the patient at higher risk for several chronic illnesses: peptic ulcer, osteoporosis, psychoses, hypertension, and diabetes mellitus.

Adrenal tumors may also cause oversecretion of the other adrenal hormones. Aldosterone excess will produce hypokalemia, hypernatremia, and hypertension from fluid volume excess. Excess androgen will result in masculinizing effects in the female.

MEDICAL MANAGEMENT

Effective treatment is dependent on identifying and removing the cause of hypersecretion. Surgical treatment may involve transsphenoidal hypophysectomy of a pituitary tumor, or unilateral or bilateral adrenalectomy. Drug treatment, which may be used as an adjunct to surgery or radiation, uses mitotane, aminoglutethimide, or metyrapone, which block cortisol synthesis. Adrenalectomy will necessitate lifelong hormone replacement. Skilled supportive care is essential while hormonal balance is being reestablished. Care in iatrogenic Cushing's syndrome is aimed at reducing the steroid dose or controlling symptoms.

TABLE 12-5 Hormones of the adrenal gland

Portion of Gland	Hormones	Functions
Adrenal cortex	Glucocorticoids (cortisol)	Overall effect is to maintain blood glucose level by increasing gluconeogenesis and decreasing rate of glucose utilization by cells
		Increase protein catabolism
		Promote lipolysis
		Promote sodium and water retention
		Antiinflammatory, decrease new antibody release
		Decrease T-lymphocyte participation in cell-mediated immunity by decreasing circulating level of T-lymphocytes
		Increase neutrophils by increasing release and decreasing destruction
		Decrease scar tissue formation, degrade collagen
		Increase gastric acid and pepsin production, stimulate appetite
		Maintain emotional stability
	Mineralocorticoids (aldosterone)	Major stimulus in renin-angiotensin system
		Primarily responsible for maintenance of normovolemic state by increasing sodium and water retention in distal tubules
		Cause potassium excretion
	Androgens	Same functions as gonadal sex hormones
Adrenal medulla	Epinephrine and norepinephrine	Necessary for maintenance of neuroendocrine integrating functions of body
		Elevate blood pressure, increase heart rate, and cause vasoconstriction
		Stimulate conversion of glycogen to glucose for emergency fuel
		Stimulate gluconeogenesis
		Increase lipolysis

Modified from Long BC and Phipps WJ: Essentials of medical-surgical nursing: a nursing process approach, ed 2, St Louis, 1989, The CV Mosby Co.

TABLE 12-6 Effects of excess adrenocortical secretion

Hormone	Characteristic and Effect
Cortisol	Appearance
	Moon face
	Altered fat metabolism
	Deposits of adipose tissue on back of neck and shoulders
	Truncal obesity
	Muscles and bones
	Thin extremities from muscle wasting
	Easy fatigability
	Osteoporosis, depletion of protein matrix of bone
	Skin
	Loss of collagen support
	Thinning of the skin
	Pale purplish striae
	Bruises and petechiae
	Flushed face
	Cardiovascular
	Excess fluid volume, sodium and water retention
	Hypertension
	Gastrointestinal
	Increased secretion of HCl
	Metabolism
	Postprandial hyperglycemia
	Immune system
	Inhibition of immune response and inflammation, decreased lymphocytes, impaired wound healing
	Emotions
	Euphoria or irritability
	Excitability or depression
Aldosterone	Fluid and electrolytes
	Severe sodium and water retention
	Severe hypokalemia
Androgens	Skin
	Hirsutism in females
	Reproductive
	Menstrual irregularities
	Changes in libido

NURSING MANAGEMENT

Assessment

Subjective

History and severity of symptoms

Patient's perception of the problem

Perceived changes in body appearance and proportions: skin, hair, body weight

Patient's complaints of the following:

   Fatigue—onset, severity, interference with activities of daily living

   Edema or weight gain

   Changes in appetite and thirst; indigestion

   Mood swings or instability

   Menstrual irregularities

Recent infections, slowed wound healing

Change in normal dietary pattern

Medications in use

History of other chronic health problems

Objective

Daily weights

Vital sign patterns, hypertension

Intake and output balance, daily food intake

Urine and blood glucose levels

Body appearance (see Table 12-6)

Muscle mass and strength

Energy level, self-care abilities

Skin integrity

Laboratory values showing increased cortisol; hypokalemia

Secondary sex characteristics

Nursing Diagnoses

Diagnoses may vary according to the severity of the disorder but commonly include the following:

   Activity intolerance related to muscle fatigability

   Fluid volume excess related to sodium and water retention

   Potential for infection related to skin changes and decreased immune response

   Knowledge deficit related to mechanisms of the disorder and measures to control symptoms

   Altered nutrition: more than body requirements, related to decreased activity, increased appetite, and altered metabolism

   Potential for injury related to bone demineralization and muscle weakness

   Body image disturbance related to changes in appearance

   Anxiety related to the physical and emotional changes produced by excess glucocorticoids

Expected Outcomes

Patient will balance rest and activity while muscle strength and endurance improve.

Patient will maintain a stable weight and show no signs of peripheral edema.

Patient will take measures to avoid exposure to infection.

Patient will be knowledgeable about disorder and treatment and comply with treatment regimen.

Patient will adjust diet pattern to compensate for hyperglycemia and fluid excess characteristic of the disease.

Patient will maintain a positive body image while waiting for physical changes to reverse or lessen.

Patient will maintain positive control and coping during diagnostic and treatment period.

Patient will not experience injury or fracture during acute period.

Nursing Interventions

Monitor vital signs frequently.

Maintain accurate intake and output records.

Measure blood glucose and urinary sugar and acetone as ordered every 4 to 8 hours.

Protect patient from staff, other patients, and visitors with infections.

Teach patient importance of good hygiene. Assess for early signs of infection.

Teach patient principles of, and purpose of, diet modification. Diet should be low in calories, high in protein, low in sodium, and high in potassium. Restrict fluids if prescribed.

Record daily weights.

Administer antacids as prescribed. Guaiac test stools for blood.

Encourage patient to verbalize feelings about body changes.

Provide ongoing support. Teach and reassure about reversibility of most symptoms.

Balance rest and activity.

Encourage patient to take short walks to combat osteoporosis.

Assist patient with activities of daily living as needed.

CARE OF THE PATIENT EXPERIENCING ADRENALECTOMY

PREOPERATIVE

Teach patient about proposed surgery and care routines to be followed postoperatively.

Teach usual coughing and deep breathing exercises.

POSTOPERATIVE

Monitor vital signs frequently as adrenal function tends to be very labile. Vasopressors may be needed.

Maintain infusions of cortisol as prescribed.

Maintain accurate records for intake and output, blood glucose, urine glucose, and ketones.

Observe patient for signs of hypoglycemia.

Monitor for signs of adrenal crisis, which include severe weakness, nausea and vomiting, and hypotension.

Monitor adequacy of urine output regularly.

Monitor wound healing.

Maintain strict asepsis.

Introduce activity gradually and assess patient's response.

Maintain adequate pain relief and effective splinting to facilitate coughing.

Initiate teaching concerning medication regimen prescribed:

Medication may be needed for lifelong replacement.

Close supervision is needed during initial months to adjust dose.

Patient should be alert for signs of hormone excess or deficit.

Patient should be cognizant of situations that will increase need for hormone, such as physical or emotional stress or illness.

Keep environmental stimuli at low levels.

Decrease physical and emotional stressors where possible.

Assist patient to control and understand mood swings.

Teach patient about widespread disease effects and proposed treatment.

Monitor patient for edema or early symptoms of congestive heart failure and hypertension.

Modify diet.

Follow good hygiene practices.

Patient should avoid infection.

Teach patient signs and symptoms of complications.

Teach patient with iatrogenic Cushing's syndrome measures that will minimize effects of steroid therapy:

Always take steroids with food or antacid as the risk of peptic ulcer is high.

Weigh daily and report any abrupt weight gain or edema.

Exercise and walk regularly to reduce bony demineralization.

Have regular follow-up and eye exams (drugs stimulate cataract formation).

Obtain and wear a Medic Alert bracelet.

Teach patient that steroid drugs must be withdrawn slowly; it takes time for the adrenal glands to recover from suppression.

NOTE: Interventions for patients being treated with adrenalectomy are outlined in the box on this page.

Evaluation

Patient is able to engage in normal activities without the onset of fatigue.

Patient exhibits no signs of fluid excess; blood pressure is in normal range.

Patient maintains scrupulous personal hygiene and is free of preventable infection.

Patient is knowledgeable about the disease and treatment and can discuss prescribed diet and medication regimen.

Patient follows a controlled-calorie, low-sodium diet and is able to maintain a stable weight.

Patient incorporates changes in body image into a positive sense of self.

Patient is free of anxiety and is knowledgeable about long-term disease management.

Patient follows a regular weight-bearing exercise program and is free of injury or fracture.

HYPOSECRETION OF THE ADRENAL CORTEX

A decrease in adrenocortical secretions may result from idiopathic atrophy of the gland, insufficient ACTH secretion by the pituitary, or glandular atrophy from long-term suppression with glucocorticoid therapy. Deficiencies in glucocorticoids lead to impairments in metabolism and an inability to maintain a normal glucose level.

Deficiencies in mineralocorticoids produce fluid and electrolyte problems. Early symptoms are often vague and insidious. Table 12-7 lists the common symptoms of deficiency. Adrenocortical hormones are essential to life and must be replaced.

Adrenal crisis (Addisonian crisis) occurs when there is a severe exacerbation of the insufficiency. It is a sudden, life-threatening condition that may be precipitated by the sudden cessation of steroid therapy or situations that create a sudden need for more cortisol than is available, usually in a previously undiagnosed individual who experiences a major stressor. The syndrome is characterized by severe hypotension, cardiovascular collapse (shock), hyperpyrexia (extremely high fever), hypoglycemia, hyponatremia, and coma.

Adrenal insufficiency is treated by administration of the deficient hormones, which are given and adjusted until symptoms abate. Patients must be helped to understand the serious nature of the disorder and the importance of taking their medications regularly and avoiding situations of undue stress. Periods of stress may necessitate doubling or tripling of the usual dosage.

HYPERSECRETION OF THE ADRENAL MEDULLA: PHEOCHROMOCYTOMA

Pheochromocytoma is a rare catecholamine-producing tumor that occurs in individuals in middle age. It is usually unilateral and benign. It produces malignant hypertension that may be labile or persistently elevated. Diagnosis is usually made during a workup for hypertension that is unresponsive to traditional therapy.

Initial treatment is aimed at controlling blood pressure through alpha- and beta-adrenergic blocking agents. Surgical resection of the tumor is the treatment of choice for a stabilized patient. Blood pressure instability is a common problem in the postoperative period, and the patient requires careful monitoring. The remainder of the care is similar to that for any adrenalectomy patient. Most individuals have a complete recovery.

PANCREATIC HORMONE DYSFUNCTION: DIABETES MELLITUS

Diabetes is a complex chronic disease involving disorders in carbohydrate, fat, and protein metabolism that lead to the development over time of microvascular and macrovascular complications and neuropathies. With over 6 million known diabetics it is a major health problem and, despite extensive research, remains a major cause of death and disability. Although it occurs at all ages, diabetes occurs most commonly in adults over 40. The incidence rate increases steadily with age. Although the cause remains unknown, diabetes is thought to be a group of disorders with various precipitating causes. Viral and autoimmune factors are believed to contribute plus a genetic or inherited base, which may play a permissive role. Environmental factors may trigger the onset in susceptible persons. A current classification system for diabetes is presented in Table 12-8.

PATHOPHYSIOLOGY

The primary function of insulin is to promote the transport of serum glucose across the cell membrane where it may be used for energy, stored as glycogen, or converted into fat. In diabetes there is an absolute or relative deficiency of insulin and its action. The pathology of IDDM and NIDDM are quite different.

In IDDM there is an absolute deficiency of insulin secretion from beta cell destruction. Hyperglycemia develops as the serum glucose increases beyond the 110 mg/100 ml normal limit. When the glucose level exceeds the renal threshold (usually about 180 mg/100 ml), glucose is excreted in the urine, producing glycosuria. Since glucose is hyperosmolar, it creates an osmotic diuresis and carries large amounts of water and electrolytes with it, producing polyuria, which can lead to dehydration and electrolyte imbalance. This fluid loss triggers thirst in the patient and polydipsia.

Amino acid transport into the cells also requires insulin. In its absence the metabolism of fatty acids is impaired and lipolysis occurs rapidly. A cellular starvation occurs, leading to increased mobilization of fats and proteins for energy. Ketone bodies, the acidic metabolites of fats, accumulate in the blood, causing ketosis and ketonuria. This inefficient energy source produces weak-

TABLE 12-7 Signs of adrenal insufficiency

Characteristic	Signs and Symptoms
Appearance	Patient has lost weight; appears fatigued
Skin	Bronze coloration of skin and mucous membranes from increased levels of melanocyte-stimulating hormone
Musculoskeletal	Severely weak and fatigued muscles
Cardiovascular	Hypotension
	Risk of complete vascular collapse
Gastrointestinal	Anorexia
	Cramping abdominal pain
	Diarrhea
	Nausea and vomiting, weight loss
Metabolism	Hypoglycemia
Fluid and electrolytes	Hyponatremia
	Hyperkalemia
	Fluid deficit
Mental-emotional	Lethargy, depression
	Loss of vigor

TABLE 12-8 Classification system for diabetes mellitus

Class	Characteristics
Insulin-dependent diabetes mellitus (IDDM): type 1	Persons are insulinopenic and depend on exogenous insulin to prevent ketoacidosis and sustain life.
	Onset of symptoms is abrupt, usually occurring while a youth and almost always before age 30.
	With certain HLA types, an autoimmune mechanism and precipitation by an environmental factor, such as a viral infection, have been associated with susceptibility and onset.
Non–insulin-dependent diabetes mellitus (NIDDM): type 2	Persons do not depend on insulin to sustain life but may be treated with insulin in special circumstances; they are resistant to ketoacidosis except during periods of excessive stress.
	Onset is usually after age 40, without classic symptoms.
	Associated with endogenous insulin levels that may be mildly depressed, normal, or high and with tissue insensitivity to insulin.
	Obesity and heredity have been associated with susceptibility and onset.
Gestational diabetes mellitus (GDM)	Person has onset of glucose abnormality during pregnancy.
	Women with known diabetes mellitus who become pregnant are not classified in this group.
	After delivery, the woman is reclassified on the basis of blood or plasma glucose testing.
Malnutrition-related diabetes mellitus	Persons require insulin.
	Diabetes mellitus found in tropical areas.
	It occurs in young adults with histories of nutritional deficiencies.
	Ketosis is not usually present.
Other types of diabetes mellitus	Diabetes mellitus may be associated with other disorders such as pancreatic disease, other endocrine diseases, drugs, and genetic syndromes.

From Phipps WJ, Long BC, and Woods NF: Medical-surgical nursing: concepts and clinical practice, ed 4, St Louis, 1990, Mosby–Year Book, Inc.

ness and hunger in the patient, resulting in polyphagia (excessive eating).

In NIDDM the serum insulin levels may be increased, decreased, or normal. Insulin release may be slowed or delayed, and the number of insulin receptors may be decreased. A postreceptor defect may also be present. There appears to be impaired suppression of hepatic glucose production.

The individual with diabetes is susceptible to a number of long-term complications resulting from macrocirculatory and microcirculatory changes and neuropathies.

Macrovascular Changes

Diabetics develop the same atherosclerotic vessel changes as do nondiabetics, but the incidence and severity of the changes are both earlier and more rapid. These macrovascular changes significantly increase the risk for coronary artery disease, cerebrovascular disease, and hypertension, and contribute to the development of peripheral vascular disease.

Microvascular Changes

Microvascular changes appear to be related to thickening of the capillary basement membranes. Nephropathy and retinopathy are very common, and renal failure is a frequent outcome. Microvascular changes contribute to widespread peripheral vascular disease; these vessel changes do not occur in nondiabetic persons.

Neuropathy

Changes in nerve structure and function are pervasive among diabetics. The sensory fibers are usually affected in a bilateral and symmetrical pattern. Sensory loss in the distal lower extremities is the most common form of involvement. The impairments occur slowly and are progressive. The diabetic foot is of particular concern. Autonomic changes are also common and may involve control of the bladder, sexual functioning, and the gastrointestinal tract.

Other Changes

Diabetics are more susceptible to infection because of the accumulation of glucose in the skin and impairments in the response of white blood cells in a glucose-rich environment.

MEDICAL MANAGEMENT

The goal of therapy is to establish adequate daily control and to delay or prevent the development of complications. Adjusting to and controlling the disease require a carefully planned program. Controversy exists over exactly how strict the control needs to be, and the treatment goals should be planned with the patient. Elements include the following:

1. *Diet.* A diabetic's diet is calculated to distribute nutrients effectively over a 24 hour period. Carbohydrates account for about 50% to 60% of the daily calories, proteins 20%, and fats about 30%.

The American Diabetes Association (ADA) exchange system diet has been most commonly utilized (Tables 12-9 and 12-10).

2. *Medications.* Subcutaneous insulin administration is used for all patients with IDDM. Oral hypoglycemic agents may be prescribed for patients with NIDDM who cannot be managed by diet and weight control alone (Tables 12-11 and 12-12).

3. *Exercise.* A regular planned activity and exercise program maximizes general health and can improve glucose utilization as well as help in weight loss. (See box on this page.)

4. *Teaching and support.* An individualized approach to teaching is used to maximize the individual's knowledge of the disorder and thus enhance intelligent self-management.

NURSING MANAGEMENT

Assessment

Subjective: newly diagnosed patient

Presence of classic signs of hyperglycemia:
Polyuria, nocturia
Polydipsia, polyphagia (excessive eating)

GUIDELINES FOR EXERCISE IN DIABETES

Exercise decreases the need for insulin.
Use aerobic exercise and start slowly. All patients with NIDDM should have a cardiovascular evaluation before starting an exercise program.
Exercise three to five times each week.
Always carry a rapid-acting glucose source during exercise.
Be sure to eat or snack prior to exercise.
Monitor carefully for signs of hypoglycemia.
Be sure to wear shoes that fit properly while exercising.
Avoid strenuous exercise during peak insulin action.

Nausea, abdominal discomfort
Weight loss
Fatigue, weakness, lethargy
Presence of other chronic diseases involving the kidneys, blood vessels, or metabolism
Presence or history of obesity
Current dietary and activity pattern
Coping pattern and history

TABLE 12-9 Exchange system for meal planning

Meat Exchange

Lean Meat
1 oz lean beef, pork, veal, or poultry without skin
2 oz fish
¼ C dry cottage cheese
¼ C tuna, mackerel
1 oz diet cheese (<55 calories/oz)

Medium-Fat Meat
1 oz 15%-fat beef, boiled ham, or liver
1 egg†

High-Fat Meat
1 oz 20%-fat beef, ground pork, duck, or regular cheeses
1 frankfurter
1 oz lunchmeat
1 T peanut butter (contains unsaturated fats)

Fat Exchange‡
1 t margarine
⅛ avocado
1 t oil
1 strip crisp bacon
1 t regular mayonnaise
1 T reduced-calorie mayonnaise
1 T cream cheese

Free Exchanges
Unsweetened gelatin
Calorie-free beverages
Coffee, tea, spices, bouillon

Milk Exchange
1 C skim or nonfat milk
1 C plain nonfat yogurt
½ C skim powdered milk
1 C skim buttermilk
1 C lowfat yogurt
1 C lowfat (2%) milk

Vegetable Exchange* (Nonstarchy)
½ C COOKED, 1 C RAW
beets, carrots, brussel sprouts, onions, sauerkraut, eggplant, asparagus, cabbage, celery, green or wax beans, or mustard greens
1 medium tomato

Fruit Exchange
1 small apple, orange, peach, tangerine, or pear
½ C applesauce
½ banana or grapefruit
⅓ cantaloupe
⅛ honeydew melon

Bread Exchange (Includes Starchy Vegetables)

1 slice bread	½ C oatmeal
½ bagel, 1 tortilla	½ C cooked pasta
½ hamburger bun	⅓ C rice
½ small baked potato	6 saltines
⅓ C corn, ½ C peas	

---

*Some vegetables, such as lettuce, raw spinach, radishes, and watercress, can be used as desired.
†Eggs and other foods high in cholesterol need to be restricted.
‡Margarine and oil should be made from corn, cottonseed, safflower, soy, or sunflower oil.

TABLE 12-10 Sample of two menu plans using the exchange list*

Exchanges	Menu I	Menu II
Breakfast		
1 Fruit	½ Glass orange juice	½ Grapefruit
1 Milk (skim)	1 Glass skim milk	1 Glass skim milk
1 Meat (medium-fat)	1 Egg, poached	1 Scrambled egg
3 Bread	2 Toast, ½ C oatmeal	1 English muffin, ½ C bran flakes
2 Fat	2 tsp Margarine	2 tsp Margarine
Lunch		
1 Fruit	½ Banana	1 Peach
1 Milk (skim)	1 Glass skim milk	1 Glass skim milk
2 Meat (lean)	Tuna salad sandwich (½ C water-packed tuna	1 MacDonald's cheeseburger (2 bread, 2 meat,
2 Bread	with celery, 2 slices of bread, 3 tsp mayonnaise	1 fat)
3 Fat	and lettuce)	1 Lettuce salad with 2 tbsp French dressing
Afternoon Snack		
1 Bread	6 Saltine crackers	¾ oz Pretzels
1 Fruit	1 Pear	15 Grapes
Dinner		
1 Fruit	¾ C strawberries or 1 apple	½ C Applesauce
2 Vegetable (nonstarchy)	1 C green beans	Sliced tomatoes
4 Meat (lean)	4 oz Round steak	4 oz Chicken
1 Milk (skim)	1 Glass skim milk	1 Glass skim milk
2 Bread	1 Small baked potato, 1 roll	½ C Rice, 1 slice bread
3 Fat	2 tbsp Sour cream/2 tsp margarine	3 tsp Margarine
Evening Snack		
1 Bread	3 Rye wafers	6 Saltine crackers
1 Milk	1 C Nonfat yogurt	1 Glass skim milk

*Distributed over three meals and two snacks. Diet based on 2100 calories with 48% CHO (253 g), 31% fats (71 g), 21% protein (112 g).

TABLE 12-11 Hypoglycemic agents (insulins)

Type of Insulin	Time of Onset (hr)	Peak of Action (hr)	Duration of Action (hr)
Rapid acting			
Regular	<1	2-4	4-6
Crystalline zinc	<1	2-4	4-6
Semilente	<1	4-7	12-16
Intermediate acting			
NPH	1-4	8-14	16-20
Globin zinc	2-4	6-10	12-18
Lente	1-4	8-14	16-20
Slow acting			
Protamine zinc	4-8	16-18	36+
Ultralente	4-8	8-20	36+

TABLE 12-12 Oral hypoglycemic agents

Drugs	Duration of Action (hr)	Dosage Range
Acetohexamide (Dymelor)	12-24	500 mg-1.5 g
Chlorpropamide (Diabinese)	24-48	100 mg-500 mg
Tolazamide (Tolinase)	12-24	100 mg-1 g
Tolbutamide (Orinase)	6-12	500 mg-3 g
Glipizide (Glucotrol)	12-24	5 mg-40 mg
Glyburide (Micronase)	24	2.5 mg-20 mg

Adapted from: Phipps WJ, Long BC, and Woods NF: Medical-surgical nursing: concepts and clinical practice, ed 4, St Louis, 1990, Mosby–Year Book, Inc.

Subjective: formerly diagnosed patient
Knowledge of and attitude toward diabetes and regimen adherence
Normal dietary pattern
  Patient's knowledge of prescribed diet
  Family shopping and cooking patterns
Presence of paresthesias or pruritus
Hypoglycemic agents in use
Self-care knowledge and skills:
  Insulin administration/site rotation
  Blood or urine testing and record keeping
  Foot care
  Use of ADA exchange system

Knowledge of hypoglycemia and ketoacidosis and
their prevention and treatment

Knowledge of need to adjust regimen with illness
or exercise

Changes or problems in sexuality—libido or impotence

Objective
Body weight
Vital signs
Blood and urine glucose concentrations
Skin turgor and condition of mucous membranes
Urine volume and specific gravity
Intake and output balance
Assessment for ketoacidosis if applicable (see box on
p. 193)
Neurovascular changes in lower extremities:
Changes in touch, pain, and temperature sensation
Peripheral pulses
Temperature of extremities
Skin appearance: color, intactness, and texture
Visual changes

Nursing Diagnoses

Diagnoses depend on the recency of diagnosis and the
extent of complications but commonly include the following:

Actual or potential fluid volume deficit related to the
hyperosmolar fluid loss that occurs with hyperglycemia

Potential for injury and infection related to circulatory and nerve impairment in the extremities

Potential for noncompliance related to the diet and
life-style modifications prescribed for diabetes
treatment

Altered nutrition: potential for less than or more than
body requirements, related to impaired glucose utilization or the presence of obesity

Sensory/perceptual alteration (tactile) related to paresthesias and peripheral neuropathies

Knowledge deficit related to the self-care skills necessary for successful self-management of diabetes

Potential for ineffective individual coping related to
the life-style changes mandated by the treatment
of diabetes

Potential for sexual dysfunction related to autonomic
nervous system impairment

Expected Outcomes

Patient will return to a normal fluid and hydration status as blood glucose is normalized.

Patient will practice scrupulous hygiene and foot care to
prevent the development of extremity complications.

Patient will maintain effective control of diabetes and
maintain a normal occupational and social life-style.

Patient will maintain desired weight and meet body's

DIETARY RECOMMENDATIONS FOR DIABETIC PATIENT

Calorie allotment should be sufficient to promote normal
growth and development in the child and maintenance
of ideal weight in the adult.

Most of the carbohydrate calories should come from
starches. Sharp limitations are placed on refined sugars.

Diet should contain 15 to 40 g of plant fibers from natural
sources each day. Fiber decreases both fasting and post-
prandial glucose levels. Increase water intake as well.

The amount of saturated fat in use should be less than
10%.

Consistency in the timing and distribution of nutrients
and meals is very important in IDDM.

Achieving and maintaining desired weight is very important in NIDDM.

Special or "dietetic" foods are not required; their content
should be analyzed carefully if they are used.

Small amounts of alcohol may be planned into the diet if
this will help to foster patient's adjustment and compliance. Avoid high-calorie drinks like beer and cordials.

nutritional needs through proper diet and medication
usage.

Patient will take measures to compensate for sensory
losses in the extremities to prevent injury.

Patient will have adequate knowledge of diabetes and its
treatment and demonstrate the necessary self-care
skills.

Patient will demonstrate positive coping behaviors and
meet age-specific developmental tasks while maintaining effective disease control.

Patient will not develop skin infections and ulcerations.

Patient will maintain satisfactory patterns of sexuality
and have knowledge of options for implants.

Nursing Interventions: Diet

Initiate diet teaching (see the box on this page for
guidelines).

Patient's diet plan should take the following into consid-
eration:
Personal and cultural preferences where possible
Life-style and occupational considerations
Exercise and activity pattern
Timing of medication usage

Teach patient to calculate menus using the ADA exchange system (see Tables 12-9 and 12-10 for examples).

Teach patient how to adapt food choices to shift work,
eating in restaurants, vacation and business travel,
and social events.

Teach patient about the relationship of exercise to diet
and how to establish a safe exercise program (see box
on p. 188).

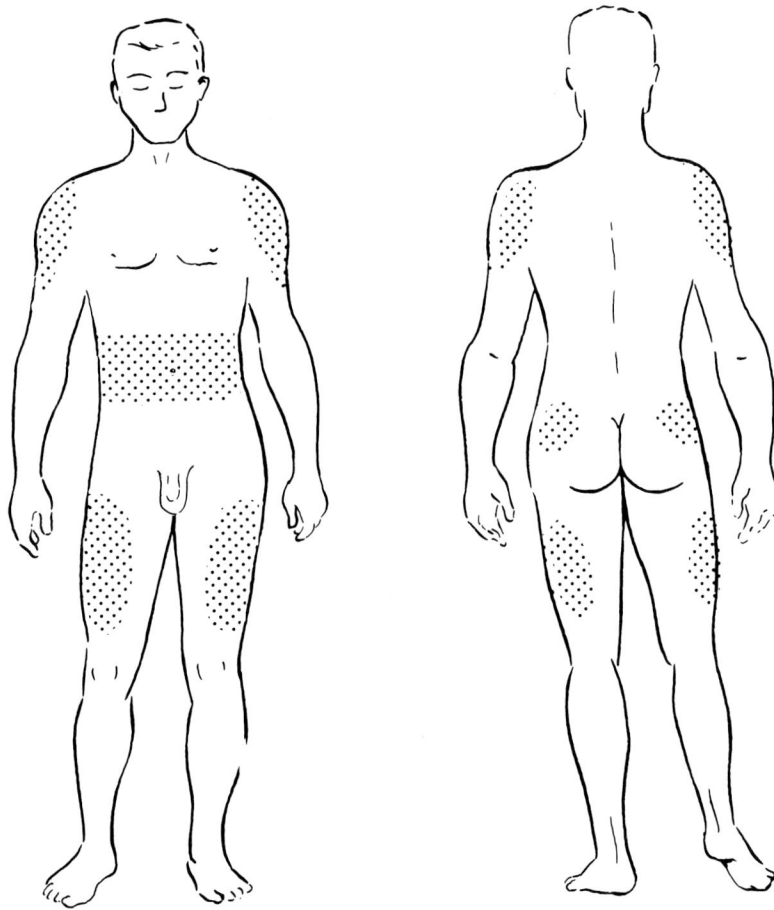

FIGURE 12-2 Arms, legs, buttocks, or abdomen can be used for insulin injections. A different site (indicated by each dot) should be used for each injection. (From Phipps WJ, Long BC, and Woods NJ: Medical-surgical nursing: concepts and clinical practice, ed 4, St Louis, 1990, Mosby–Year Book, Inc.

Teach patient how to adapt diet during gastrointestinal upset or illness.

Encourage patient to verbalize and discuss perceived effects of diet restrictions on normal desired life-style.

Nursing Interventions: Medications

Teach patient and family about prescribed insulin.

Explain onset, peak, and duration of action.

Explain that food must be taken within the time of onset for insulin prescribed.

Explain importance of planning a snack for time of peak action of insulin.

Explain importance of bedtime snack for patients on long-acting insulin to provide glucose coverage for the night.

Teach patient relationship of insulin need and illness.

Insulin needs are greater during illness; patient should never skip a dose.

Patient should adjust diet to liquids if necessary but maintain intake.

Patient should increase frequency of blood and urine testing and contact physician if hyperglycemia worsens.

Teach patient the proper preparation and administration of insulin (see box on next page).

Encourage patient to utilize all available sites to avoid the development of lipodystrophies (see Figure 12-2 for acceptable insulin sites).

Minimize antigenicity with the use of highly purified pork or human insulins.

GUIDELINES FOR INSULIN ADMINISTRATION

Always use an insulin syringe calibrated in the same unit/ml scale that matches the scale of the insulin.

Select insulin according to type, strength, species, and brand name as specified by the prescription.

Rotate or gently roll the bottle if it is other than regular or globin insulin.

Examine *intermediate* and *long-acting* insulin vials for appearance and expiration dates; do not use unless solution is cloudy.

Check for and remove any air bubbles after insulin is drawn into the syringe (do not use an air bubble to clear the needle after injection).

When mixing insulins, do not vary the sequence in which two insulins are drawn into the same syringe; usually air is injected into both bottles (regular and intermediate); the insulin is withdrawn first from the regular vial and then from the longer acting insulin vial.

Rotate injection sites using all sites in one geographic area before moving to another. Document sites on rotation grid (see Figure 12-2).

Do not use one geographic area more than once every 4 to 6 weeks. Injection sites should be 1 to 1½ inches apart.

Insert the needle into the area beneath the fatty tissue using a 45 to 90 degree angle as appropriate.

Store currently used insulin at room temperature; refrigerate extra supplies.

Keep extra supplies on hand and immediately available when traveling.

GUIDELINES FOR DIABETIC FOOT CARE

Wear well-fitting shoes and clean stockings at all times when ambulating; never walk barefooted.

Bathe feet daily and dry them well, paying particular attention to areas between the toes. Keep skin softened with bland cream or petroleum jelly.

Do not self-treat calluses, corns, or ingrown toenails; a podiatrist should be consulted if these are present.

Cut toenails straight across, and smooth with emery board.

Bath water should be 29.5 to 32° C (85 to 90° F) and should be tested with a bath thermometer or the elbow before immersing the feet.

Heating pads and hot water bottles should be avoided.

Measures that help increase circulation to the lower extremities should be instituted:
  Avoid smoking.
  Avoid crossing legs when sitting.
  Protect extremities when exposed to cold.
  Avoid immersing feet in cold water.
  Use socks or stockings that do not apply pressure to the legs at specific sites.
  Institute a regimen of regular exercise.
Inspect feet daily and report any cuts, cracks, redness, blisters, or other signs of trauma so early treatment can be instituted.

From Long BC and Phipps WJ: Essentials of medical-surgical nursing: a nursing process approach, ed 2, St Louis, 1989, The CV Mosby Co.

Nursing Interventions: Testing

Teach patient technique of blood or urine testing:
  Describe method to use and number of times it should be done per day or week.
  Explain importance of accurate record keeping.
ALERT: Patients who do blood glucose testing should still test their urine for ketones, especially when ill.

Explain importance of recording urine results by percent since the scales vary with different brands of equipment.

Explain how to interpret the results.

Tell when to notify the physician.

Explain importance of increasing the frequency of testing during illness.

Nursing Interventions: Hygiene

Teach patient importance of scrupulous hygiene. Keep skin supple and dry.

Explain importance of meticulous care for even minor trauma to skin.

Describe methods for prevention of peripheral vascular disease (see box on next page for foot care principles).

Nursing Interventions: Adjustment

Encourage patient to discuss feelings and frustrations about treatment regimen.

Include appropriate family members in teaching sessions.

Explain importance of wearing Medic Alert tag or bracelet.

Assist patient to problem solve for control of difficult periods in daily life-style.

Support and reinforce all positive coping behaviors.

Support involvement in self-help groups.

Nursing Interventions: Complications

Teach patient to recognize signs of hypoglycemia, blood glucose < 50 mg/100 ml (see box on next page).
  Hypoglycemia is usually related to too much insulin or exercise, and too little food.
  Reverse effects with 10 to 15 g of a rapidly absorbed glucose source, such as:
    ½ cup fruit juice or sugar cola
    4 cubes or 2 packets sugar
    2 squares graham crackers
    2 or 3 pieces of hard candy
  When symptoms resolve, offer additional food, either a scheduled meal or a complex carbohydrate and protein such as cheese or crackers and peanut butter.

Teach patient to recognize symptoms of ketoacidosis (see box on next page).

SIGNS AND SYMPTOMS OF HYPOGLYCEMIA

SYMPATHETIC NERVOUS SYSTEM ACTIVITY
(usually precedes CNS manifestations)

Pallor	*Perspiration
Piloerection	Hunger
Tachycardia	Palpitation
*Nervousness	Irritability
*Weakness	Trembling

CENTRAL NERVOUS SYSTEM ACTIVITY

Headache	Blurred vision
Diplopia (double vision)	Incoherent speech
Emotional changes	Fatigue
*Mental confusion	Numbness of lips, tongue
Convulsions	Coma

*Four most commonly reported by patients (Paulk, 1983).
From Long BC and Phipps WJ: Essentials of medical-surgical nursing: a nursing process approach, ed. 2, St Louis, 1989, The CV Mosby Co.

Ketoacidosis is usually related to insufficient insulin, too much food, or the presence of illness or infection, which increases insulin requirements.

Emphasize importance of taking insulin when ill and increasing frequency of glucose testing.

Treatment requires hospitalization (see box on this page).

NOTE: Another complication—hyperglycemic, hyperosmolar, nonketotic coma (HHNC)—may occur in diabetics with NIDDM or in elderly persons with no history of diabetes. The serum glucose becomes extremely high, but the condition is not associated with ketosis. The signs and symptoms and treatment principles for HHNC are outlined in the box on this page. This complication has a high mortality.

Evaluation

Patient maintains an adequate fluid and electrolyte balance and maintains blood glucose within desired levels.

Patient can discuss importance of good hygiene to prevent complications and practices good preventive foot care.

Patient maintains good control of diabetes while participating fully in occupational, social, and recreational pursuits.

Patient can describe basic prescribed meal plan, chooses and follows a balanced diet, makes correct adjustments to maintain control while traveling or eating out, maintains desired weight, and properly adjusts diet to changes in activity and occurrence of illness.

Patient compensates for sensory losses in extremities by

KETOACIDOSIS

Onset of ketoacidosis is slow.

SYMPTOMS
Increased thirst
*Nausea and vomiting, anorexia
Abdominal cramping
*Lethargy

SIGNS
Increased temperature
*Kussmaul breathing (deep and rapid)
*Fruity acetone odor to breath
*Hot, dry, flushed skin
Loss of skin turgor
Decreasing level of consciousness to coma

MEDICAL AND NURSING CARE
Restore fluid balance with isotonic saline
Reduce plasma glucose with low-dose continuous infusion of regular insulin.
Replace potassium and other electrolytes after adequate urine volume is restored and on the basis of serum values.
Monitor vital signs, intake and output, level of consciousness, and peristalsis.
Reassure patient and provide comfort measures

*Classic signs and symptoms.

SIGNS AND TREATMENT OF HYPERGLYCEMIC, HYPEROSMOLAR, NONKETOTIC COMA (HHNC)

SIGNS
Fluid deficit

Dehydration	Circulatory collapse
Hypotension	Elevated body temperature
Anuria	

Neurologic changes

Sensory deficits	Aphasia
Motor deficits	Coma
Focal seizures	

TREATMENT
IV fluid and electrolyte replacement as indicated by serum values
Low-dose regular insulin by infusion
Careful monitoring of the following:
Intake and output
Vital signs
Level of consciousness
Electrolytes
Vascular response to fluid

practicing preventive foot care and inspection; patient scrupulously treats all skin abrasions.

Patient is knowledgeable about diabetes and its complications, correctly prepares and administers insulin, rotates injection sites, stores equipment and insulin properly, correctly and consistently tests urine or blood and maintains accurate records, can identify signs of hypoglycemia and ketoacidosis, states correct treatment to follow, wears Medic Alert tag, and receives adequate medical supervision.

Patient demonstrates effective coping behaviors and expresses desire and commitment to maintain adequate disease control.

REFERENCES

Anderson JW and others: Fiber and diabetes (review), Diabetes Care **2:**369-379, 1979.

Paulk LH: Hypoglycemic reactions: from the diabetic's perspective, unpublished thesis, Kent, Ohio, 1983, Kent State University.

BIBLIOGRAPHY

Anderson JW and others: Dietary fibers and diabetes; a comprehensive review and practical application. J Am Dietetic Assoc **87:**1189-1197, 1987.

Ball P: The diabetic patient, AORN J **43:**485-491, 1986.

Butts DE: Fluid and electrolyte disorders associated with diabetic ketoacidosis and hyperglycemic hyperosmolar nonketotic coma, Nurs Clin North Am **22:**827-836, 1987.

Byrnes CA: What's new in the diabetic diet, Nursing **17**(8):58-59, 1987.

Cagno J: Diabetes insipidus, Crit Care Nurse **9**(6):86-93, 1989.

Chandler W and others: Surgical treatment of Cushing's Disease, J Neurosurg Nurs **6**(2):204-290, 1987.

Christman C and Bennett J: Diabetes, new names, new test, new diet. Nursing **7**(8):34-41, 1987.

German K: Fluid and electrolyte problems associated with diabetes insipidus and syndrome of inappropriate antidiuretic hormone, Nurs Clin North Am **22:**785-796, 1987.

Hernandez CM: Surgery and diabetes, minimizing the risks, Am J Nurs **87:**788-792, 1987.

Kruger LB: Complications of transsphenoidal surgery, J Neurosci Nurs **17**(3):179-183, 1985.

Lockhart J: Action stat, Nursing 88, **18:**33, 1988.

Lumey W: Controlling hypoglycemia and hyperglycemia, Nursing **18:**34-41, 1988.

Nath C and others: Lessons in living with Type II diabetes mellitus, Nursing **18:**44-49, 1988.

O'Neil J: Thyroid crisis, Nursing 87, **17**(11):335-338, 1987.

Sarsany S: Thyroid storm, RN **51**(7):46-48, 1988.

Schira M: Steroid dependent states and adrenal insufficiency, Nurs Clin North Am **22:**837-841, 1987.

Staren E et al: Surgical intervention for pheochromocytoma, AORN J **44**(5):764-767, 1986.

CHAPTER 13

Disorders of the Urinary System

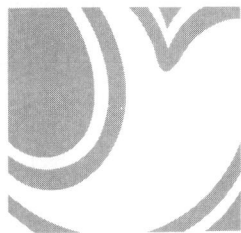

The kidneys and other structures of the urinary system play a major role in regulating the body's internal environment. Functions include regulating the fluid and electrolyte balance, excreting metabolic wastes, maintaining the acid-base balance, producing or modifying the level of hormones responsible for regulation of blood pressure, metabolizing calcium, and synthesizing red blood cells.

Major health problems of the urinary system include infections and inflammatory disorders, congenital disorders, urinary incontinence, and vascular and obstructive disorders. Infections and obstructions are the most common. Figure 13-1 shows the anatomical structure of the urinary system and kidney.

URINARY TRACT INFECTIONS

Infections within the urinary tract are extremely common health problems, especially in women. They may occur at any point in the urinary system and are commonly associated with urinary retention and stasis, intrusive procedures, obstruction, and the presence of chronic illnesses such as diabetes. The two most common forms are cystitis and pyelonephritis.

Cystitis involves infection of the bladder or urethra. Bacterial contamination from the rectum or during intercourse is frequently a predisposing factor. Pyelonephritis involves infection of the kidney tissue and may occur when bacteria ascend the urinary tract following cystitis. It may be acute or chronic. Infection usually starts in the medulla and in chronic forms spreads to the cortex. It can produce kidney fibrosis and scarring and in rare cases may advance to renal failure. Table 13-1 summarizes two other common inflammatory conditions affecting the urinary system.

PATHOPHYSIOLOGY

Most infections result from gram-negative bacteria that originate in the intestinal tract and ascend to the bladder and urethra. They are most likely to occur when host resistance is compromised and in the presence of stasis plus an alkaline urine, which encourages bacterial growth. Reflux of urine into the ureters may facilitate movement of the organisms upward to the kidney itself.

MEDICAL MANAGEMENT

The treatment of cystitis and pyelonephritis revolves around identification of the infecting organism through urine cultures and sterilization of the urine with appropriate antibiotic therapy. Follow-up cultures are indicated in pyelonephritis to identify and treat chronic forms. Medications commonly prescribed include the following:

Urinary antiseptics—nitrofurantoin (Furadantin)
Sulfonamides—cotrimoxazole (Bactrim, Septra)
Urinary analgesics—phenazopyridine (Pyridium)
Systemic antibiotics—ampicillin, cephalosporins

NURSING MANAGEMENT

Assessment

Subjective

History of urinary tract infection or disease
History of chronic disease
History of renal stones, prostatic enlargement, stasis, or intrusive procedure
Patient's complaints of the following:
  Dysuria (painful urination): urgency, frequency, burning sensation
  Fatigue or malaise
  Flank pain or tenderness (pyelonephritis)

Objective

Hematuria (blood in urine)
Urine sample: odor, cloudiness, pH

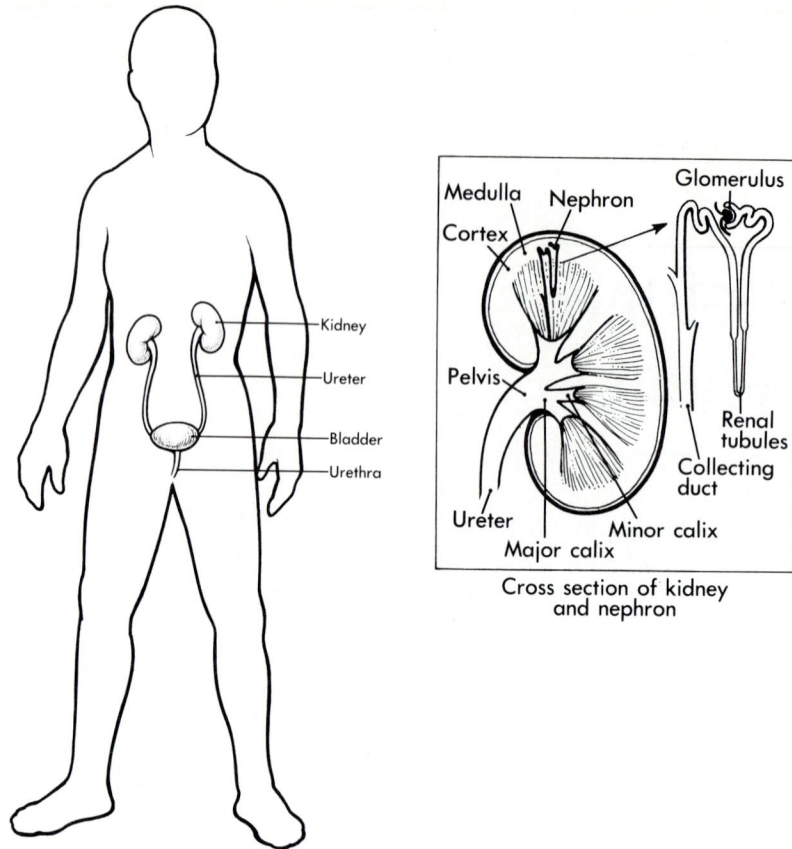

FIGURE 13-1 Urinary system.

Chills and fever

Positive laboratory reports from urine culture; elevated white blood cell count

Nursing Diagnoses

Frequently encountered diagnoses include the following:

Pain and burning on urination related to bladder inflammation and irritation

Altered patterns of urinary elimination related to urgency and frequency

Knowledge deficit related to health promotional activities that prevent the recurrence of urinary tract infection

Expected Outcomes

Patient's urinary symptoms will gradually decrease.

Patient will reestablish a normal urination schedule.

Patient will be knowledgeable about measures that can help prevent recurrences of urinary tract infection.

Nursing Interventions

Administer prescribed medication.

Teach patient importance of taking full course of antibiotics.

Maintain high fluid intake during infection. Give 3000 to 4000 ml per day if not contraindicated.

Encourage patient to take warm sitz baths for comfort if urethral burning is present.

Monitor patient's vital signs until infection is resolved.

Encourage increased rest during acute phase.

Teach patient health promotion activities to decrease chance of reoccurrence.

Explain importance of scrupulous perineal hygiene to female patients.

Patient should wipe carefully from front to back after urination or defecation.

Patient should empty bladder and cleanse self and partner before and after intercourse.

Patient should avoid use of bubble baths, contraceptive jellies, and other products that may alter vaginal pH.

Explain importance of maintaining high fluid intake (approximately 3 L daily).

Patient should modify diet to ensure urinary acidity (fish and poultry, whole grains) and monitor urine pH regularly.

Explain importance of responding promptly to urge to void. Empty bladder every 2 to 3 hours.

Describe signs and symptoms of reinfection.

TABLE 13-1 Inflammatory conditions affecting urinary system function

Condition	Description	Signs and Symptoms	Medical Management
Glomerulonephritis Acute Chronic	An inflammatory process involving the glomerulus, which results from a disordered immune response: Poststreptococcal reaction Autoantibody production to glomerular basement membrane Most patients experience complete recovery; some go on into renal failure	Glomerular porosity increases, causing proteinuria and hematuria Scarring produces gradual loss of glomerular function Fluid retention may cause massive edema and hypertension	Treatment is based on relief of symptoms and management of renal failure. Maintain patient on bed rest. Restrict sodium and fluids. Administer diuretics. Administer antihypertensives. Provide high-carbohydrate, low-protein diet.
Nephrosis (nephrotic syndrome)	A clinical syndrome that may result from many causes; basement membrane becomes very porous, allowing massive excretion of protein in the urine	Massive proteinuria and pitting edema Albuminuria	Administer diuretics. Provide low-sodium, high-protein diet. Corticosteroid therapy is effective for certain causes.

Evaluation

Patient is free of symptoms of burning and urgency.

Patient reestablishes normal pattern of urinary elimination.

Patient maintains an adequate fluid intake, practices optimal hygiene, and is free of recurrent infection.

CONGENITAL DISORDERS

Structural malformations of the urinary system occur in about 10% to 15% of the population. They range from minor and inconsequential to conditions that are incompatible with life. Common congenital problems are outlined in the box on this page.

STRUCTURAL MALFORMATIONS OF URINARY SYSTEM

Duplication of ureters (partial or complete)
  Usually requires no intervention unless complications occur
Hydroureters
  Dilation of ureters
  May require surgical repair
Exstrophy of bladder
  Eversion of bladder on outer abdominal wall
  Requires extensive surgical correction in infancy
Epispadias or hypospadias
  Opening of urethra on dorsum or underside of penis
  Usually necessitates surgical correction
Polycystic disease
  Inherited disease in which kidneys are enlarged and fill with cysts
    When it develops in adulthood, it typically results in end-stage renal disease in about 10 to 15 years

URINARY INCONTINENCE

Urinary incontinence is the involuntary loss of urine from the lower urinary tract. It produces hygiene, social, and emotional consequences that can be profound for the patient. Medical and nursing management involve the identification of the nature of the problem and exploring diet changes, weight loss, and exercise strategies with the patient. Bladder retraining and surgical interventions are options for complex cases. The major forms of incontinence are summarized in the box on this page.

TYPES OF INCONTINENCE

Stress
  Involuntary loss of <50 ml of urine with increased abdominal pressure
  Related to obesity and relaxed pelvic muscles
Reflex
  Involuntary loss of urine when a specific volume is reached
  Related to neurologic impairment such as spinal cord injury or lesion
Urge
  Involuntary loss of urine occurring soon after a strong sense of urgency to void
  Related to infection, decreased bladder capacity, overdistention of bladder
Functional
  Involuntary unpredictable loss of urine
  Related to sensory, cognitive, or mobility deficits
Total
  Continuous and unpredictable loss of urine
  Related to neurologic dysfunction, spinal nerve disease, or trauma

OBSTRUCTIVE DISORDERS

RENAL CALCULI

The development of renal stones is a relatively common problem that can result in the eventual destruction of and loss of the kidney. Renal calculi produce urinary tract problems that reflect the stones' size and position. Large stones may produce obstruction of urine flow, pressure destruction of kidney tissue, and infection. Small stones may be successfully excreted from the urinary tract but cause severe local pain spasm and inflammation in the process. Rough stone edges may cause hematuria.

PATHOPHYSIOLOGY

Urinary stones may develop at any level in the urinary system but are most commonly found within the kidney. Stones are crystallizations of minerals around an organic base. Calcium stones account for about 75% of stones. No cause can be found in many cases, but urinary tract infection, alkaline urine, and urinary stasis are precipitating factors for stone development. Any condition that increases the mineral content of the urine can lead to stone formation.

MEDICAL MANAGEMENT

Since about 90% of renal calculi are passed spontaneously, the patient receives symptomatic support with hydration and analgesics. Larger stones may need to be treated with extracorporeal shock wave lithotripsy, which bombards the stone with multiple ultrasonic shock waves. The procedure is typically performed under spinal or general anesthesia and prevents the need for surgery. Surgery will be used if other treatment approaches fail or if the kidney itself must be removed.

NURSING MANAGEMENT

Assessment
   Subjective
   Patient's complaint of the following:
      Pain (classic feature)
      Constant, dull pain if stone is in kidney
      Excruciating pain if stone is in ureter; pain may radiate to genitals or thigh
      Nausea and vomiting
   Prior history of stones or urinary tract infection
   Family history of stones
   Objective
   Hematuria
   Changes in vital signs—fever or mild shock
   Positive results from intravenous pyelogram (IVP)
   Serum mineral levels

Nursing Diagnoses
Intense pain related to spasm and pressure in kidney or ureter

Alteration in patterns of urinary elimination related to symptoms of dysuria
Knowledge deficit related to measures to prevent stone reoccurrence

Expected Outcomes
Patient's pain will be reduced to manageable levels; nausea and vomiting will be relieved.
Patient will return to a normal pattern of urinary elimination.
Patient will be knowledgeable concerning measures that can prevent the reoccurrence of calculi.

Nursing Interventions
Administer analgesics liberally as prescribed (morphine is usually ordered).
Assess effectiveness of pain relief.
Administer antispasmodics as ordered (Pro-Banthine)
Instruct patient to strain all urine.
Force fluids orally, or administer intravenously to at least 3000 to 4000 ml daily.
Encourage patient to ambulate as tolerated once pain is controlled.
Monitor intake and output.
Assess urine for blood.
Teach patient measures to prevent reoccurrence of stones.
   Patient should maintain high daily fluid intake—approximately 3000 ml daily.
   Patient should engage in active exercise and avoid constipation and immobility.
   Patient should modify diet if appropriate. Possible modifications include the following:
      Restrict calcium, found in milk and milk products, beans, dried fruit, chocolate, and cocoa.
      Restrict oxalate found in coffee, tea, chocolate, spinach, and beans.
      Restrict purines, found in organ meats, legumes, sardines, and herring; moderate amounts are present in most meats.
      Take measures to acidify the urine, by eating meat and fish, whole grains, cheese, and cranberries.
Monitor urine pH at regular intervals.
Explain purpose and side effects of prescribed medications.
Provide appropriate preoperative teaching if surgery is planned.
(Care of the patient following kidney surgery is outlined in the box on the next page.)

Evaluation
Patient passes stone and is free of pain, nausea, and tenderness.
Patient voids at regular intervals and is free of hematuria or dysuria.
Patient can discuss appropriate diet modification for

CARE OF THE PATIENT FOLLOWING UROLOGIC SURGERY

PREOPERATIVE

Reinforce teaching about procedure and aftercare as needed.

Teach coughing and deep breathing methods. Emphasize importance of effective coughing to patients with high flank incision since the incision's proximity to diaphragm will make coughing difficult.

POSTOPERATIVE

Provide adequate analgesia to facilitate deep breathing and coughing.
Use incentive spirometer every 2 hours.
Help patient to splint incision.
Change positions frequently.
Monitor urine output every 1 to 2 hours; should be at least 50 ml/hr.
Record output separately for each drainage tube.
Estimate urine drainage on dressings.
Observe urine's color and consistency.
Weigh patient daily.
Encourage patient to ambulate if ureteral catheters are not in place.
Assess patient for return of bowel sounds, passage of flatus.
Ensure IV hydration until patient tolerates food and fluids orally.
Monitor patient carefully for signs of bleeding.
Risk is high if parenchyma has been incised.
Risk is greatest on day of surgery and 8 to 12 days after surgery.
Change dressing aseptically frequently to keep site of incision dry. Use of Montgomery straps will facilitate dressing changes.
Stoma bags may be utilized for large amounts of drainage.
Keep skin clean and odor free.
Maintain patency of all drainage tubes.
Position patient so kinking or obstruction does not occur.
Never clamp or irrigate ureteral catheters or nephrostomy tubes without specific orders.

---

type of stone; patient understands importance of hydration and exercise to avoid reoccurrence.

Patient who is treated surgically recovers without complications.

CANCER OF THE BLADDER

Tumors of the urinary system affect both the kidney and bladder. Nephrectomy is the treatment of choice for renal tumors, and the associated care is similar to that provided for other renal or abdominal surgery. Bladder tumors are the most common form, occurring primarily in men in late middle age and frequently with multiple tumor sites. The incidence of bladder cancer is associated with chronic exposure to cigarette smoke, chemicals, and dyes.

PATHOPHYSIOLOGY

Most bladder tumors begin as benign papillomas and occur in multiple locations. Most arise from transitional epithelium cell types. Painless hematuria is a common early sign. Advanced disease may cause infection, fistula development, or ureteral obstruction leading to renal failure.

MEDICAL MANAGEMENT

Benign papillomas and small tumors are treated with transurethral fulguration or excision. The definitive diagnosis is established first with cystoscopic visualization and biopsy. Cystectomy is performed only if the disease appears to be curable. External radiation treatment may be given before surgery to slow tumor growth. The ileal conduit is the most common form of permanent urinary diversion. One variation, the Kock or Indiana pouch, inserts a valve that permits the patient to self-catheterize and be continent rather than wear a permanent drainage bag.

NURSING MANAGEMENT

The nursing care for patients with urinary diversions is similar to that provided after any major abdominal surgery. It may necessitate short-term hemodynamic monitoring. The care is outlined in the box on the next page.

RENAL FAILURE

The kidneys have a tremendous ability to adapt to a decreasing number of functioning nephrons and still maintain adequate function. Renal failure is a state of severe impairment or total lack of renal function, and it does not occur until the number of functioning nephrons falls below 25%. The patient is then unable to maintain the internal equilibrium of the body fluids.

ACUTE RENAL FAILURE

Acute failure is a sudden and frequently reversible decrease or cessation of kidney function. It generally follows contact with a nephrotoxic agent, trauma, or surgical procedures. The box on the next page lists some of the common causes.

PATHOPHYSIOLOGY

Renal ischemia occurs when blood flow to the kidneys is decreased. The kidney responds with vasoconstriction, which further reduces blood flow and worsens ischemia. Prolonged ischemia produces death of renal tubular tissue and triggers the failure. The kidneys are then unable to excrete fluid loads, regulate electrolytes, or excrete metabolic wastes. Acute failure commonly occurs in three phases:

Oliguric phase. Output falls to 400 ml or less per day, reflecting damage to nephrons. Urine may also be

CARE OF THE PATIENT WITH A URINARY DIVERSION (ILEAL CONDUIT)

DESCRIPTION OF OPERATION

Ureters are excised from the bladder and transplanted into a section of ileum resected from the intestinal tract with blood supply intact. One end is closed and the other is brought to the surface of the abdomen to form a stoma to drain urine.

PREOPERATIVE CARE

Provide accurate information about procedure and care.
Provide introduction to self-care materials if patient exhibits readiness.
Introduce enterostomal therapist to begin teaching plan.
Encourage patient to verbalize feelings about change in body image and function.
Initiate bowel preparation as ordered.
   Provide clear liquids.
   Administer enemas, intestinal antibiotics, and oral bowel cleansing solutions.

POSTOPERATIVE CARE

Use standard interventions to identify and prevent complications.
Provide TED stockings; encourage patient to do range of motion exercises, make position changes, and ambulate as permitted to prevent thrombophlebitis (risk is high after pelvic surgery).
Assess for Homans' sign every shift.
Maintain patency of nasogastric tube until peristalsis returns (3 to 5 days). Auscultate abdomen for bowel sounds.
Observe stoma for complications.
   Stoma should be healthy bright pink or red.
   Observe for bleeding or erosion.
   Assess surrounding skin.
Maintain high fluid intake. Teach patient symptoms of urinary tract infection.
   Stent tubes will be placed initially to promote drainage.
   Urine will contain mucus from bowel.
   Empty bag every 2 hours; attach to Foley drainage bag at night.
Provide meticulous care to surrounding skin.
   Ensure proper fit of appliance; remeasure carefully as stoma shrinks.
   Maintain an acid pH.
   Teach patient skills for self-care of appliance (assembly, application, emptying and changing of the pouch).
Encourage patient to verbalize feelings about surgery. Discuss impact of surgery on work, leisure, clothing, and sexual activity.
Put patient in touch with support groups and agencies in the community to facilitate adjustment.

dilute because of the tubules' loss of concentrating ability.
Diuretic phase. Second phase begins in days or weeks. Increasing output indicates healing of the nephrons. Inability to excrete proportional amounts of wastes or concentrate urine reflects continued tubular damage. Large amounts of fluids and electrolytes are lost.

CAUSES OF ACUTE RENAL FAILURE

TOXIC SUBSTANCES

Solvents (carbon tetrachloride, methanol, ethylene glycol)
Heavy metals (lead, arsenic, mercury)
Antibiotics (kanamycin, gentamicin, polymyxin B, amphotericin B, colistin, neomycin, phenazopyridine)
Pesticides
Mushrooms
Drug overdose

ISCHEMIA

Hypovolemia
Blood loss (surgery, trauma)
Plasma loss (burns, surgery, acute pancreatitis)
Sodium and water loss (prolonged diarrhea or vomiting, gastrointestinal tract drainage, sustained high fever)
Cardiac failure
Myocardial infarction
Cardiac arrhythmias
Congestive heart failure
Septic shock
Bilateral occlusion of renal arteries

OTHER FACTORS

Acute glomerular disease
Acute, severe infection of kidney tissue
Hemoglobinuria (from hemolysis, for example, a transfusion reaction)
Myoglobinuria (from massive muscle insult, for example, a crush injury)
Mechanical obstructions in the urinary tract

Modified from Phipps WJ, Long BC, and Woods NF: Medical-surgical nursing: concepts and clinical practice, ed 4, St Louis, 1990, Mosby–Year Book, Inc.

Recovery phase. Recovery may take months as kidneys gradually return to normal or near normal levels of functioning. Fluid and electrolyte levels are at or near normal levels.
Table 13-2 lists the major symptoms of and physiologic changes occurring in renal failure.

MEDICAL MANAGEMENT

The treatment of acute renal failure is specific to the problems of each stage. In the oliguric phase, dialysis is used to control fluids, regulate electrolytes, and excrete rising metabolic wastes. Diet is modified to reduce protein, sodium, and potassium, and provide carbohydrates for energy. Careful monitoring is employed to maintain appropriate electrolyte levels; the patient should be observed for signs of fluid overload and other complications.

In the diuretic phase, fluid replacement may be necessary to prevent dehydration. Dialysis is continued as needed to maintain acceptable levels of electrolytes and excretion of wastes until adequate kidney function returns.

TABLE 13-2 Symptoms caused by physiologic changes in acute renal failure

Symptoms	Physiologic Effects	Findings
Oliguric Phase		
Nausea, vomiting, drowsiness, confusion, coma, gastrointestinal bleeding, asterixis, pericarditis	Inability to excrete metabolic wastes	Increased serum urea nitrogen and creatinine levels
Nausea, vomiting, cardiac arrhythmias, Kussmaul's breathing, drowsiness, confusion, coma	Inability to regulate electrolytes	Hyperkalemia, hyponatremia, acidosis
Edema, congestive heart failure, pulmonary edema, hypertension	Inability to excrete fluid loads	Fluid overload, hypervolemia
Diuretic Phase		
Urinary output of up to 4-5 L/day, postural hypotension, tachycardia	Increased production of urine	Hypovolemia, loss of sodium and potassium in urine
Increasing mental alertness and activity	Slowly increasing excretion of metabolic wastes	Initially, high BUN (fluid loss greater than solute loss); gradual return of BUN to normal

From Long BC, and Phipps WJ: Essentials of medical-surgical nursing: a nursing process approach, ed 2, St Louis, 1989, The CV Mosby Co.

NURSING MANAGEMENT

Assessment

Subjective (onset of failure)
History of precipitating factors
Use of drugs—prescription or recreational
Patient's complaints of the following:
    Change in voiding pattern
    Abrupt weight gain, edema
    Weakness, fatigue, nausea
    Confusion or drowsiness

Objective
Signs of fluid overload
    Congestive heart failure, pulmonary edema
    Hypertension
    Peripheral edema
Accurate intake and output records; low specific gravity of urine
Daily weights
Level of consciousness
Laboratory reports demonstrating hyperkalemia, elevated creatinine and BUN (blood urea nitrogen), metabolic acidosis, hyponatremia

Nursing Diagnoses
Diagnoses will depend on the extent and duration of failure and the adequacy of therapy. Common diagnoses include the following:
    Fluid volume excess related to failure of the renal regulatory mechanism
    Potential impairment of skin integrity related to alterations in skin turgor associated with edema
    Altered patterns of urinary elimination related to falling urine production
    Altered thought processes related to the accumulation of waste products
    Potential for altered nutrition: less than body requirements, related to diet restrictions, anorexia, and nausea

Expected Outcomes
Patient will maintain a fluid and electrolyte balance that is within an acceptable range.
Patient will maintain an intact skin; edema will decrease.
Patient will return to normal urinary elimination patterns without need for dialysis.
Patient will be fully oriented and able to problem-solve effectively.
Patient will ingest a diet that conforms to needed restrictions yet meets all nutritional needs.

Nursing Interventions: Oliguric Phase
Fluid and electrolytes
Maintain accurate intake and output records.
Restrict fluids as prescribed (usually 500 ml daily plus output).
    Plan with patient to distribute fluids effectively throughout the day.
    Teach the rationale and importance of fluid restrictions.
    Employ comfort measures for thirst (mouth care, ice chips, moist cloth for mouth).
Assess status of edema.
Weigh patient daily.
Monitor vital signs frequently.
Assess for signs of sodium and potassium imbalance.

Teach patient rationale for dialysis and mechanisms of action.

Monitor patency of vascular access site for dialysis.

Diet

Maintain flow of patient's IV, if any, at prescribed rate.

Explore use of simple foods rich in carbohydrates as tolerated.

Add high biologic value protein to diet to prevent tissue wasting as tolerated.

Administer antiemetics if prescribed.

Explore food preferences and encourage adequate intake.

Activity and comfort

Promote maximal rest to lower metabolic load during acute phase. Assist patient with activities of daily living as needed.

Encourage use of deep breathing during immobility.

Turn patient frequently and provide excellent skin care.

Encourage patient to ambulate as condition stabilizes.

Maintain safe environment during period of lethargy. Use side rails and check patient frequently. Assess mental status every 8 hours.

Administer measures to combat pruritus.

Protect patient from exposure to infection.

Monitor patient's level of consciousness frequently.

Keep patient oriented to environment and reassure patient about reversible nature of mental changes.

Nursing Interventions: Diuretic Phase

Maintain interventions outlined above.

Monitor patient for fluid and electrolyte depletion. Monitor output hourly. Assess skin turgor and mucous membranes. Assess mental status every 8 hours.

Provide replacement fluid as prescribed.

Teach patient rationale for ongoing dialysis in face of rising urine output.

Teach patient about diet restrictions and medications for long-term rehabilitation, and explain importance of avoiding infection.

Evaluation

Patient is relieved of anorexia and nausea through dialysis or returning renal function; patient eats diet within ongoing restrictions.

Patient follows prescribed fluid restriction; laboratory reports and clinical signs demonstrate an adequate fluid and electrolyte balance.

Patient's skin is intact, edema is minimal or absent, and pruritus is relieved.

Patient experiences a gradual return of renal function, has a normal pattern of urinary elimination, and no longer needs dialysis.

Patient returns to preillness levels of intellectual functioning and personality.

NURSING CARE PLAN

ACUTE RENAL FAILURE

Nursing Diagnoses	Expected Patient Outcomes	Nursing Interventions
Altered patterns of urinary elimination related to falling urine production	Patient returns to a normal urinary elimination pattern without need for dialysis.	1. Measure output carefully. Check urine specific gravity. 2. Teach patient about dialysis procedures.
Fluid volume excess related to failure of renal regulatory mechanism	Patient's fluid and electrolyte values are within normal limits. Patient maintains a stable weight.	1. Maintain IV at prescribed rate; restrict fluids as prescribed. 2. Keep accurate intake and output records. Weigh patient daily. 3. Monitor vital signs (including postural signs) frequently. 4. Assess neck veins, skin turgor, and mucous membrane; note peripheral edema. 5. Monitor for and report signs of hyperkalemia, hyponatremia, or acidosis during oliguric phase. 6. Administer prescribed medications.
Potential impairment of skin integrity related to decreased mobility and tissue edema	Patient maintains an intact skin.	1. Assess skin each shift. 2. Keep skin clean and dry. 3. Put pressure devices on bed—special attention to heels and sacrum. 4. Turn every 2 hours. 5. Avoid shearing force when moving patient. 6. Bathe patient frequently, using bland soap and tepid water. 7. Administer prescribed antipruritics as needed.
Altered nutrition: less than body requirements, related to anorexia and multiple diet restrictions	Patient's diet conforms to needed restrictions and meets body needs for nutrients.	1. Assess nutrient intake. Perform calorie counts. 2. Give good mouth care prior to oral feedings. 3. Encourage eating of prescribed diet. 4. Restrict protein content as prescribed—ensure high biologic value. 5. Use measures to decrease nausea (e.g., antiemetics, deep breathing). 6. Give mouth care. 7. Provide patient with a moist cloth to keep lips moist. Offer ice chips if allowed. 8. Plan with patient to distribute allowed fluid intake effectively throughout the day. 9. Plan with patient to include food preferences where possible. 10. Give prescribed antipruritics as needed.
Alteration in thought processes related to the accumulation of waste products	Patient is fully oriented and able to problem-solve effectively.	1. Assess mental status for changes (confusion, somnolence). 2. Orient to person, place, and time as necessary. 3. Provide simple explanations and repeat instructions as necessary. 4. Ensure a safe environment. Keep siderails up and supervise ambulation. 5. Reassure patient that mental capacities will return with recovery. 6. Explain reasons for behavior to family and friends.

Continued.

NURSING CARE PLAN

ACUTE RENAL FAILURE—cont'd

Nursing Diagnoses	Expected Patient Outcomes	Nursing Interventions
Fatigue related to waste product accumulation	Patient gradually resumes normal pattern of activities of daily living.	1. Promote maximal rest to lower metabolic load. 2. Assist with activities of daily living as needed. 3. Employ active nursing measures to prevent complications related to immobility. 4. Encourage ambulation as condition stabilizes. 5. Avoid exposing patient to persons with infections.

Knowledge deficit related to treatment and progression of disease process	Patient understands nature of disorder and therapeutic regimen.	1. Teach patient the following:
		  a. Basis of symptoms and therapy.
		  b. Avoidance of preventable factors, if appropriate.
		  c. Prescribed medications and dietary regimens.
		  d. Signs of returning renal problems or infections.
		  e. Need for follow-up care.

CHRONIC RENAL FAILURE

Chronic renal failure is a significant health care problem, causing nearly 60,000 deaths each year and leaving an additional 100,000 dependent on lifelong dialysis. Chronic failure exists when the kidneys are unable to maintain the body's internal environment and recovery is not expected. The development of chronic failure is usually a slow process, occurring over a period of years. Recurrent infections, obstruction, and blood vessel destruction from diabetes and hypertension are common predisposing causes. Repeated episodes of tissue death and scarring may trigger insufficiency and finally total failure.

PATHOPHYSIOLOGY

In chronic failure the nephrons are selectively destroyed. Intact nephron units hypertrophy and allow the kidney to compensate until about 75% of the nephrons are destroyed. Initially, the heavy solute load may trigger an osmotic diuresis, but eventually, with the loss of more nephrons, oliguria and retention of waste products occur. The signs and symptoms are the result of fluid and electrolyte disturbances, altered regulatory mechanisms, and waste product retention. Table 13-3 summarizes these effects.

MEDICAL MANAGEMENT

In early stages the failure may be controlled by strictly limiting the intake of fluid and substances that require kidney excretion. Most patients progress to the point at which dialysis or transplantation is essential to preserve life.

NURSING MANAGEMENT

Assessment
Subjective
History/duration of disease and its treatment
Knowledge of disease and treatment
Medications in use and patient's knowledge of their purpose
Usual dietary patterns, adherence to restrictions
Impact of disease and treatment on preferred lifestyle
Effect of disease on relationships, sexual functioning

TABLE 13-3 Summary of major organ system involvement in patients with chronic renal failure

System	Manifestation	Cause
Integumentary		
Skin	Pallor	Anemia
	Gray/bronze pigmentation	Pigment retained
	Dry and scaly	Decreased size and activity of sweat and oil glands
	Pruritus	Dry skin; phosphate deposits
Nails	Thin, brittle	Protein wasting
Hair	Dry	Decreased activity of oil glands
	Brittle	Protein wasting
Gastrointestinal		
Oral cavity	Halitosis (fetor uremicus)	Urea converted to ammonia by saline
	Bleeding of gums	Change in platelet activity
Stomach	Nausea, vomiting, anorexia	Serum uremic toxins
	Gastritis, ulceration	Serum uremic toxins and electrolyte imbalances
Lower bowel	Constipation	Aluminum hydroxide given as phosphate binder, elevated ammonia levels
Cardiovascular	Hypertension	Fluid overload, renin-angiotensin mechanism
	Congestive heart failure	Fluid overload, anemia
	Arteriosclerotic heart disease	Chronic hypertension
	Pericarditis	Calcification of soft tissues, uremic toxins in pericardial fluid, fibrin formation on epicardium
Neurologic	Fatigue, headache, sleep disturbance	Uremic toxins
	Seizures	Electrolyte imbalances
Hematologic	Anemia	Suppression of RBC production, decreased survival time of RBCs, loss of blood through bleeding or dialysis
	Bleeding	Mild thrombocytopenia, decreased platelet activity
Skeletal	Renal osteodystrophy	Decreased calcium absorption
	Joint pain, renal	Decreased phosphate excretion
Endocrine	Glucose intolerance	Decreased sensitivity to insulin
	Infertility, change in menstrual cycle	Mechanism unknown
	Sexual dysfunction, impotence	Mechanism unknown

Adapted from Long BC and Phipps WJ: Essentials of medical-surgical nursing: a nursing process approach, ed 2, St Louis, 1989, The CV Mosby Co.

Patient's complaints of the following:
    Lethargy, fatigue, irritability, or depression
    Headaches and anorexia, nausea
    Paresthesias, muscle twitching, pruritus
    Weight loss
    Bone pain with ambulation, neuropathies

Objective

Skin changes—sallow, brownish, pale, dry
Evidence of petechiae, bruising
Edema
Hypertension, signs of congestive heart failure
Intake and output—oliguria or anuria
Daily weights
Dry hair and nails
Evidence of calcium deposits in skin
Ammonia odor to breath
Laboratory reports showing hyperkalemia and elevated BUN, creatinine, and phosphate levels; metabolic acidosis; anemia

Nursing Diagnoses

Diagnoses will depend on the degree of disease and the effectiveness of treatment control but commonly include the following:

Fatigue related to anemia and decreased nutrition
Activity intolerance related to generalized weakness
Bone pain and muscle cramping related to uremia and electrolyte imbalance
Actual or potential fluid volume excess related to the failure of renal regulatory mechanisms
Potential for ineffective individual or family coping related to life-style restrictions and dependence on dialysis for sustaining life
Knowledge deficit related to the treatment protocol necessary to sustain healthy functioning
Altered nutrition: potential for less than body requirements, related to multiple restrictions, anorexia, and nausea
Powerlessness related to the demands of the dialysis regimen
Sexual dysfunction related to physiologic changes and stresses of chronic illness

Expected Outcomes

Patient's energy level will improve to the point where patient can complete normal daily activities without undue fatigue.
Patient will have less pruritus, anorexia, and nausea as condition stabilizes with dialysis. Patient's pain will not interfere with normal activities.
Patient will maintain an acceptable fluid and electrolyte balance on dialysis.
Patient and family will make adequate adjustments to the life-style changes caused by dialysis.
Patient will be knowledgeable about all aspects of treatment protocol: medications, diet, dialysis.

Patient will plan and consume a daily food intake that meets the body's nutritional needs and stays within prescribed restrictions.
Patient will maintain a sense of control over his or her life and participate in all care decisions.
Patient will maintain open communication with partner about sexual changes and reestablish a satisfactory pattern of sexual expression.

Nursing Interventions: Fluid and Electrolytes

Maintain accurate intake and output records. Monitor for imbalances.
Weigh patient daily.
Restrict fluids as prescribed. Plan with patient to distribute fluids effectively throughout the day.
Teach patient principles of sodium-restricted diet.
Encourage patient to read product labels carefully.
Monitor patient for edema; assess thirst.
Assess vital signs for signs of fluid overload.
Teach patient importance of restricting potassium in diet. Explain which foods are high in potassium.
    Teach patient to avoid trauma and infection, as tissue breakdown liberates potassium.
ALERT: Caution patient that most salt substitutes are high in potassium and should not be used.
Administer aluminum hydroxide with meals to bind excess phosphorus.
Administer vitamin D and calcium as prescribed to combat bone demineralization.

Nursing Interventions: Azotemia and Acidosis

Teach patient dietary protein restrictions as prescribed.
    Ensure use of high biologic value protein.
    Restriction usually is not below 40 g daily.
    Ensure adequate intake of carbohydrates and fats for energy.
Ensure adequate pulmonary function to assist in excretion of CO_2.
Assess patient for changes in level of consciousness.
Ensure environmental safety.
Use stool softeners as needed to avoid constipation.

Nursing Interventions: Activity and Comfort

Help patient plan and space activities to conserve energy.
    Plan for adequate rest.
    Assist patient with activities of daily living as needed.
    Assess patient for dyspnea and tachycardia, peripheral perfusion, and other symptoms of activity intolerance.
    Provide adequate warmth.
Institute measures to control pruritus.
    Teach patient importance of maintaining skin integrity. Administer antipruritics.
    Control heat and humidity in environment.
    Use oils and lotions to keep skin soft.

Attempt to relieve muscle cramps with use of heat and massage.

Provide frequent gentle oral hygiene.

Assess regularly for bleeding or bruising. Avoid use of aspirin.

Make meals and environment as pleasant as possible.

Nursing Interventions: Coping

Encourage patient to verbalize feelings about restrictions and treatment regimen.

Help patient maintain open communication with family and sexual partner.

Help patient explore financial and social resources in community.

Support all positive coping strategies employed by patient and family.

Support maintenance of family structure and desired roles.

Provide patient with opportunities to discuss issues involving sexuality and reproduction. Provide patient with accurate information.

Encourage patient to maintain hope and positive feelings about dialysis.

Nursing Interventions: Dialysis

Assess for patency of vascular access (see Table 13-4 and Figure 13-2).

Teach patient about peritoneal dialysis or hemodialysis if in use.

Evaluation

Patient has sufficient energy to participate in normal activities of daily living; hemoglobin and hematocrit levels are stable.

Anorexia, nausea, and pruritus are absent or controlled; skin is intact.

Patient's fluid and electrolyte balance is stabilized; there are no signs of peripheral edema; blood pressure is controlled.

Patient expresses positive attitude toward integrating successful dialysis regimen into life-style.

Patient can knowledgeably discuss treatment protocol and takes medications on schedule.

Patient plans and eats a diet that meets baseline nutritional needs and follows prescribed restrictions; positive nitrogen balance is maintained.

Patient acts as informed decision maker in all aspects of care planning and is consulted about proposed changes in treatment regimen.

Patient adjusts to changes in sexual functioning and expresses satisfaction with sexuality.

DIALYSIS

Dialysis involves the movement of fluid and particles across a semipermeable membrane. It can help restore normal fluid and electrolyte balance, control acid-base balance, and remove waste and toxic material from the body through the processes of diffusion, osmosis, and ultrafiltration. It is used temporarily in acute failure and as a permanent substitute for the loss of renal function in patients with chronic end-stage disease. There are two main types: hemodialysis and peritoneal dialysis.

Hemodialysis

Hemodialysis shunts the patient's blood from the body through a dialyzer in which diffusion and ultrafiltration occur. Hemodialysis requires access to the patient's

TABLE 13-4 Indications and nursing interventions associated with vascular access for hemodialysis

Type	Indication for Use	Advantages	Nursing Interventions
External shunt	Long-term access Need for immediate access	Ease of access Can be used immediately	Do not start IVs or take blood pressure on affected arm or leg. Assess for bleeding from insertion sites. Assess patency by observing color of blood flow through shunt. Listen for bruit. Assess adequacy of perfusion to extremity. Assess for infection; change dressing frequently, using institution's protocol. Keep clamps or tourniquet at bedside.
Arteriovenous fistula/graft	Permanent access needed	Easy access once graft has matured Least likely to develop infection or dislodge	Assess for patency by palpating for thrill or auscultating bruit. Teach patient to avoid compression caused by tight clothing or positioning with arm bent. Assess adequacy of perfusion to extremity. Teach patient to assess site for signs of infection. Do not start IVs or take blood pressure on affected arm.

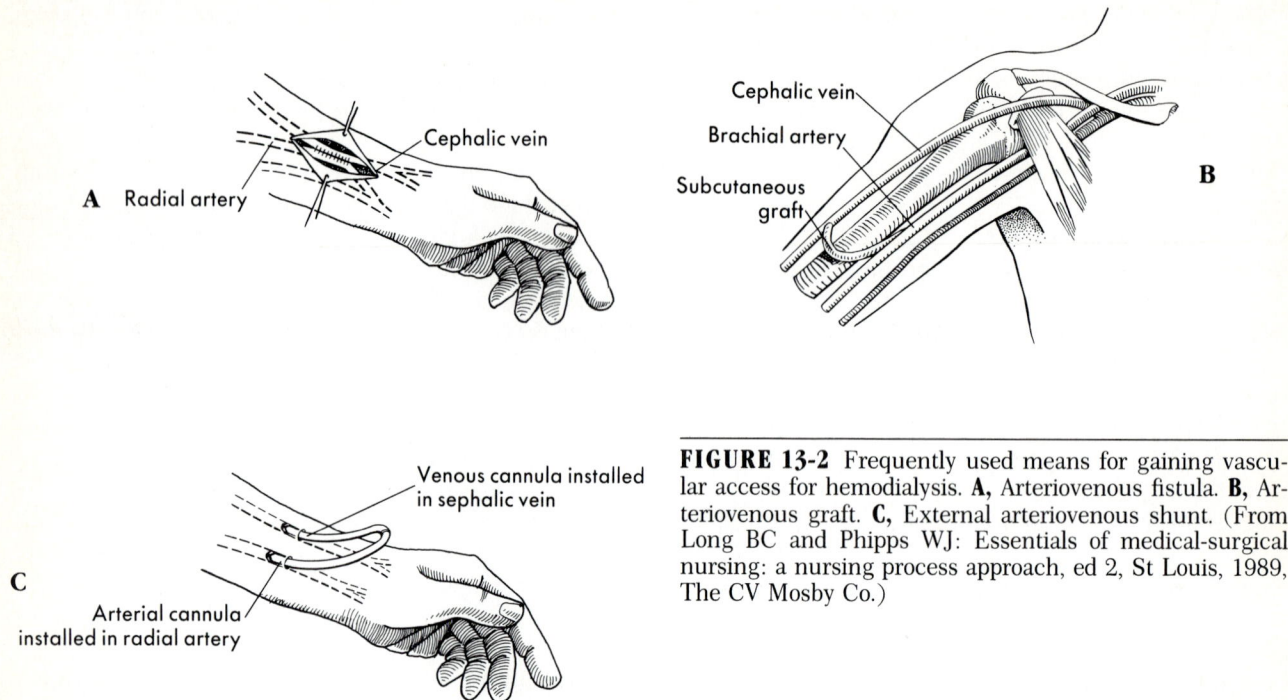

FIGURE 13-2 Frequently used means for gaining vascular access for hemodialysis. **A,** Arteriovenous fistula. **B,** Arteriovenous graft. **C,** External arteriovenous shunt. (From Long BC and Phipps WJ: Essentials of medical-surgical nursing: a nursing process approach, ed 2, St Louis, 1989, The CV Mosby Co.)

blood. The primary methods of vascular access include the following:

The external cannula or shunt, in which a Silastic cannula is implanted into an artery and adjacent vein in the forearm or elsewhere; the two ends are connected by a U-shaped external connector. (See Figure 13-2).

The internal arteriovenous fistula, in which a subcutaneous anastomosis is made between an artery and a vein. Fistulas may also be created using bovine or synthetic grafts.

Dialysis nursing is a specialty area of practice. The major nursing responsibilities for nondialysis nurses include the following:

Protecting the vascular access site (see Table 13-4)

Teaching the patient and family ways to manage the disease effectively

Assisting the patient to plan a work and activity schedule that is minimally disrupted by dialysis routine

Peritoneal Dialysis

The dialyzing fluid is instilled into the peritoneal cavity, and the peritoneum becomes the dialyzing membrane. It may take up to 36 hours to complete the treatment. Dialysis may be done intermittently or on a continuous daily ambulatory basis with the insertion of a permanent peritoneal catheter. The procedure is relatively simple and allows the patient more control over daily life. Fewer medications and dietary restrictions are usually necessary. The placement of a permanent catheter,

NURSING INTERVENTIONS FOR PATIENTS RECEIVING PERITONEAL DIALYSIS

PREDIALYSIS
Take baseline weight and vital signs.
Have patient empty bladder before catheter insertion.
Provide meticulous skin and catheter prep per institution's protocol before connecting dialysis fluid line.

DURING DIALYSIS
To initiate each cycle:
Run prescribed amount of solution (usually 2 L) into peritoneal cavity over about 10 minutes.
Clamp tubing for prescribed time (usually 20 to 30 minutes).
Drain cavity by gravity (usually takes 20 minutes).
Repeat procedure with fresh dialysate solution as many times as prescribed.
Make sure solution is at body temperature during instillation.
Maintain sterility during bottle changes.
Monitor patient continuously for the following:
Changes in vital signs indicating hypotension or hypovolemia
Pain
Respiratory distress
Signs of peritonitis
Turn patient side to side to facilitate drainage of fluid.
Maintain accurate intake and output records.
Record amount of fluid instilled.
Record amount of fluid drained.
Note net gains or losses of fluid.
Discontinue dialysis following institution's protocol, keeping strict asepsis.
Send fluid cultures as ordered.

however, presents a continual potential route for organisms to enter the peritoneum, and strict asepsis and careful monitoring for infection are essential. Nursing interventions are summarized in the box on the preceding page.

KIDNEY TRANSPLANTATION

Kidney transplants are being performed with increasing frequency, and ongoing developments in surgical techniques, tissue typing, and antirejection drug therapy have made transplant a viable treatment alternative for most patients. Its use is primarily limited at this time by the availability of acceptable donor organs.

Control of the body's tendency to reject the organ has improved but has not been completely achieved. A lifelong protocol of immunosuppression is required. The nursing care associated with renal transplant is similar to that for other renal surgery, with substantial additional teaching concerning immunosuppressive therapy. The boxes on this page describe the major types of rejection and the drugs most commonly used for immunosuppression.

KIDNEY TRANSPLANT REJECTION

TYPES

Acute rejection—usually occurs 4 days to 4 months after transplant. May be successfully treated with immunosuppressive drugs. Most patients experience at least one episode.

Chronic rejection—usually occurs over months or years and is associated with gradual occlusion of renal blood vessels. There is no definitive treatment.

SIGNS AND SYMPTOMS

Decreasing urine output, oliguria, or anuria
Fever >37.7° C
Pain or tenderness over transplant site
Elevated serum creatinine and BUN levels
Edema, sudden weight gain—2 to 3 lb over 24 hours
Hypertension
Proteinuria
Slowly rising creatinine and BUN levels
Malaise
Gradually deteriorating condition

IMMUNOSUPPRESSIVE DRUG THERAPY

Cyclosporine (Sandimmune)
  Strongly inhibits the antibody production that leads to graft rejection but does not affect the systems that protect against general infection; drug of choice for cadaver transplants
Azathioprine (Imuran)
  Suppresses antibody synthesis by inhibiting RNA and DNA synthesis
Cyclophosphamide (Cytoxan)
  Often used in combination with azathioprine; also destroys the circulating lymphocytes.
Adrenal corticosteroids
  Cause general suppression of the immune/inflammatory response.

BIBLIOGRAPHY

Alt D, Balduf R, and Thompson E: When a vascular access site complicates care, RN **49**(10):36-39, 1986.

Bellinger MF: The history of diversion and undiversion, J Enterostomal Ther **16**:39-41, 1989.

Booth S and Dobberstein K: Living without kidneys, Am J Nurs **89**:270, 1989.

Brogna L and Lakaszawski ML: The continent urostomy, Am J Nurs **86**:160-163, 1986.

Chambers JK: Fluid and electrolyte problems in renal and urologic disorders, Nurs Clin North Am **22**:815-816, 1987.

Conti MT and Eutropius L: Preventing UTI's: what works?, Am J Nurs **87**:307-309, 1987.

Harwood C: Pulverizing kidney stones: what you should know about lithotripsy, RN **48**(7):32-37, 1985.

Petillo MH: The patient with a urinary stoma, Nurs Clin North Am **22**:263-279, 1987.

Plawecki HM and others: Chronic renal failure, J Gerontol Nurs **13**(12):14-17, 1987.

Prevention and treatment of kidney stones (Kidney Stone Consensus Conference), JAMA **260**:977-981, 1988.

Solomon J: Does renal failure mean sexual failure?, RN **49**(8):41-43, 1986.

Strangio L: Believe it or not: peritoneal dialysis made easy, Nursing 88 **18**(1):43-46, 1988.

Watt RC: Nursing management of a patient with a urinary diversion, Semin Oncol Nurs **2**(4):265-269, 1986.

Disorders of the Reproductive System and Sexually Transmitted Diseases

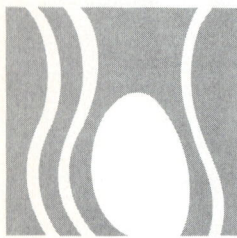

Human sexuality involves a complex interplay of biologic, psychologic, and sociocultural variables. Sexual self-concept includes the images individuals have of themselves as men or women and is as integral a component of sexual health as sexual functioning and relationships. There are significant variations in the range of sexual expression reflecting personal, cultural, and religious norms and attitudes.

The impact of aging, illness, surgery, and hospitalization on sexuality has received a great deal of attention in recent years. It is now clearly recognized that most cardiovascular, endocrine, neurologic, and orthopedic conditions have the potential to significantly interrupt a patient's view of himself or herself as a man or woman as well as indirectly or directly affect sexual functioning. It is essential that the nurse be sensitive and alert to these influences as she assesses and plans care. The continued specter of traditional sexually transmitted diseases and the continuing growth of the AIDS epidemic make it crucial that every nurse possess the ability and commitment to assess sexual health and include it in care planning with all patients, not just those experiencing reproductive disorders.

ASSESSING SEXUAL HEALTH

Many nurses are unfamiliar with the techniques of sexual assessment and uncomfortable about learning them. The increased openness in our society about sexual matters has resulted in patients who expect to be able to approach their health care providers to discuss issues of sexual concern. A brief sexual assessment may be incorporated into the nursing data base with three simple questions:

Has your (illness, hospitalization, etc.) affected your being a (wife, husband, mother, etc.)?

Has your (illness, surgery, etc.) affected the way you see yourself as a (man, woman)?

Has your (surgery, heart attack, etc.) affected your ability to function sexually (or your sex life)?

These brief questions invite the patient to share sexual concerns with the nurse. If used in an environment of privacy, incorporating language the patient can relate to, then permission is conveyed to the patient to add sexuality concerns to the overall discussion.

The remainder of this chapter discusses specific reproductive health problems that may significantly impact on the individual's sexuality.

FEMALE REPRODUCTIVE SYSTEM

The most common problems of the female reproductive system are problems of menstruation and menopause, contraception, and vaginal infection. With the exception of pelvic inflammatory disease, these disorders are usually treated on an outpatient basis. Nursing interventions involve careful teaching of patients to prevent recurrence where possible. Figure 14-1 illustrates the female internal organs of reproduction. Table 14-1 summarizes commonly encountered vaginal infections and their treatment.

Problems of the female reproductive system that necessitate hospital and frequently surgery include structural problems, benign tumors, and cancer. Table 14-2 describes common structural problems and their treatment. Table 14-3 describes common benign tumors other than fibroid tumors, which are discussed in the text. Cancers of the reproductive tract are also covered in the text. Breast disorders, both benign and malignant, are also significant health problems for women. These disorders are discussed at the end of this section.

FIBROID TUMORS (MYOMAS)

Fibroid tumors are quite common, particularly in black women and women who have never been pregnant. It is

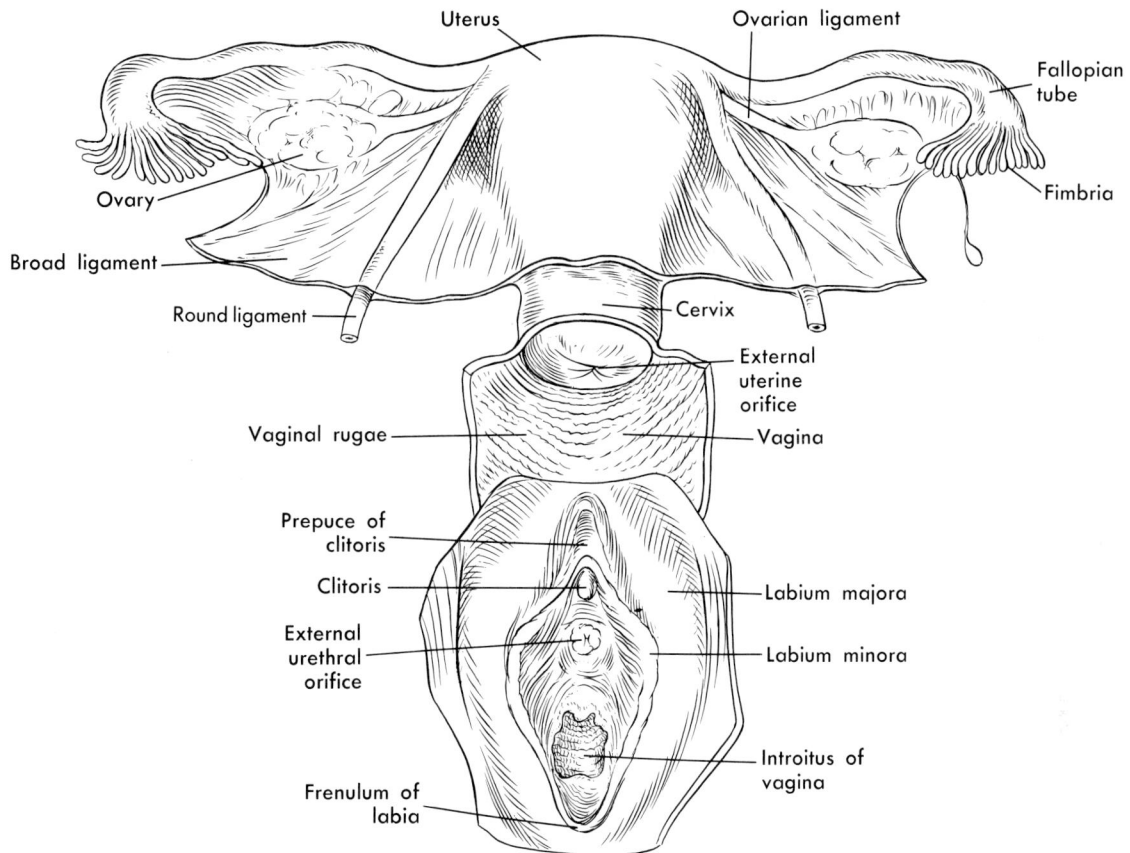

FIGURE 14-1 Female internal organs of reproduction. Major ligaments are shown. (From Long BC and Phipps WJ: Essentials of medical-surgical nursing: a nursing process approach, ed 2, St Louis, 1989, The CV Mosby Co.)

TABLE 14-1 Common infections of the female reproductive system

Condition	Symptoms	Medical Management
Candidiasis	Vaginal itching and irritation Thick, white, cheesy discharge Frequent recurrence	Nystatin (Mycostatin) vaginal suppositories Miconazole (Monistat) vaginal cream
Trichomoniasis	Severe vulvar itching, burning, excoriation Yellowish to greenish discharge that is thick, foamy, and malodorous	Metronidazole (Flagyl) orally Floraquin vaginal tablets preceded by white vinegar douching
Simple vaginitis	Vulvar irritation Yellowish mucoid discharge	Appropriate antibiotic applied locally or taken systemically
Bartholinitis	Erythema around Bartholin's gland Swelling, edema, and pain	Appropriate antibiotics Surgical drainage or gland excision

Pelvic inflammatory disease (PID)	Ascending infection, which may affect ovaries, fallopian tubes, and other pelvic tissue. Acute symptoms include the following:
	Severe lower abdominal pain
	Fever and chills
	Purulent discharge
	Malaise, nausea, and vomiting
		Appropriate antibiotics orally or IV
		Bed rest for acute cases
		Analgesics and local comfort measures as needed
		General care:
		  Sitz baths
		  Sexual abstinence while symptomatic
		  Careful personal hygiene

TABLE 14-2 Structural problems of the female reproductive tract

Disorder	Signs and Symptoms	Medical Management
Uterine displacement or prolapse	Dysmenorrhea Chronic backache, pelvic pressure	Minor displacement may be treated with pelvic exercises Prolapse is treated by hysterectomy
Cystocele (weakening of anterior wall causes bladder to herniate into vagina)	Dragging pain in back and pelvis, worsened by prolonged standing or walking Stress incontinence	Surgical repair through tightening of the vaginal wall (anterior colporrhaphy)
Rectocele (weakening of the posterior wall causes rectum to herniate into vagina)	Dragging pain in back and pelvis, worsened by prolonged standing or walking Constipation and hemorrhoids	Surgical repair through tightening of the vaginal wall (posterior colporrhaphy)

TABLE 14-3 Benign tumors of the female reproductive tract

Disorder	Signs and Symptoms	Medical Management

Ovarian tumors and cysts (numerous varieties develop)	Early stages:
	  Asymptomatic or nonspecific
	Later stages:
	  Increasing abdominal size
	  Pelvic fullness or pressure
	  Menstrual irregularities
	  Pain if cyst twists
		Surgical removal, usually involving oopherectomy

Endometriosis (seeding of endometrial cells throughout the pelvis)	Pain and discomfort with menstruation Fullness in abdomen Menstrual irregularities Infertility	Oral contraceptives to produce endometrial atrophy In advanced cases with widespread adhesions, surgery may be necessary—hysterectomy, oopherectomy, or salpingectomy
Cervical polyps (proliferation of an area of cervical mucosa)	Small episodes of bleeding between menstrual cycles Contact bleeding with intercourse, examination, or douching	Removal of the polyp with biopsy forceps or sharp curette

estimated that 20% to 25% of women over 30 years of age develop myomas. Their growth is believed to be stimulated by hormones so they tend to disappear at menopause and rarely become malignant.

PATHOPHYSIOLOGY

The cause of myomas is unknown. They vary significantly in size and primarily affect the body of the uterus but also can affect the cervix or the broad ligament. Larger tumors may cause actual uterine enlargement, impinge on the blood supply, or cause bleeding or obstruction.

MEDICAL MANAGEMENT

Treatment depends on the severity of symptoms and the age of the patient. Close supervision may be all that is necessary if symptoms are not severe, although women nearing menopause who have completed their families are frequently treated by hysterectomy.

NURSING MANAGEMENT

Assessment

Subjective

History of the condition

Presenting symptoms and severity: menorrhagia or pain

Feelings about hysterectomy

Knowledge of procedure and its effects

Constipation

Menstrual history

Objective (postoperative)

Vital signs

Urinary output

Vaginal bleeding

Peripheral circulation

Nursing Diagnoses

Diagnoses depend on the surgical approach used and the patient's response to surgery but commonly include the following:

Pain related to surgical incision and gaseous distention

Potential for ineffective individual coping related to the situational crisis of abrupt loss of childbearing potential

Potential for altered tissue perfusion (peripheral) related to pelvic vessel congestion

Expected Outcomes

Patient will experience decreasing discomfort and resume normal activity.

Patient will make a positive adjustment to the loss of reproductive function and maintain a positive body image.

Patient will maintain adequate venous return and be free of phlebitis or thrombosis.

Nursing Interventions: Preoperative

Teach patient about planned procedure.

Explain importance of early ambulation and leg exercises to prevent complications.

Administer douche or enema as ordered.

Nursing Interventions: Postoperative

Maintain use of thigh-high TED stockings.

Encourage patient to ambulate and perform ankle and leg exercises. Assess for Homans' sign.

Maintain patency of urinary catheter if used.

     Ensure adequacy of output after removal.

     Keep accurate intake and output records.

     Provide regular perineal care after each void or defecation.

     Catheterize for residual if ordered.

Assess incision frequently if abdominal approach used.

Maintain perineal pad count. Assess for excess bleeding.

Auscultate abdomen for return of active peristalsis.

     Restrict food and fluid until patient passes flatus.

     Encourage ambulation to stimulate peristalsis.

     Offer rectal tube for excess flatus if ordered.

Encourage patient to verbalize feelings and concerns.

Offer support if depression occurs.

Teach patient the following before discharge:

     Patient should avoid driving for first weeks after surgery.

     Patient should avoid lifting, straining, or constipation.

     Patient can resume sexual intercourse after 4 to 6 weeks. Vaginal sensation may be decreased initially.

Ensure that patient understands changes that will result from onset of menopause, as appropriate.

Explain precaution for estrogen replacement if ordered.

Evaluation

Patient is free of discomfort and gradually resumes all preoperative activities.

Patient integrates body changes into a positive body image and resumes preoperative familial and sexual roles.

Patient experiences no complications in the postoperative period.

CANCER OF THE REPRODUCTIVE TRACT

Cancer involving the reproductive tract may affect the cervix, uterus, or ovaries and is a significant cause of death. Women with gynecologic cancers are faced with multiple threats—to survival, body image, gender role, and sexuality. The nurse must be sensitive to the potential effects of these disorders and their treatment. The nurse's approach to care needs to be both individual and holistic.

CANCER OF THE CERVIX

Early detection through the routine and regular use of Papanicolaou smears has helped to produce a steady decline in the mortality associated with cancer of the cervix. The disease is now considered to be virtually 100% curable when detected in the early stages.

Invasive cervical cancer occurs primarily in women of age 45 or older. Associated risk factors include first coitus at an early age, multiple sex partners, low socioeconomic status, and exposure to herpes virus type 2. Because the disease is virtually asymptomatic in the early stages, it is essential that screening efforts be directed at the high-risk populations.

Cervical cancer is treated according to the stage of the disease and the woman's age and general health status. Carcinoma in situ may be treated by excisional conization, cryosurgery, or simple hysterectomy. More invasive disease is treated with simple or radical hysterectomy, radiotherapy, or radiation implants. See Chapter 2 for a discussion of care associated with radiotherapy and page 212 for a discussion of hysterectomy.

NURSING CARE PLAN

FOLLOWING HYSTERECTOMY

Nursing Diagnoses	Expected Patient Outcomes	Nursing Interventions
Self-esteem disturbance related to loss of childbearing function	Patient verbalizes concerns about loss of uterus and maintains a positive view of herself.	1. Give patient opportunities to express feelings and concerns about loss of uterus. 2. Be empathetic of patient's feelings that may include grief, guilt, shame, or remorse. 3. Encourage patient to continue activities associated with femininity, such as putting on makeup, arranging hair, wearing own apparel. 4. Help patient identify personal strengths. 5. Help partner understand rationale for behaviors expressed by patient and encourage him to demonstrate continued affection. 6. Correct any misconceptions about effect of surgery on sexual intercourse (normal relationships may be resumed after 4 to 6 weeks).
Pain related to surgical incision and gaseous distention	Patient experiences decreasing discomfort and successfully passes flatus.	1. Use analgesics as needed during early postoperative period. 2. Encourage progressive ambulation to prevent abdominal distention. 3. If abdominal distention occurs, try a heating pad or rectal tube; administer any prescribed enemas.
Potential for altered patterns of urinary elimination related to pelvic edema and discomfort	Patient resumes a normal urinary elimination pattern.	1. Monitor intake and output for at least 48 hours; assess for urinary retention, if appropriate. 2. Use measures to facilitate voiding if urinary retention occurs. Monitor frequency and amount of voidings. 3. Provide catheter care if patient has an indwelling catheter.
Potential for altered tissue perfusion (peripheral) related to venous congestion in the pelvis	Patient maintains an adequate venous return and is free of thrombosis or phlebitis.	1. Monitor patient for leg or chest pain or for sudden dyspnea; assess for Homans' sign. Apply thigh-high TED stockings. 2. Encourage leg exercises and frequent turning in bed during early postoperative period. Encourage ambulation. 3. Avoid elevating bottom of bed or placing pillows under knees; encourage patient to keep knees flat while in bed.

Knowledge deficit related to onset and management of menopause	Patient is knowledgeable about the effects of surgery and makes informed decisions about estrogen replacement.	1. Teach patient the following:
		  a. Physiologic effects of the hysterectomy
		  b. That psychologic reactions may continue for a few weeks
		  c. Possibility of slight vaginal discharge for 1 to 2 weeks
		  d. To avoid driving a car for 2 to 4 weeks (especially with standard shift drive)
		  e. To avoid heavy activities and active sports for 4 to 6 weeks
		  f. To report to physician excessive or persistent vaginal drainage or signs of thrombophlebitis
		  g. Pros and cons of estrogen replacement therapy

CANCER OF THE ENDOMETRIUM

Cancer of the uterus primarily affects postmenopausal women between the ages of 50 and 65. Associated risk factors include obesity, late menopause, and nulliparity. Risks associated with the use of exogenous estrogens are under intense scrutiny. The tumor usually grows slowly and is responsive to treatment if identified early. There are few early symptoms—spotting and bleeding are the most common. Postmenopausal bleeding should always be carefully evaluated to rule out cancer.

Endometrial cancer is treated according to the stage of the disease but most commonly includes total abdominal hysterectomy and bilateral salpingo oophorectomy. Treatment for advanced disease may also include the use of postoperative radiation.

CANCER OF THE OVARY

Ovarian cancer is the most deadly form of female genital cancer. It can occur at any age, although the greatest number of cases occur in women between 50 and 59. There are no identified risk factors, and early diagnosis usually occurs by chance. Symptoms include abdominal enlargement, pain, pressure, and constipation. The disease is staged during an initial laparotomy, which usually includes total abdominal hysterectomy and bilateral salpingo oophorectomy. Depending on the stage of the disease, chemotherapy and radiation may also be used as adjuvant therapy, but the prognosis is generally poor.

BENIGN BREAST DISORDERS

Fibrocystic disease causes thickened nodules, often bilateral, that become painful before or during menstruation and are believed to be related to cyclic hormonal imbalance. One distressing factor about fibrocystic disease is that it makes malignancies much more difficult to detect. Meticulous breast self-examination is particularly important.

Fibroadenomas are tumors thought to result from hyperestrinism (excess estrogen). The tumor is usually removed locally and carefully analyzed for malignant cells.

MALIGNANT BREAST DISORDERS

The prevalence of breast cancer makes the disease of enormous concern to women of all ages. Breast cancers are the most common malignancies in women and are the second leading cause of cancer-related deaths in women. The reason breast cancers occur is not known, although some risk factors have been identified and are listed in the box on this page. The incidence is increasing in virtually all populations. Breast cancer can occur at virtually any age, but two thirds of the cases are in women over age 50. Despite significant advances in therapy, the mortality rate has remained almost un-

---

RISK FACTORS ASSOCIATED WITH BREAST CANCER

Menarche before age 11
Menopause after age 50
Family history of breast cancer—especially mother or sister
Nulliparity or birth of first child after age 30
History of uterine cancer
Link with obesity, high consumption of fat and alcohol
Presence of benign breast disease
Link with the use of oral contraceptives, remains unproven

---

changed over the last 40 years and is primarily dependent on the size of the lesion at diagnosis.

Prevention of breast cancer is not possible at this time, but early diagnosis is essential to successful treatment. Ninety percent of cancers are identified through breast self-examination, which should be taught to and practiced by all women beginning at high school age. The technique is summarized in the box on this page. Mammography is about 80% to 97% accurate in detecting breast cancer, and the American Cancer Society recommends a baseline mammogram between the ages of 35 and 40, with annual exams after age 50. Thermography, xeroradiography, ultrasound, computed tomography (CT), and magnetic resonance imaging (MRI) scans are other diagnostic options. A biopsy, however, is necessary to accurately diagnose the tumor.

PATHOPHYSIOLOGY

Breast cancer is not a single disease but many related ones, with its exact nature dependent on the tissue of

---

BREAST SELF-EXAMINATION (BSE)

Perform BSE regularly each month.
  Premenopausal women: shortly after conclusion of the menstrual period
  Postmenopausal women: at a set time each month (such as the first day of the month)
Use a systematic approach (*one* of the three listed below)
  Palpate in concentric circles, beginning at outer rim of breast tissue and moving toward nipple.
  Divide breast into quadrants and examine area in each quadrant from outer perimeter toward nipple.
  Palpate inner half then outer half of breast.
Examine the entire breast tissue, including the tail and the nipple.
Carry out examination in both the horizontal and vertical body positions.
Use the flat parts of the fingers for palpation.

From Long BC and Phipps WJ: Essentials of medical-surgical nursing: a nursing process approach, ed 2, St Louis, 1989, The CV Mosby Co.

the breast involved, its estrogen dependency, and the age of the patient at onset. Premenopausal and post-menopausal patients in particular show different treatment responses and prognoses. Prognosis depends on the extent of disease present at the time of diagnosis. Classic symptoms that define breast cancers include the following:

Firm, nontender, nonmobile masses

Solitary, irregularly shaped mass

Adherence to muscle or skin, causing dimpling effect

Involvement of upper outer quadrant or central nipple portion of breast

MEDICAL MANAGEMENT

Major changes are currently being made in modes of treatment for women with breast cancer. The nurse plays a major role in assisting the patient to make informed choices and assume a partnership role in planning her own care. A variety of treatment plans are available, and controversy persists over the use of the various protocols.

In the past the treatment of choice for breast cancer was consistently surgical, but today a combination of treatments is frequently used to meet the primary goal of effecting local and regional disease control. Several surgical options are available:

Lumpectomy (believed to be sufficient treatment in combination with irradiation for small lesions up to 5 cm in size)

Partial mastectomy

Simple mastectomy

Modified radical mastectomy

Radiation therapy may be administered externally or through the implantation of iridium needles. This implantation treatment was initiated in Europe and initially has shown outcomes similar to those of modified radical surgery. Chemotherapy is typically given as adjuvant therapy after treatment. Breast reconstruction is an option being offered to increasing numbers of women.

NURSING MANAGEMENT

Assessment

Subjective

Presence of risk factors

Breast self-examination routine

Symptoms and time period since discovery

Knowledge of treatment options

Patient's procurement of a second opinion

Knowledge of treatment protocol planned

Support systems and their adequacy and response

Usual coping patterns

Current state of anxiety

Feelings about surgery and future

Attitudes and knowledge of husband or partner

Objective

General health status

Breast inspection (symmetry, skin dimpling)

Presence of breast mass confirmed by mammography or biopsy

Nursing Diagnoses

Diagnoses will depend on the extent of surgery and the woman's response, but commonly include the following:

Anxiety related to uncertainty of diagnosis or decisions about treatment protocol

Potential for ineffective individual or family coping related to body changes and perceived loss of attractiveness

Body image disturbance related to mutilating aspects of the surgical procedure

Knowledge deficit related to postoperative rehabilitation and support groups

Pain related to surgical incision and alteration in chest wall musculature

Anticipatory grieving related to loss of body part

Expected Outcomes

Patient's anxiety will be reduced to a level that allows informed decision making and ongoing self-care.

Patient and family will verbalize their feelings concerning the diagnosis and treatment, providing mutual support.

Patient will gradually integrate body changes into an altered but positive body image.

Patient will be knowledgeable concerning the exercises and self-care practices that will facilitate rehabilitation.

Patient will experience decreasing levels of discomfort and maintain full use of affected arm and shoulder.

Patient will express feelings of grief over needed surgery and loss of breast.

Nursing Interventions: Preoperative

Assist patient to verbalize feelings about meaning of impending surgery. Include husband and family as appropriate.

Encourage family to express fears and love to patient.

Support patient in whatever decisions she makes about treatment protocol. Repeat all teaching as needed.

Provide simple explanations of impending surgery and expected postoperative care.

Describe size and appearance of postoperative dressing.

Explain use of Hemovac if planned.

Teach exercises that will be used postoperatively.

Evaluate suitability of preoperative visit by Reach to Recovery volunteer.

Nursing Interventions: Postoperative (Mastectomy)

Place patient in semi-Fowler's position, with arm elevated on pillows.

Monitor Hemovac output.

Check dressing frequently for bleeding or excess serous drainage.

Check behind patient for bleeding.

Post signs warning against taking blood pressure, starting IVs, or drawing blood on affected side.

Initiate exercises to prevent stiffness and contracture of shoulder girdle.

Immediate:

Flex and extend fingers.

Pronate and supinate forearm.

Day 1 after operation:

Squeeze rubber ball as tolerated.

Brush teeth and hair.

Teach special mastectomy exercises as prescribed (see box on this page). Exercise bilaterally, using both arms.

POSTMASTECTOMY ARM EXERCISES

EXERCISE: CLIMBING THE WALL

1. Stand facing wall with toes close to wall.
2. Bend elbows and place palms of hands against wall at shoulder level.
3. Move both hands parallel to each other up the wall as far as possible until incisional pull or pain occurs.
4. Move both hands down to starting position.
5. Goal is complete extension with elbow straight.
6. Activities that utilize the same action, reaching top shelves, hanging out clothes, washing windows, hanging curtains, setting hair.

EXERCISE: ARM SWINGING

1. Bend forward from waist, permitting both arms to relax and hang naturally.
2. Swing arms together left to right (motion comes from shoulder).
3. Swing arms in circles parallel to floor, clockwise and counterclockwise.
4. Stand up slowly.

EXERCISE: ROPE PULL

1. Attach a rope over a shower rod or hook.
2. Grasp each end of rope, alternately pulling on each end, raising affected arm to a point of incisional pull or pain.
3. Shorten rope over time until affected arm is raised almost directly overhead.

EXERCISE: ELBOW SPREAD

1. Clasp hands behind neck.
2. Raise elbows to chin level, holding head erect. Move slowly and rest when incisional pull or pain occurs.
3. Gradually spread elbows apart. Rest when pull or pain occurs.

From American Cancer Society: Reach to recovery, New York, The Society.

Provide adequate analgesia to promote ambulation and exercise. Pain may be referred to arm and shoulder.

Encourage regular coughing and deep breathing exercises.

Continue to assist patient to explore and verbalize her feelings and grief. Prepare for easy fatigability.

Prepare patient for size and appearance of the incision. Provide support when incision is viewed for first time.

Help family to show patient appropriate love and support.

Arrange visit by Reach to Recovery volunteer.

Provide patient with detailed information concerning breast prostheses.

Fitting is not possible for 4 to 6 weeks.

A temporary prosthesis or lightly padded bra is worn until healing is complete.

Teach patient to avoid constrictive clothing and report persistent edema, redness, or infection of incision.

Teach patient to protect arm from minor injury, particularly if lymphedema is present.

Teach patient importance of continuing monthly breast examination on remaining breast (see box on p. 215).

Refer to Chapter 2 for appropriate interventions related to chemotherapy or radiation therapy.

Assist patient to explore available options for breast reconstruction.

Evaluation

Patient's anxiety is controlled; patient participates in decision making and acquires self-care skills.

Patient and family verbalize feelings with each other and provide mutual support.

Patient integrates mastectomy into body image, speaks positively of self, and resumes normal social and sexual activity.

Patient practices postmastectomy exercises and maintains full range of motion and strength on affected side.

Patient is free of discomfort and edema.

Patient successfully resolves grief related to diagnosis and surgery.

MALE REPRODUCTIVE SYSTEM

Disorders of the male reproductive system may affect any structure, but by far the most commonly affected site is the prostate gland. Other disorders include a wide range of infectious, obstructive, and malignant processes. Figure 14-2 illustrates the male organs of reproduction.

BENIGN PROSTATIC HYPERTROPHY
PATHOPHYSIOLOGY

Prostatic enlargement affects more than 50% of men over age 50 and 75% of those over 70. Benign prostatic

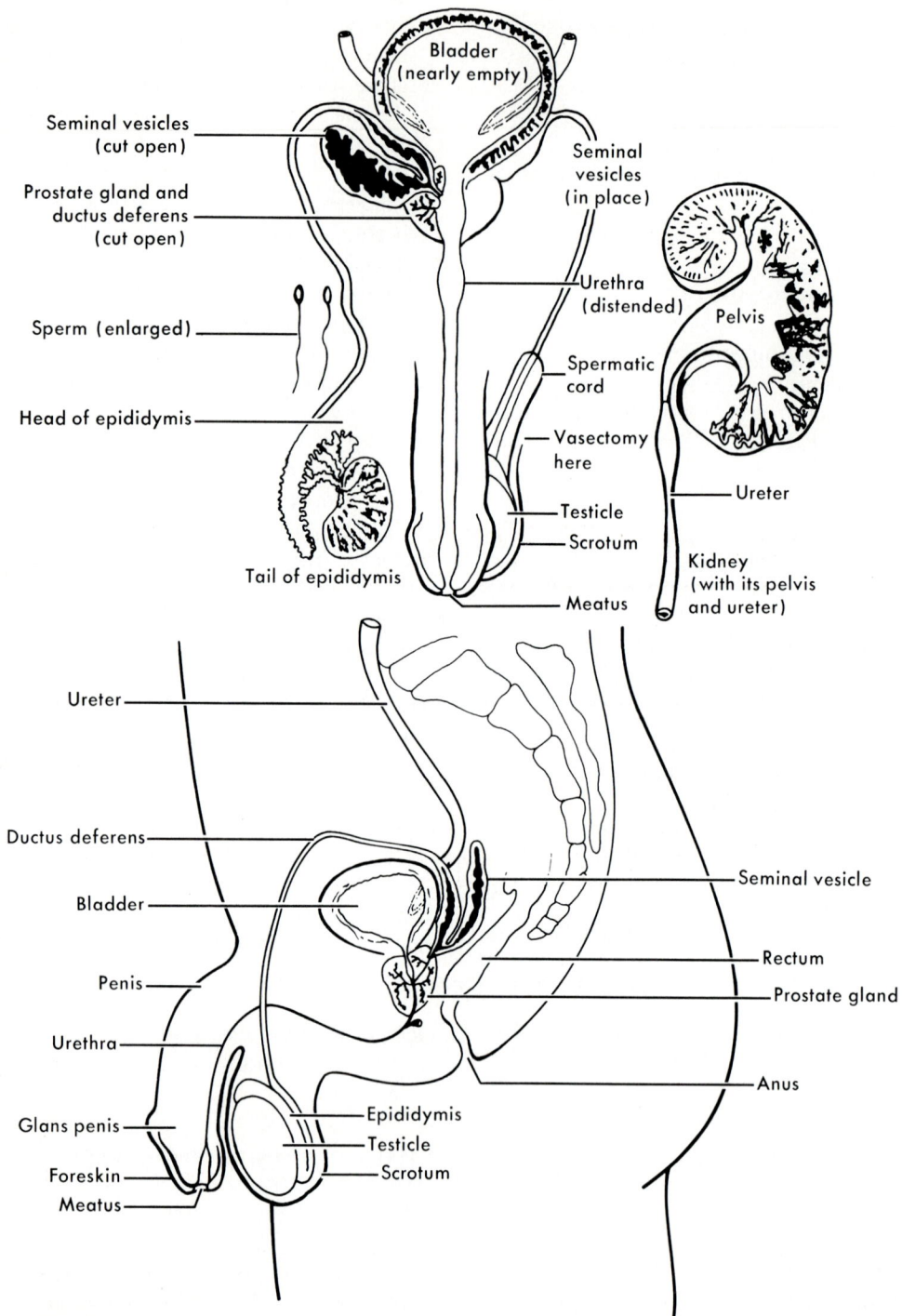

FIGURE 14-2 Male organs of reproduction. Note relatively large size of seminal vesicle as compared with testicle. (From Long BC and Phipps WJ: Medical-surgical nursing: a nursing process approach, ed 2, St Louis, 1989, The CV Mosby Co.)

hypertrophy or hyperplasia (BPH) is an adenomatous enlargement of the prostate gland. The cause is unknown, but the condition appears to be related to the presence of a hormone imbalance that occurs with aging. There is overgrowth of smooth muscle and connective tissue and an increase in glandular tissue. The enlargement produces compression of the urethra and symptoms of progressive urinary obstruction.

MEDICAL MANAGEMENT

Prevention of BPH is not possible, but early detection and effective treatment can successfully prevent complications. Surgery is the primary treatment. The various procedures used are described in Table 14-4. The transurethral resection (TUR) is the most common. In this procedure the capsule is left intact while the adenomatous soft tissue overgrowth is removed.

NURSING MANAGEMENT

Assessment

Subjective
History of the disorder and symptoms
Patient's knowledge of cause and proposed treatment
Patient's feelings about proposed surgery
    Impact on sexuality and self-concept
Patient's complaints of the following:
    Urinary frequency, nocturia
    Difficulty starting urinary stream
    Decrease in size or force of stream
    Symptoms of cystitis

Objective
Hematuria
Acute urinary retention
Evidence of prostatic enlargement with rectal digital examination and/or cystoscopy

---

TABLE 14-4 Comparison of types of prostatic surgery

Type of Surgery and Reason for Use	Location of Incision	Drainage Tubes	Bladder Spasms	Dressing	Complications
Transurethral resection Enlargement of medial lobe surrounding urethra	No incision; removal by way of urethra	Three-way Foley catheter with 30 ml bag in urethra, constant irrigation for 24 hr	Yes	No dressing	Hemorrhage; water intoxication; incontinence
Suprapubic resection Extremely large mass of obstructing tissue	Low midline abdominal incision through bladder to prostate gland	Cystotomy tube or drain through incision; Foley catheter with 30 ml bag in urethra	Yes	Abdominal dressing; easily soaked with urinary drainage	Hemorrhage; wound infection
Retropubic resection Large mass located high in pelvic area	Low midline incision into prostate gland (bladder not incised)	Foley catheter with 30 ml bag in urethra, constant irrigation for 24 hr	Few	Abdominal dressing; no urinary drainage	Hemorrhage; wound infection
Perineal resection Large mass located low in pelvic area	Incision between scrotum and rectum	Foley catheter with 30 ml bag in urethra	Few	Perineal dressing; no urinary drainage	Hemorrhage; wound infection
Radical perineal resection Cancer of prostate gland	Large perineal incision between scrotum and rectum	Foley catheter with 30 ml bag in urethra; drain in incision	Few	Perineal dressing; urinary drainage	Urinary incontinence; wound infection; impotence; sterility

Modified from Phipps WJ, Long BC, and Woods NF: Medical-surgical nursing: concepts and clinical practice, ed 4, St Louis, 1990, Mosby-Year Book, Inc.

BENIGN PROSTATIC HYPERTROPHY FOLLOWING TUR PROSTATECTOMY

Nursing Diagnoses	Expected Patient Outcomes	Nursing Interventions

Altered patterns of urinary elimination related to obstruction of urine outflow or presence of Foley catheter	Urinary output is unobstructed and bleeding gradually decreases.
	Patient returns to a normal continent pattern of urinary elimination.
		1. Monitor urinary output and characteristics frequently.
		2. Maintain constant bladder irrigation as prescribed during first 24 hours at a rate sufficient to keep output pink to light red in color.
		3. Monitor patient for signs of bladder spasms. Ensure patency of system if spasms occur.
		4. Teach patient not to try to void around the catheter.
		5. Administer prescribed antispasmodics and reassure patient that spasms diminish in 24 to 48 hours.
		6. Maintain patency of indwelling urinary catheter:
		  a. Irrigate manually as prescribed to keep catheter free of clots.
		  b. Maintain straight-line closed drainage system.
		7. Encourage high fluid intake (2500 to 3000 ml/day) to promote increased urinary flow.
		8. After catheter is removed, monitor for signs of retention. Assess patient for dribbling. If dribbling occurs:
		  a. Tell patient this is a common occurrence but that continence will return.
		  b. Teach patient perineal exercises.

Potential for sexual dysfunction, related to perceived effects of prostatectomy on sexual functioning	Patient returns to his preillness pattern of sexual activity and satisfaction.	1. Provide information as necessary:
		  a. TUR procedure does not affect sexual functioning but does cause sterility.
		  b. Retrograde ejaculation will occur and urine may have a milky appearance.
		2. Give patient opportunities to discuss feelings about the effects of prostatectomy on sexual potency.
		3. Avoid sexual intercourse for 4 to 6 weeks after surgery.

Knowledge deficit related to activity restrictions for the postdischarge period	Patient understands activity restrictions to be followed and need for medical follow-up.	1. Teach patient the following:
		  a. Avoidance of heavy activities for 4 to 6 weeks.
		  b. Avoidance of straining at stool for 4 to 6 weeks; use stool softeners or laxatives as necessary; avoid Valsalva maneuver.
		  c. Patient should not drive a car or sit for prolonged periods for 4 to 6 weeks.
		  d. Ambulation is encouraged.
		  e. Fluid maintenance of at least 2500 ml/day to prevent complications.
		  f. Urine should remain clear; report onset of fresh bleeding to physician.
		  g. Instructions for medical follow-up.

Nursing Diagnoses

Altered patterns of urinary elimination related to obstruction of urine outflow

Knowledge deficit related to the functions of the prostate gland and its role in sexual performance

Potential for sexual dysfunction related to the perceived effects of prostatectomy on sexual potency

Expected Outcomes

Patient will gradually return to a normal continent pattern of urinary elimination.

Patient will be knowledgeable about the role of the prostate gland and the impact of prostatectomy.

Patient will return to his preillness pattern of sexual activity and satisfaction.

Nursing Interventions (for TUR): Preoperative

Monitor intake and output.

Teach patient about procedure and expected care routines after surgery.

Encourage patient to express concerns about surgery and its impact on sexuality. Reassure patient that procedures other than radical prostatectomy do not affect sexual potency.

Nursing Interventions (for TUR): Postoperative

Maintain patency of continuous bladder irrigation if utilized (usually for first 24 hours).

Solution should run rapidly enough to maintain urinary drainage of light pink-red color.

Monitor carefully for clot formation.

Maintain accurate intake and output records.

Maintain traction on catheter as prescribed.

Monitor vital signs frequently.

Teach patient that 30 ml catheter balloon triggers constant urge to void and bladder spasms.

Sensations decrease after 24 to 48 hours.

Instruct patient not to strain to void around the catheter.

Administer analgesics and antispasmodics as needed (belladonna and opium).

Manually irrigate catheter if prescribed.

Encourage liberal fluid intake by mouth unless contraindicated.

Avoid use of rectal thermometer or tube and enemas.

Provide or teach patient scrupulous catheter care. Monitor carefully for signs of infection.

Measure and record time and amount of each voiding.

Assess for adequacy of voiding and bladder emptying when catheter is removed.

Teach patient perineal exercises to aid in full return of urinary control. Dribbling is a common temporary problem.

Teach patient about postdischarge care.

Patient should refrain from lifting, vigorous exercise, driving, and sexual activity for 3 to 6 weeks.

Patient should use stool softener to avoid straining.

Patient should keep fluid intake high.

Patient should contact physician if hematuria or signs of infection or cystitis occur. Rebleeding after 2 weeks is possible.

Instruct patient to avoid alcohol, which may cause burning during healing.

Evaluation

Patient voids comfortably at regular intervals and does not experience dribbling.

Patient is knowledgeable about procedure, its effects on sexuality, and activity restrictions in postoperative period.

Patient returns to presurgical sexual functioning.

TUMORS

Tumors of the male reproductive tract are almost always malignant. Except for tumors of the prostate gland, they occur quite rarely. Cancer of the testes and penis is described in Table 14-5. These disorders and their treatment may have devastating effects on the man's body image and sexual role. Testicular self-examination is considered an important health promotion technique to be taught to young adult males. The steps are outlined in the box on the next page and illustrated in Figure 14-3.

TABLE 14-5 Cancer of the testes and penis

Site	Incidence Rate (%)	Usual Age of Onset (yr)	Signs and Symptoms	Medical Management
Testes	1-2	18-35	Painless enlarged testis and scrotum Gynecomastia (breast development)	Surgery (orchiectomy) plus radiation and/or chemotherapy
Penis	1	50-70	Nodular growth on foreskin Fatigue, weight loss	Surgery—partial or total penectomy followed by plastic repair if feasible

TESTICULAR SELF-EXAMINATION

Perform testicular self-examination (TSE) after a bath or shower when scrotum is warm and most relaxed.

Grasp testis with both hands and palpate gently between thumb and fingers.

The testis should feel smooth, egg-shaped, and firm to touch.

The epididymis, found behind the testis, feels like a soft tube.

Report any abnormal lump or swelling to the physician.

From Long BC, and Phipps WJ: Essentials of medical-surgical nursing: a nursing approach, ed 2, St Louis, 1989, The CV Mosby Co.

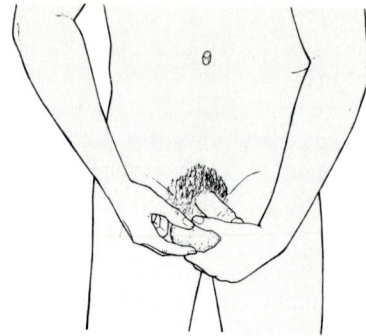

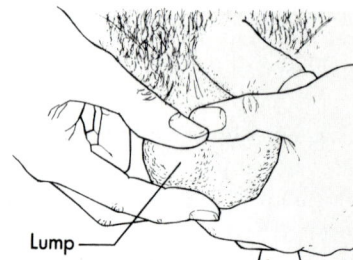

CANCER OF THE PROSTATE

Cancer of the prostate, the third leading cause of cancer-related death in men, typically occurs in men over the age of 60. The reason cancer of the prostate develops remains unknown, but it is clearly related to the aging process. The actual disease prevalence is unknown as it is frequently found undiagnosed at autopsy.

Most tumors are multifocal and arise as one or more palpable hardened nodules. The tumors may invade adjacent anatomic structures and metastasize through vascular and lymph pathways. Tumor growth gradually obstructs the bladder outlet, interfering with urinary elimination. There are often no early symptoms, but advanced disease may mimic BPH.

Treatment varies and is based on the type of tumor and its stage. Radical prostatectomy may be used when the tumor is confined to the prostatic capsule. Radiotherapy administered externally or through implantation of irradiated seeds and hormonal therapy are other treatment options. Urinary incontinence and sexual impotence are common complications of treatment.

FIGURE 14-3 Self-examination of the testis. (From Phipps WJ, Long BC, and Woods NF: Medical-surgical nursing: concepts and clinical practice, ed 4, St Louis, 1990, Mosby–Year Book, Inc.)

INFLAMMATORY DISORDERS

Urethritis, prostatitis, epididymitis, and orchitis are the most common infections affecting the male reproductive tract. The infecting organisms may reach the genital tract by direct spread up the urethra or be borne by blood or lymph. Table 14-6 describes these conditions.

STRUCTURAL DISORDERS

Structural disorders of the testes and scrotum are described in Table 14-7. Immediate medical attention is crucial because the degree of testicular damage may be influenced by the promptness of intervention.

TABLE 14-6 Inflammatory disorders of the male reproductive tract

Disorder	Signs and Symptoms	Medical Management
Urethritis	Urgency, frequency, and burning with urination Purulent urethral discharge	Appropriate antibiotics
Prostatitis	Perineal pain, fever, dysuria Urethral discharge	Appropriate antibiotics Rest, hydration, sitz baths, stool softeners
Epididymitis	Sudden scrotal pain and edema	Appropriate antibiotics Bed rest with scrotal elevation Analgesics
Orchitis	Same as for epididymitis Nausea and vomiting Pain radiating to inguinal canal	Same as for epididymitis

TABLE 14-7 Structural disorders of the testes and scrotum

Disorder	Description	Medical Management
Hydrocele	Benign, nontender collection of clear amber fluid within the outer covering of the testes; leads to scrotal swelling	Aspiration of the fluid
Spermatocele	Benign, nontender cystic mass attached to epididymis; contains milky fluid and sperm	Usually no treatment is needed—aspiration or excision
Varicocele	Dilation of spermatic vein, usually on the left side	Ligation of the vein
Torsion of spermatic cord	Kinking and twisting of spermatic cord and artery	Surgical fixation of testes to scrotal wall; excision of testes if gangrenous Spermatogenesis is usually destroyed, although hormone production may continue

SEXUALLY TRANSMITTED DISEASES

Sexually transmitted diseases (STDs) are disorders that are usually transmitted from one person to another during sexual contact with the genitals, mouth, or rectum. The category includes classic venereal diseases such as syphilis and gonorrhea as well as a wide variety of other diseases including genital herpes, nonspecific urethritis, scabies, and venereal warts. The addition of AIDS to the roster of STDs has refocused attention on these ancient health problems.

Changing sexual behavior patterns and improved laboratory methods for diagnosis have resulted in many of the STDs reaching epidemic proportions. The more recently recognized effects of these diseases on fertility and maternal and infant mortality makes their prompt identification and treatment of significant concern to nurses. The highest incidence is typically in the 15- to 29-year-old age group, but any sexually active person may be at risk, particularly individuals with multiple sex partners. Table 14-8 outlines the symptoms and treatment of syphilis and gonorrhea. Table 14-9 lists other common STDs and their causative features.

NURSING MANAGEMENT

Assessment

Subjective
History of sexual activity—number of partners
Prior history of STD and treatment
Knowledge of disease—risks, mode of transmission
Complaints of the following:
    Vulvar or vaginal itching
    Dysuria and urgency
    Rectal symptoms
    Abdominal discomfort

Objective
Vaginal or penile discharge
Genital lesions
Skin rashes

Nursing Diagnoses
Knowledge deficit related to transmission of STD and prevention
Pain related to the presence of genital or rectal lesions
Self-esteem disturbance related to guilt or anger over acquiring a sexually transmitted disease

Expected Outcomes
Patient understands means of transmission of STDs and methods to prevent them.
Patient experiences decreased pain from effective local treatment.
Patient resolves feelings of anger and guilt associated with diagnosis.

Nursing Interventions
Encourage patient to verbalize feelings about acquisition of the disease.
Teach patient about etiology, transmission, treatment, and prevention of infection (see box on p. 225).
Teach patient principles of safer sex.
Encourage patient to complete full course of treatment.
Teach importance of refraining from sexual activity until treatment is complete.
Teach patient local care of skin lesions as appropriate:
    Frequent bathing
    Keeping lesions dry
    Use of cotton underwear to improve air circulation
    Local treatment as prescribed by physician
Encourage patient to inform sexual partners and assist them to seek appropriate treatment
Reinforce importance of basic hygiene in prevention

Evaluation
Patient is knowledgeable about treatment and prevention of STDs.
Patient is free of pain and itching from lesions.
Patient regains previous positive attitude toward self.

TABLE 14-8 Syphilis and gonorrhea

Disease	Incubation Period	Signs and Symptoms	Medical Management
Gonorrhea	Men: 3-30 days Women: 3 days to indefinite period	Men: purulent urethral discharge, dysuria, prostatitis, epididymitis; rectal and pharyngeal forms are usually asymptomatic Women: asymptomatic in early stages; slight purulent discharge, aching or discomfort in pelvis or abdomen	Intramuscular penicillin G and probenicid by mouth or ampicillin and probenicid Problems with resistant organisms have developed. Salpingitis, PID, and sterility are potential complications in women
Syphilis	3 weeks (9 days to 3 months)	Positive serologic tests Stage I: chancre (hard sore or pimple that breaks and forms painless, draining erosion on vulva, penis, mouth, or rectum) Stage II: fever, headache, malaise accompanied by sores or generalized body rash No signs during latent period Stage III: tumorlike masses, damage to heart valves and vessels, CNS involvement with paresis, loss of judgment and memory	Penicillin G benzathine intramuscularly or tetracycline for 7 days Amoxicillin with probenicid as single-dose therapy.

TABLE 14-9 Sexually transmitted diseases

Disease	Causes and Effects	Treatment
Chlamydial infection	The most prevalent STD in the United States; causes urethritis, epididymitis, cervicitis, PID, and lymphogranuloma venereum	Tetracycline or doxycycline for 7 days
Lymphogranuloma venereum	Usually caused by chlamydia organism; affects lymph nodes, often in inguinal area, which may suppurate; often accompanied by urethritis symptoms	Tetracycline for 2 weeks; erythromycin for 2-6 weeks
Chancroid	Rare disease caused by gram-negative bacilli; produces lesions on genitals—ragged irregular ulcers that are highly infectious	Erythromycin for 10 days; local cleansing and comfort measures
Candidiasis	Monilial infection caused by a yeast form; produces thick white vaginal discharge	Fungicidal creams, ointments and tablets—nystatin, miconazole; local measures to control itching
Human papillomavirus infection	Recently linked with development of cancer of the cervix; characterized by single or multiple painless growths in genital area	Application of podophyllin in tincture of benzoin; several treatments may be necessary.
Herpes genitalis	Caused by infection with herpesvirus type 2; 15% to 20% of Americans are estimated to suffer from the disease; causes primary lesions that develop into clear fluid-filled vesicles that form ulcerations when they rupture; causes pain and local inflammation and may produce general symptoms of infection	Symptomatic treatment of lesions; acyclovir ointment to limit duration of initial attack (does not prevent recurrences)

ACQUIRED IMMUNE DEFICIENCY SYNDROME (AIDS)

The phenomenon of AIDS emerged in this country in 1981 and has since grown to become the most significant and deadly of the sexually transmitted diseases. Over 100,000 cases have been identified in the United States since 1981, and the disease presents enormous medical, epidemiological, and social challenges to our society. Although once primarily confined to the homosexual male population, the disease has now made significant inroads into other populations, particularly IV drug abusers (see Table 14-10). Nurses must be knowledgeable about the disease process, skillful in the delivery of needed care, and strongly committed to efforts designed to educate the general population and reduce the spread of the disease.

PREVENTION OF STDS

Reduce the number of sex partners and avoid contact with persons with multiple partners.

Examine genital area regularly for sores, rashes, or discharge.

Wash hands and genital/rectal area before and after sex.

Use a condom as a barrier.

Use water-based lubricants to reduce spread of organisms.

Void before and after intercourse.

Avoid frequent douching.

Seek medical help promptly if symptoms develop. Abstain from sex until treatment is fully complete.

PATHOPHYSIOLOGY

AIDS is caused by the human immunodeficiency virus (HIV), which is classified as a retrovirus. The virus attacks the body's immune system, primarily the T cells, which are found in the bone marrow, develop in the thymus, and are responsible for all mediated immunity that protects the body from malignant cells, viruses, and parasites. The T_4 helper cells are particularly affected by the virus that invades the host cell, lives within it, and replicates itself.

The HIV is able to remain dormant in the body for years, producing no clinical symptoms. Although they are asymptomatic, persons infected with HIV are contagious and able to transmit the virus to others. At present, it is not known how many of these seropositive asymptomatic persons will eventually develop clinical AIDS.

Two tests are currently used to diagnose HIV infection. The most common is the enzyme-linked immunosorbent assay (ELISA), which was developed as a screening tool for blood donors. False positive results are possible in persons who have had multiple transfusions as are false negative results when the test is run after exposure to the virus but before the buildup of antibodies. The Western blot test may be used to confirm the diagnosis. When both tests are used, their combined accuracy is about 99%.

The HIV virus has been found in a variety of body fluids, including blood, semen, cerebrospinal fluid, urine, stool, and saliva. The highest concentrations are found in the blood and cerebrospinal fluid. The virus is transmitted by three major methods:

1. Intimate contact with body secretions during intercourse
2. Contact with infected blood during venipuncture, transfusion, or needle stick, or when sharing drug paraphernalia
3. Maternal-infant transmission via placental exchange or breast milk

MEDICAL MANAGEMENT

There is at present no known cure for AIDS. Treatment therefore is aimed at slowing the progression of the disease, managing symptoms, and dealing with complications. AIDS produces few characteristic symptoms. Treatment is instead directed at the opportunistic infections and tumors that are the outcomes of the immunodeficiency. Frequently encountered problems are summarized in Table 14-11. Patients may also exhibit the AIDS-related complex (ARC), which is a serious debilitating syndrome of fever, weight loss, and fatigue without the classic infections and malignancies.

Azidothymidine (AZT, Zetrovir, Zidovudine) was first introduced for experimental treatment in 1987. It acts by inhibiting the replication of the virus and has been successful in reducing the number of opportunistic infections and prolonging lives. Research is ongoing in a variety of other directions.

NURSING MANAGEMENT

Assessment

Subjective

Knowledge of disease, seropositivity

Sexual history, drug history

Recent health status

Exposure to blood products, equipment

Knowledge of transmission, safe sex practices

Complaints of the following:

    Fatigue and lethargy

    Chills and night sweats

    Anorexia

    Headache

Objective

Weight loss

Abdominal discomfort and diarrhea

Fever

Cough and dyspnea

Lymphadenopathy

Oral lesions or skin rashes

TABLE 14-10 Distribution of AIDS by exposure category as of August 31, 1989

Risk Group	Percentage
Homosexual and bisexual males	60
Heterosexual IV drug abusers	20
Homosexual and bisexual IV drug abusers	7
Heterosexual men and women	3
Users of blood products	3
Hemophiliacs	1
Parents with/at risk of AIDS	1
Other/unknown	4

Data from Centers for Disease Control.

TABLE 14-11 AIDS complications and their management

Complication	Description	Medical Management
Pneumocystis carinii pneumonia	Caused by a protozoan; the most common HIV complication; not airborne and not transmitted person to person	Intravenous or aerosolized antibiotic treatments; respiratory support and mechanical ventilation; symptom management
Candidiasis	Fungal infection caused by a yeast, usually presenting as oral thrush; can extend to involve the entire gastrointestinal system	Drug therapy with nystatin and clotrimazole; supportive nutritional care
Cryptosporidiosis	Protozoan infection causing massive abdominal cramping and diarrhea with weight loss and fluid and electrolyte imbalance	Currently no effective treatment; symptomatic care and replacement of fluids
Cytomegalovirus infection	A herpesvirus infection that may affect the lung, intestines, and eye; can lead to blindness	No effective treatment available but derivatives of acyclovir are showing promise; symptomatic care
Herpes zoster	Chicken pox in children and shingles in adults, with vesicular eruptions and painful tingling and itching	Local care of lesions; symptomatic relief; acyclovir
Herpes simplex	Oral, genital, and rectal lesions occur that may become ulcerated, bleed, and be extremely painful	Symptomatic relief; acyclovir; prevention of spread
Mycobacterium tuberculosis infection	Incidence is on the upswing; may present with traditional respiratory symptoms or involve the lymph, meninges, bone, etc.	Drug therapy with antituberculosis drugs (see Chapter 9); symptom management
Toxoplasma gondii infection	A protozoan infection that causes a focal encephalitis which can lead to confusion, seizures, memory loss	Culture-specific antibiotics; symptomatic care
Meningitis	Usually fungal in nature but causes traditional meningitis symptoms such as fever, stiff neck, nausea, and vomiting	Antifungal medications such as amphotericin B; symptom management
HIV encephalopathy	Invasion of the central nervous system by the virus itself causing progressive loss in cognitive, motor, or behavioral functioning; eventually leads to dementia	Treatment is primarily palliative and supportive; AZT may be useful in early stages
Tumors		
Lymphomas	Malignant lymphomas frequently develop in the central nervous system and are associated with a poor prognosis	Radiotherapy may be used for palliative purposes; symptomatic and supportive care
Kaposi's sarcoma	Affects the vascular epithelium, creating purplish cutaneous lesions	Symptomatic and supportive care; surgical excision occasionally used.

Nursing Diagnoses

Diagnoses will depend on the specific patient symptoms and disease severity but may include the following:

Activity intolerance related to generalized weakness and persistent fatigue

Body image disturbance related to excessive weight loss and the presence of skin lesions

Ineffective individual coping related to societal rejection and personal vulnerability

Hopelessness related to failing physical condition

Potential for infection related to decreased immune response

Knowledge deficit related to transmission of disease and safe sex practices

Altered nutrition: less than body requirements, related to chronic anorexia, nausea, or diarrhea

Social isolation related to societal rejection, changed personal appearance, and chronic fatigue

Expected Outcomes

Patient will have sufficient energy to remain independent in activities of daily living.

Patient will accept changes in appearance and maintain a positive body image.

Patient will strengthen usual coping strategies and explore alternatives.

Patient will express feelings about condition and prognosis and maintain hope.

Patient will not develop secondary infections.

Patient will be knowledgeable about AIDS and its transmission and practice safe sex.

Patient will ingest balanced nutrients and maintain a stable body weight.

Patient will maintain social involvement with family and friends.

Nursing Interventions (Asymptomatic Patient with HIV Infection)

Teach patient about HIV infection:

Disease transmission (see box on this page)

Safe sex practices (see box on this page)

Assess and support all effective coping mechanisms.

Assist patient to deal with responses of family and friends to seropositivity.

Reinforce importance of informing all known sex partners of seropositivity.

Facilitate patient participation in community support groups.

Encourage patient to keep home environment clean and damp mop daily to reduce dust.

Avoid environmental microbes.

Reinforce importance of meticulous personal hygiene and frequent hand washing.

Shower daily with mild soap.

Use soft toothbrush for regular oral care.

Teach patient to seek immediate medical assistance for any infection.

Teach patient to use household bleach to clean any articles or areas contaminated with blood or other body fluids.

Encourage patient to follow a high protein balanced diet, washing all fresh fruits and vegetables well and cooking meats thoroughly.

Nursing Interventions (Symptomatic AIDS)

Take routine vital signs. Assess carefully for signs of new infection.

Monitor for fever. Provide comfort measures (tepid baths, linen changes) and ensure additional fluids.

Administer acetaminophen if ordered.

Assist patient with daily hygiene and oral care as needed.

PREVENTING TRANSMISSION OF AIDS

Hand washing remains the most crucial factor—before and after contact and after removal of gloves.

Gloves should be worn whenever there will be contact with body secretions:

Skin and incontinence care

Dressing changes

Drawing blood or starting IVs

Dispose of soiled dressings, wet linen, and respiratory equipment in heavy plastic bags.

Discard all needles in puncture resistant containers. *WARNING:* Do not recap.

Emergency equipment such as airways should be accessible near all patients.

Use mask and goggles for tracheal or endotracheal suctioning.

SAFE SEX PRACTICES

Maintain a mutually monogamous relationship with an uninfected partner or limit the number of sex partners.

Avoid sexual partners with a history of promiscuity.

Explore history and risks honestly with any new sex partner.

Low-risk sexual activities include hugging, massage, body contact, dry kissing, and masturbation.

Unless certain that the partner is free of infection, use a latex condom for vaginal and anal intercourse and oral penile contact.

Keep environment clean and dust-free.

Maintain scrupulous hand-washing routines and protect patient from care givers and visitors with infections.

Provide meticulous skin care. Utilize pressure-relieving devices on bed as appropriate.

Provide frequent cleansing and moisture barriers if diarrhea is present.

Encourage deep breathing, coughing, and position changes hourly while awake.

Encourage patient to be as active and independent as possible. Use energy conservation techniques, and space activities to allow for needed rest.

Monitor daily weight and maintain accurate intake and output records.

Provide oral hygiene prior to meals.

Enrich the diet with potassium if diarrhea is present.

Use viscous xylocaine prior to meals if oral lesions are present.

Maintain a safe environment. Use side rails as needed if confusion is present.

Support ongoing patient coping.

Explore new coping strategies with patient.

Assist family and friends to provide needed support to patient.

Encourage use of community support system.

Support involvement in religious activities as desired.

Evaluation

Patient is independent in the activities of daily living.

Patient has accepted changes in appearance and speaks positively of self.

Patient utilizes effective coping strategies to deal with disease and prognosis.

Patient has realistic understanding of disease process but maintains an attitude of hope.

Patient is knowledgeable about disease process, takes measures to avoid infections, and practices safe sex.

Patient eats a balanced diet and maintains a stable weight.

Patient maintains involvement with and receives support from family and friends.

NURSING CARE PLAN

AIDS

Nursing Diagnoses	Expected Patient Outcomes	Nursing Interventions
Potential for ineffective individual coping related to the persistent stress of the AIDS diagnosis and prognosis	Patient utilizes effective coping strategies to deal with diagnosis and prognosis.	1. Give patient opportunities to discuss feelings about having AIDS. 2. Give friends and family opportunities to discuss their feelings and concerns related to AIDS. 3. Provide appropriate factual information. 4. Assist patient to identify usual coping mechanisms. 5. Assist patient to explore alternative coping strategies. 6. Reinforce all positive coping behaviors. 7. Teach relaxation techniques if appropriate.
Anticipatory grieving related to uncertainty of disease course and prognosis	Patient, family, and friends make realistic plans for the future and appropriately resolve grief feelings.	1. Assist patient and friends or family to explore and share their concerns about the future probabilities. 2. Support grief responses. 3. Help the involved persons identify personal strengths. 4. Help patient identify specific support persons and facilitate interactions with these persons. 5. Maintain realistic hopes. 6. When patient and others are ready, help them discuss plans for the immediate future.
Potential for social isolation related to stigma of the disease	Patient maintains contacts with family and friends and is not ostracized.	1. Help patient identify feelings about interacting with or being rejected by others. 2. Help other persons to identify their concerns about acquiring AIDS; provide data about modes of transmission (blood products and needles, sexual relationships, and mother-to-fetus, but *not* casual contact). 3. Help patient explore ways of maintaining contacts with others at desired level. 4. Facilitate interaction of patient with others when possible. Encourage link with local support groups.
Potential for infection related to incompetent immune system and frequent hospitalization	Patient is free of opportunistic infections.	1. Encourage patient to follow scrupulous personal hygiene. Emphasize importance of good skin care and oral care. 2. Patient should avoid contact with persons with infections. 3. Patient should avoid activities that may result in minor skin trauma. 4. Teach ways to prevent spread of AIDS to others. 5. Teach patient to report early signs of infection. 6. Monitor hospitalized patient daily for signs of new infection, particularly respiratory, gastrointestinal, or skin. Employ protective isolation if appropriate.

NURSING CARE PLAN

AIDS—cont'd

Nursing Diagnoses	Expected Patient Outcomes	Nursing Interventions
Alteration in nutrition: less than body requirements, related to anorexia and effects of chronic illness	Patient maintains a stable weight.	1. Monitor weight and nutritional intake. 2. Provide a high-protein, high-calorie diet. 3. Plan frequency of meals to promote increased intake; several small meals may be better tolerated. 4. Provide between-meal snacks. Offer supplements as appropriate 5. Use measures to encourage eating. 6. Provide oral hygiene before meals. 7. Provide total parenteral nutrition care, if needed. 8. Ensure adequate fluids and bulk to prevent constipation. 9. Wash all fresh fruits and vegetables carefully. Cook all food thoroughly.

Knowledge deficit related to condition, treatment modalities, and modes of transmission	Patient understands the disease and the proposed treatment plan. Patient is knowledgeable about measures to prevent transmission.	1. Teach patient the following:
		  a. Nature of the disease process.
		  b. Treatment plan, including action and side effects of all medications.
		  c. How to maintain adequate levels of nutrition, exercise, and rest.
		  d. How to avoid infection.
		  e. To avoid smoking, drugs, and excessive alcohol.
		  f. To inform necessary persons, such as dentists, of AIDS diagnosis.
		  g. How to prevent transmission by practicing safe sex.
		  h. Resources available in community to provide financial, physical, or psychosocial assistance.

BIBLIOGRAPHY

Andrist L: Taking a sexual history and educating clients about safe sex, Nurs Clin North Am **23**:959-973, 1988.

Centers for Disease Control: Update: universal precautions for prevention of transmission of human immunodeficiency virus in health care settings, MMWR **37**:24, 1988.

DeBow M: Safer sex. Imprint **35**(1):33-34, 36, 1988.

Durham J and Cohen F: The person with AIDS: nursing perspectives, New York, 1987, Springer Publishing.

Feather BL and Lanigan C: Looking good after your mastectomy, Am J Nurs **87**:1048-1049, 1987.

Flaskerud JH: AIDS: the psychosocial dimension, J Psychosoc Nurs **25**:4-36, 1987.

Fogel CI: Gonorrhea: not a new problem but a serious one, Nurs Clin North Am **23**:885-897, 1988.

Henrich-Rynning T: Prostatic cancer treatments and their effects on sexual functioning, Oncol Nurs Forum **14**(6):37, 1987.

Hutcheson HA: New options for breast reconstruction, Nursing **86**(16):52, 1986.

Jenkins B: Patients reports of sexual changes after treatment for gynecologic cancer, Oncol Nurs Forum **15**(3):349-354, 1988.

Lamb M: Ovarian cancer: patient information booklet, Oncol Nurs Forum **12**(5):83-88, 1985.

Lewis A: Nursing care of the person with AIDS/ARC, Rockville, Md, 1988, Aspen Publishers.

Managing the patient with testicular cancer: Nursing Grand Rounds, Nursing 86 **16**(8):42-45, 1986.

National Cancer Institute: Breast cancer: understanding treatment options, Bethesda, Md, 1986, U.S. Department of Health and Human Services, 86-2675.

Robertson C and Moreland B: Overview of ovarian cancer, Dimens Oncol Nurs **1**:11, 1985.

Schain WS: Breast cancer surgeries and psychosexual sequilae: implications for remediation, Semin Oncol Nurs **1**:200, 1985.

Secor RMC: Bacterial vaginosis: a comprehensive review, Nurs Clin North Am **23**:865-875, 1988.

Smith D: Gynecologic cancers: etiology and pathophysiology, Semin Oncol Nurs **2**(4):270-274, 1986.

Strauss R and Glimp T: Sexually transmitted diseases, Top Emerg Med **7**(2):73-84, 1985.

CHAPTER 15

Pain

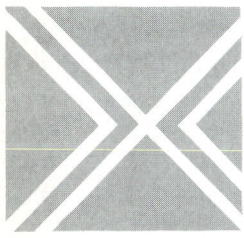

The successful management of pain is one of the greatest challenges confronting medicine and nursing today. The experience of pain is a universal one, but no phenomenon in health care is more elusive. Pain is an entirely subjective feeling that can be described only by the person experiencing it. It is a learned process that is inextricably interwoven with the personal, social, cultural, and religious situation of the individual. What is experienced as pain varies widely among people and even may differ in the same person from one time to another.

Pain serves an undeniably important role. It warns us of the presence of environmental danger, causes us to rest and allow injured parts to heal, and stimulates us to seek help for dealing with organ disease or tissue damage. Not all pain, however has apparent meaning, and its presence frequently persists long after its warning purpose has been achieved. Pain is the most dreaded aspect of the diagnosis of cancer, and in most individuals facing surgery it arouses primitive fears. As pain management strategies have, of necessity, become more holistic, nurses have assumed an integral role in its diagnosis and treatment.

TYPES OF PAIN

Pain is an abstract concept that defies accurate definition. Margo McCaffery's classic definition that "Pain is whatever the experiencing person says it is and exists whenever he says it does" provides the most useful framework for nursing. There are, however, several different types of pain, each of which challenges the nurse and patient in different ways. One common classification of pain is based on the length of time it has persisted.

Acute pain is pain that generally lasts a few days. It is typically caused by tissue injury and can be expected to end when the tissue heals.

Subacute pain is similar in nature to acute pain but persists from days to weeks.

Recurrent acute pain is episodic bouts of what is typically acute pain. The pathology underlying the pain may or may not be known.

Chronic pain is pain that persists for longer than 6 months.

The major features of acute and chronic pain are compared in Table 15-1.

Some research further subdivides the large chronic pain category into ongoing cancer pain, chronic benign pain, and chronic intractable pain in which the person is completely immobilized by the pain experience. Pain may also be classified by its presumed physiologic source. These categories are summarized in the box on the next page.

PATHOPHYSIOLOGY OF PAIN

Several theories concerning the physiology of pain have been developed over many years of active research. None, however, adequately describes all the aspects of pain transmission. The three major theories are the specificity theory, the pattern theory, and the gate control theory. These theories have the following primary features:

1. *Specificity theory.* The specificity theory contends that (a) there are specific nerve fibers that respond to noxious stimuli and (b) these stimuli are consistently interpreted as pain. It also contends that pain impulses are transmitted by two types of pain fibers—fast myelinated A-delta fibers and slower unmyelinated C fibers. Impulses are then transmitted via the corticothalamic tract to the ce-

TYPES OF PAIN

Somatic pain: Pain that originates in the superficial structures (skin and subcutaneous tissue) or in deeper structures (muscles or bones). It may be experienced as sharp and well localized, dull and diffusely aching, or poorly localized, depending on the fibers involved in transmission.

Visceral pain: Pain that originates in the viscera. It is usually poorly localized and is frequently accompanied by nausea, vomiting, and other autonomic symptoms. It frequently radiates or is referred.

Referred pain: Pain that is felt in areas other than those stimulated. It appears to occur most commonly in response to visceral injury. Although the mechanism is not well understood, the pattern of referral has been well documented and is fairly constant. Major areas of referral are shown in Figure 15-1.

Psychogenic pain: Pain that appears to have no physiologic basis, originating in the mind of the patient. No adequate explanation exists at present.

Phantom limb pain: Pain perceived to be occurring in an extremity that has been amputated. The process is poorly understood.

Neuralgia: Pain that has a segmental or peripheral nerve distribution.

Headache: Although many forms have a clear physiologic basis, it is not yet possible to explain the nature of migraine or cluster headaches fully.

rebral cortex where pain perception takes place. This mechanism is illustrated in Figure 15-2.

2. *Pattern theory.* The pattern theory contends that pain results from the combined effects of an intense stimulus and the interpretation of that stimulus in the dorsal horns of the spinal cord.

3. *Gate control theory.* The gate control theory contends that pain and pain perception result from the interplay of three systems—the substantia gelatinosa of the dorsal horn of the spinal cord, a central control system in the thalamus and cortex, and the peripheral nerves responsible for transmission. It proposes that a gate mechanism exists in the substantia gelatinosa that can be closed, partially or completely blocking the pain impulse. Factors such as conflicting impulses from the skin or impulses from the reticular formation, thalamus, or cortex are theorized to influence the gate.

Several additional features have been added to the understanding of pain perception and transmission in recent years. Each of these shows another aspect of this complex phenomenon.

Receptors that detect tissue injury are called nociceptors, and it has been determined that about 50% of all sensory fibers have this property. Neurotransmitters involved in processing pain include serotonin, histamine, bradykinin, prostaglandins, H^+ ions, and substance P. All of these have excitatory effects. Many medications have been shown to affect one or more of these neurotransmitters. The brain and spinal cord both have receptors to which morphine binds. Two groups of polypeptides, the enkephalins and endorphins, have been found to have morphinelike qualities. The enkephalins appear to be primarily concerned with pain modulation and are short-lived. The endorphins have a much longer half-life.

The exact role of each of these elements has yet to be fully determined. What is clear is the realization that the process of pain perception and transmission is even more complex than originally recognized.

TABLE 15-1 Comparison of acute and chronic pain

Characteristic	Acute Pain	Chronic Pain
Experience	An event	A situation, state of existence
Source	External agent or internal disease	Unknown; or if known, changes cannot occur or treatment is prolonged or ineffective
Onset	Usually sudden	May either be sudden or develop insidiously
Duration	Transient (up to 6 months)	Prolonged (months to years)
Pain identification	Pain versus nonpain areas generally well identified	Pain versus nonpain areas less easily differentiated; intensity becomes more difficult to evaluate (change in sensations)
Clinical signs	Typical response pattern with more visible signs	Response patterns vary; fewer overt signs (adaptation)
Meaning	Meaningful (informs person something is wrong)	Meaningless; person looks for meanings
Pattern	Self-limiting or readily corrected	Continuous or intermittent; intensity may vary or remain constant
Course	Suffering usually decreases over time	Suffering usually increases over time
Actions	Leads to actions to relieve pain	Leads to actions to modify pain experience
Prognosis	Likelihood of eventual complete relief	Complete relief usually not possible

From Phipps WJ, Long BC, and Woods NF: Medical-surgical nursing: concepts and clinical practice, ed 4, St Louis, 1990, Mosby–Year Book, Inc.

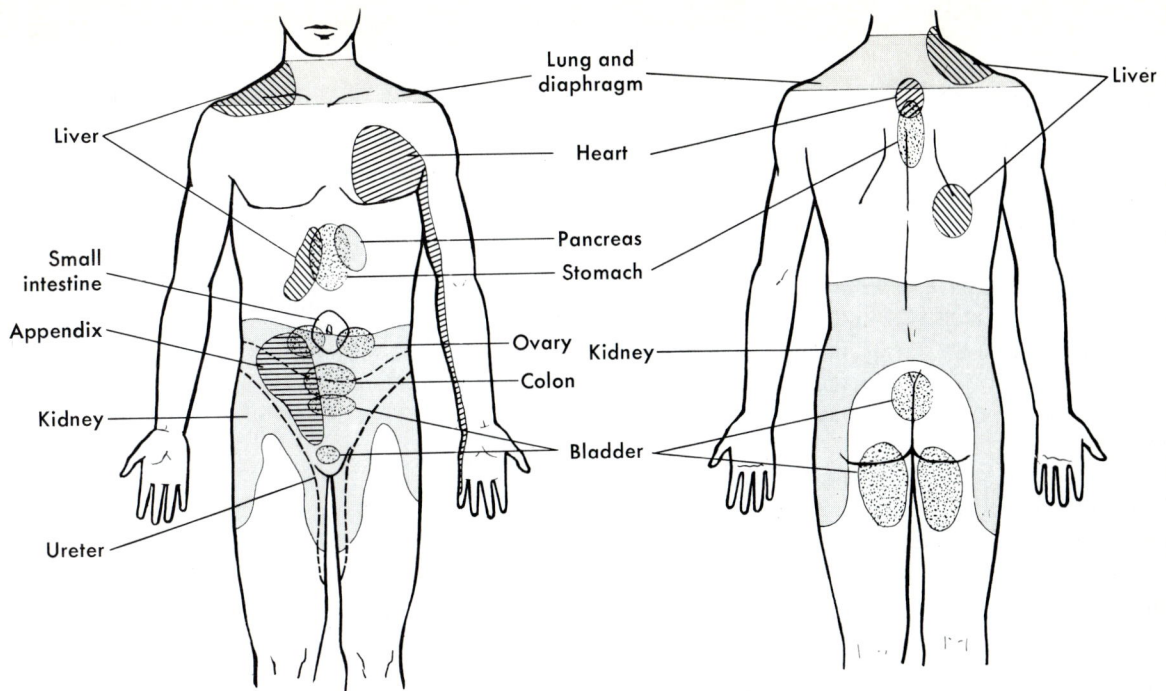

FIGURE 15-1 Patterns of referred pain, front and back. (From Phipps WJ, Long BC, and Woods NF: Medical-surgical nursing: concepts and clinical practice, ed 4, St Louis, 1990, The CV Mosby Co.)

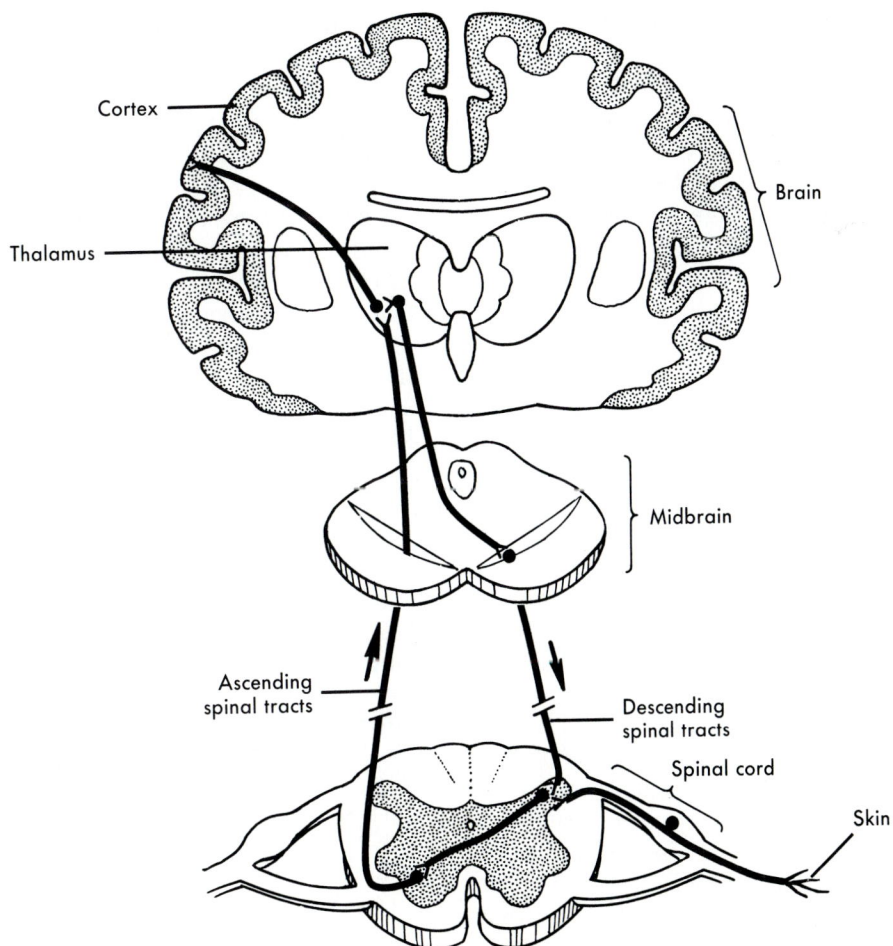

FIGURE 15-2 Pathways of pain transmission to and from cortex. (From Long BC and Phipps WJ: Medical-surgical nursing: a nursing process approach, ed 2, St Louis, 1989, The CV Mosby Co.)

MEDICAL MANAGEMENT OF PAIN

Pain is an elusive concept to define and describe. Because it has so many varied components, it is essential that its management be holistic. Some comfort strategies require the intervention of a physician for drug prescription or surgical care. Others fall in the more cognitive or noninvasive categories and may be safely employed by health care workers at all levels. As the complexity of the pain phenomenon is increasingly recognized, so is the need for creative and multifaceted management.

Appropriate management strategies depend on an understanding of the differences between pain threshold perception and tolerance. The pain threshold is the point at which an individual perceives a stimulus as painful. Although variations do exist in pain threshold from person to person, these differences are not significant. Pain tolerance, however, refers to the individual's ability to endure a stimulus perceived as painful, and this level varies enormously from person to person and can be influenced in the same person by distraction, fatigue, anger, anxiety, and conditioning. The variation reflects the fact that pain is perceived and interpreted in the cerebral cortex, leaving that perception open to a host of mediating variables. The perception and meaning attached to any pain stimulus help to determine the individual's reaction to it, which is also tremendously variable. Nurses' and physicians' responses to pain are also highly variable and reflective of the overall milieu of health care. This factor also significantly influences pain management and must be factored into any attempt at care planning.

PAIN ASSESSMENT

The assessment of the person in pain is so essential that it is discussed separately. The process requires careful and thorough data collection over time in an attempt to understand the nuances of a subjective experience from the perspective of the patient. Data to be included in the assessment are summarized in the box on this page.

Numerous tools have been developed in recent years to help health care personnel gather accurate and detailed data concerning pain. Figure 15-3 is an example of a detailed pain assessment tool. Simple tools can be easily used at the bedside and maintained by either the nurse or the patient. They provide an efficient way to track a patient's pain experience or response to medication over time. Figure 15-4 contains examples of several scales that can be easily adapted for this purpose.

Objective physical responses are also assessed when pain is present. Traditional physiologic signs of pain are the result of the activation of the sympathetic nervous system and are usually present in the face of acute severe pain. The response can be so severe as to trigger

---

ASSESSMENT OF PAIN: SUBJECTIVE DATA

Characteristics and description of the pain:

site	type
severity	intensity
duration	changes over time
location	

Measures that relieve the pain
Factors that worsen the pain
Usual coping strategies and their effectiveness
Expectations of health care team in regard to the pain
Interference of the pain with preferred life style:
　Impact on activities of daily living
　Social impact
　Occupational impact
　Impact on family and sexual life
Medications being taken for pain
　Dose
　Frequency
　Success in pain control or relief

---

neurogenic shock. These signs are less likely to accompany chronic pain, which may be manifested by behavioral responses or no discernible response at all. In these cases, the patient's subjective description is the foundation of the assessment. Common signs of pain are summarized in the box on this page.

MEDICAL MANAGEMENT STRATEGIES
ANALGESICS

Medications may be prescribed to directly relieve the cause of the patient's pain (i.e., antispasmodics) or to block or mediate its perception by the cortex. Aspirin and acetaminophen are the first-line drugs of the analgesic category and the drugs against which the effectiveness of others is measured. Commonly used analgesics are summarized in Table 15-2 and include the following categories:

Salicylates and acetaminophen: The specific action of these agents remains unknown, but they block prostaglandin production and have an additive effect when administered with a narcotic.

OBJECTIVE SIGNS OF PAIN

PHYSIOLOGIC

Tachycardia	Pallor and diaphoresis
Tachypnea	Dilated pupils
Increased blood pressure (both systolic and diastolic)	Muscle tension
	Nausea and vomiting

BEHAVIORAL

Restlessness and irritability	Frowning
Clenched teeth or fists	Crying or moaning
Rigid body posture	

PAIN ASSESSMENT TOOL

Name _____

Age _____ Diagnosis _____

Physician _____ Date first seen _____

Medications for pain _____

Location

Have patient point to or trace the area of pain

_____

_____

Intensity

Rate pain on a 0 to 5 scale (0 = no pain,
5 = worst pain imaginable):

At present: _____

1 hour after medication: _____

Worst it gets: _____

Best it gets: _____

Comfort

Rate comfort on a 0 to 5 scale (0 = no relief,
5 = complete relief:

At present: _____

1 hour after medication: _____

Worst it gets: _____

Best it gets: _____

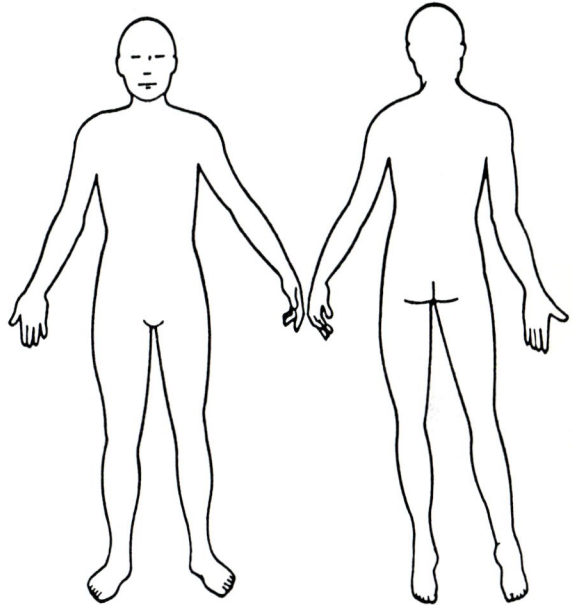

Quality

Have patient describe pain in his words: _____

Chronology

When did the pain start? _____

What time of day does it occur? _____

How often does it appear? _____

How long does it last? _____

Is it constant or intermittent? _____

Has the intensity changed? _____

Patient's view of pain

What makes the pain better? _____

What makes the pain worse? _____

Any associated symptoms? _____

Does pain disturb the patient's sleep? _____

How does the pain affect the patient's mood? _____

What has helped control pain in the past? _____

What is the pain preventing the patient from doing that he would like to do? _____

_____

Signature of person performing assessment _____

FIGURE 15-3 Sample pain assessment tool. (From Beare PG and Myers JC: Principles and practice of adult health nursing, St. Louis, 1990, The CV Mosby Co.)

Pain scales

0—No pain*	0—No pain	0—No pain
1—Mild pain	1—Mild pain	1—Slight pain
2—Discomfort	2—Moderate pain	2—Moderate
3—Distressing	3—Severe pain	pain
4—Horrible	4—As bad as it	3—Severe pain
5—Excruciating	could be	

*NOTE: The first scale is the McGill Pain Scale.

A

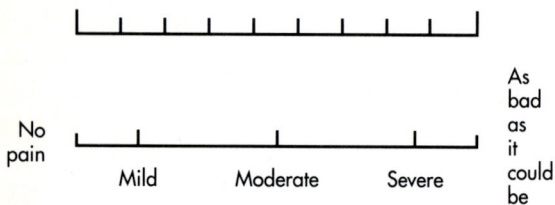

B

FIGURE 15-4 Pain assessment scales. **A,** Three numerical pain scales. **B,** Visual analog pain scales. (From Phipps WJ, Long BC, and Woods NF: Medical-surgical nursing: concepts and clinical practice, ed 4, St Louis, 1990, Mosby—Year Book, Inc.)

Nonsteroidal antiinflammatory agents (NSAIDs): This broad group of drugs have analgesic and antiinflammatory effects. They appear to act by inhibiting an enzyme that is key to the formation of prostaglandins.

Narcotics: Opium alkaloids and synthetic narcotics such as meperidine (Demerol) are narcotic agonists that have an affinity for certain receptor sites and depress brain cells involved in pain perception. The mixed agonist-antagonist group, which includes pentazocine, buprenorphine, and butorphanol, share many of the pain-relieving properties of the narcotic agonists but are less likely to induce respiratory depression, tolerance, and possibly abuse. The two categories should not be used concurrently in the same patient.

Much attention has been paid to the danger of addiction in the use of analgesics, often to the detriment of the patient. Studies have repeatedly shown that the danger of addiction from the hospital administration of narcotics is minimal. It is important that the differences between the following terms be clearly understood.

Tolerance is the need for a larger dose of a drug or increased frequency of administration to achieve the same degree of pain relief. If the level of pain remains unchanged, tolerance will *always* develop.

Physical dependence is the body's physiologic adjustment to the ongoing presence of narcotics. It will

develop in *anyone* who receives consistent doses of narcotics over a period of 5 to 7 days and should be anticipated. The use of the drugs must be tapered.

Addiction refers to the overwhelming involvement of the individual with acquiring and using a drug. It should not be a factor with hospitalized patients whose pain is effectively managed.

The proper use of analgesics is dependent on the correct drug being administered in an adequate dose by an appropriate route at appropriate intervals. Not all drugs are equally effective in all forms. Table 15-3 compares common oral analgesics and Table 15-4 compares the oral and parenteral effectiveness of several commonly used analgesics.

In recent years, new options have been developed for the administration of analgesics. Continuous IV infusion, subcutaneous infusion pumps, and the development of sustained-release forms of oral morphine have added several alternatives. Perhaps the most significant of the new approaches is patient-controlled analgesia (PCA), in which the patient self-activates a syringe pump with narcotic attached to an IV line on an as-needed basis. Patients using PCA report improved pain relief and often use less total analgesics than patients receiving narcotics by traditional methods.

ANALGESIC ADJUNCTS

Numerous drugs have been administered over the years in attempts to augment pain relief or deal with concurrent problems and thus relieve pain. Common drugs are summarized in Table 15-5.

Sedatives

Careful use of sedatives may permit sufficient relaxation and drowsiness for an analgesic to be effective. It is essential, however, that the sedated state not be automatically equated with a pain-free state.

Antianxiety and Antidepressant Agents

Antianxiety and antidepressant agents affect the mood of the patient and may assist the patient to separate pain perception and reaction. The tricyclic antidepressants have been particularly effective in augmenting pain relief and promoting restful sleep.

Antiemetic and Antihistamine Agents

The antihistamine drugs in particular are commonly administered with parenteral analgesics. They do *not* potentiate analgesic activity but do have additive effects in producing sedation and central nervous system depression.

NERVE STIMULATORS

The most common nerve stimulator is the transcutaneous electrical nerve stimulator (TENS), which involves

TABLE 15-2 Commonly used analgesics

Name	Usual Dosage*	Route	Onset	Peak	Duration
Narcotics (Opiate Agonists)					
Morphine sulfate	5-20 mg q 3-4 hr	sc, IM	5-10 min	60 min	4-6 hr
Codeine sulfate	15-60 mg q 3-4 hr	sc, oral	5-30 min	30-60 min	3-4 hr
Hydromorphone hydrochloride (Dilaudid)	2-4 mg q 4-6 hr	IV, IM, sc, oral	5-15 min	1 hr	4-6 hr
Meperidine hydrochloride (Demerol)	50-150 mg q 3-4 hr	IV, IM, sc, oral	10-15 min	30-60 min	2-4 hr
Methadone (Dolophine)	2.5-10 mg q 3-4 hr	IM, sc, oral	10 min	1-2 hr	4-6 hr
Mixed Agonist-Antagonists					
Buprenorphine (Buprenex)	0.3-0.6 mg q 6-8 hr	IM	15 min	1 hr	6 hr
Butorphanol (Stadol)	1-4 mg q 3-4 hr	IM	10-30 min	1 hr	4 hr
	0.5-2.0 mg q 3-4 hr	IV			
Nalbuphine (Nubain)	10 mg q 3-6 hr	IV, IM, sc	2-15 min	1 hr	3-6 hr
Pentazocine (Talwin)	15-30 mg q 3-4 hr	IV, IM	10-30 min	1 hr	2-3 hr
	50-100 mg q 3-4 hr	Oral			
Nonnarcotics					
Acetylsalicylic acid (aspirin)	300-1000 mg q 3-4 hr	Oral	15-30 min	1 hr	3-4 hr
Acetaminophen (Tylenol, Datril)	325-650 mg q 4-6 hr	Oral	15-30 min	1-2 hr	4-6 hr
Ibuprofen (Motrin, Advil, Nuprin)	200-600 mg q 4-6 hr	Oral	15-30 min	1-2 hr	3-4 hr

From Phipps WJ, Long BC, and Woods NF: Medical-surgical nursing: concepts and clinical practice, ed 4, St Louis, 1990, Mosby–Year Book, Inc.
*Must be individualized.

TABLE 15-3 Approximate equianalgesic doses of common analgesics

Name	Dose (mg)
Acetylsalicylic acid (aspirin)	650
Acetaminophen (Tylenol)	650
Codeine	32
Meperidine (Demerol)	50
Oxycodone	5
Propoxyphene napsylate (Darvon-N)	100

From Phipps WJ, Long BC, and Woods NF: Medical-surgical nursing: concepts and clinical practice, ed 4, St Louis, 1990, Mosby–Year Book, Inc.

TABLE 15-4 Approximate equianalgesic dose of common analgesics administered by oral and parenteral routes

Generic Name	IM Dose (mg)	Oral Dose (mg)
Codeine	120	200
Hydromorphone	1.5	7.5
Meperidine	75	300
Methadone	10	20
Morphine sulfate	10	60
Oxycodone	15	30
Pentazocine	60	180

From Phipps WJ, Long BC, and Woods NF: Medical-surgical nursing: concepts and clinical practice, ed 4, St Louis, 1990, Mosby–Year Book, Inc.

TABLE 15-5 Analgesic adjuncts

Drugs	Uses	Comments
Major tranquilizers (phenothiazines, chlorpromazine)	Nausea, anxiety	Little justification for use in pain management
Benzodiazepines (diazepam, chlordiazepoxide)	Muscle spasm, alcohol withdrawal	Not recommended for chronic pain because they cause depression
Tricyclic antidepressants (amitriptyline, doxepin)	Chronic pain, cancer pain, phantom limb pain	Direct analgesic effect and may potentiate narcotics Block reuptake of serotonin and when given at bedtime can be a sleep aid
Antihistamines (Hydroxyzine)	Nausea, anxiety	Have some analgesic effects (50 mg intramuscularly = 5 mg of morphine) Give deep intramuscularly as injections are extremely painful and irritating

a battery-powered stimulator attached to two or more electrodes that are applied around or near the pain site. The patient regulates the power source to achieve the best effect. The stimuli modify painful stimuli or block their transmission from the site. Principles for the use of TENS are outlined in the box on this page. Implanted devices for spinal cord stimulation are also available.

NEUROSURGICAL APPROACHES

Relentless intractable pain may be reduced or abolished by the use of one of the following surgical procedures.

Neurectomy: Nerve fibers to affected area are severed from the cord. Also sacrifices the fibers controlling movement and position sense.

Rhizotomy: A posterior nerve root is resected just before it enters the spinal cord. May be employed to relieve painful spasticity.

Cordotomy: The pain pathways in the spinothalamic tract of the spinal cord are severed, producing a wide sense of analgesia while preserving other sensory and motor functions.

Nerve blocks: Local anesthetics or neurolytic agents are injected close to nerves to block the transmission of impulses. Effects are not fully predictable.

ACUPUNCTURE

Acupuncture is an ancient method of pain relief that has only recently been used in Western societies. It involves the insertion and manipulation of small needles at specific body points, producing often immediate and ongoing pain relief.

OTHER STRATEGIES

Numerous other options exist for dealing with pain. Most of these are noninvasive and can be safely employed by nurses in a wide variety of situations.

Cutaneous Stimulation

The application of heat and cold are forms of cutaneous stimulation and utilize the principles of the gate control pain theory. Besides their effectiveness in controlling and resolving inflammation they also are able to modify the sensory input at the site of pain. Massage is the classic form of cutaneous stimulation and is used spontaneously by most individuals who experience mild to moderate discomfort.

Cognitive Strategies

Relaxation exercises, rhythmical breathing, distraction, and visual imagery are all techniques that attempt to deal with the anxiety that frequently surrounds the pain experience. Reducing fear and anxiety assists patients to remain in control of their overall situation. Not all of

---

GUIDELINES FOR USING TENS

Follow manufacturer's directions carefully because units vary.

Apply electrodes to clean, unbroken skin near area of pain.

Observe skin daily for signs of irritation.

Make sure the device is turned off before applying or removing electrodes.

Tape electrodes to the skin using hypoallergenic tape.

Remember to recharge the batteries or change them as needed.

Adjust the controls so that the impulse is a comfortable, pleasant sensation. If muscle contraction occurs, turn down the intensity.

Placement of electrodes should never be over the eyes, carotid sinuses, throat, or abdomen during pregnancy.

Contraindications for TENS use

People with demand cardiac pacemakers

Patients with a history of cardiac dysrhythmias or myocardial infarction

Pregnancy in the first trimester (may have some benefit for back labor during delivery)

Confused or elderly patients with decreased sensory perception

these techniques are effective with every patient, but they can help in restoring a sense of power and self-mastery. Being overwhelmed by pain can be terrifying.

Biofeedback and Autogenic Training
Some persons are able to alter body functions through mental concentration. Hypnosis helps patients to alter their perception of pain through suggestions made to the subconscious.

Pain Clinics
Pain clinics are a relatively new team approach to management of pain, particularly chronic pain. Typical goals include withdrawing patients from drugs and increasing health and physical fitness.

NURSING MANAGEMENT OF PAIN

ASSESSMENT

Subjective
History of the pain experience
Beliefs about pain origins and causes
Description of the pain (see boxes on p. 234)
Strategies in use for dealing with pain, effectiveness of strategies
Impact of pain on activities of daily living, job, social activities
Medications in use and their side effects—constipation, depression, gastric acidity
Sleep and rest pattern—complaints of fatigue or insomnia
Impact of pain on mobility
Usual coping patterns and effectiveness
Knowledge of and attitudes concerning nonpharmacologic pain management strategies

Objective
General appearance
Vital signs—presence of tachycardia, tachypnea, or elevated blood pressure
Restless, anxious, irritable behavior; tense muscles
Moist skin or pallor

NURSING DIAGNOSES

The diagnosis of pain is consistent. Other diagnoses will be dependent on the severity and duration of the pain experience and the individual patient's reaction. Diagnoses commonly include the following:
Acute or chronic pain related to disease process, surgery, trauma, or other cause
Sleep pattern disturbance related to depression or inadequate nighttime pain control
Impaired physical mobility caused by movement-related pain
Constipation related to the side effects of analgesics

Knowledge deficit related to nonpharmacologic pain control strategies
Anxiety related to inability to control the pain experience

EXPECTED OUTCOMES

Patient will experience only manageable levels of pain.
Patient will experience restful sleep free from frequent or early morning awakenings.
Patient will resume normal activity pattern and meet all self-care needs.
Patient will reestablish a regular pattern of bowel elimination.
Patient will be knowledgeable concerning the appropriate use of analgesics and other pain relief strategies.
Patient will be confident that the experience of pain is manageable with available strategies.

NURSING INTERVENTIONS

Establish a bedside tool to monitor pain and evaluate the effectiveness of interventions. Teach patient how to properly use the tool.
Reassure patient that control of pain is possible.
Assist patient to find positions that promote comfort.
    Encourage frequent position changes.
    Move patient gently, using support to affected areas.
    Use pressure-relieving aids to augment comfort.
    Offer gentle back rubs with position changes.
Maintain or establish a pleasant environment.
    Assist patient with hygiene, fresh clothes, and linens.
    Maintain comfortable temperature, eliminate odors.
Teach patient about the cause and expected duration of the pain and measures immediately available for dealing with it.
Involve patient in all plans concerning pain management, activity, and medications.
Maintain consistency in assignments if possible.
Plan activities and needed care for pain-free intervals if possible. Plan for additional rest periods.
Discuss with patient the use of distraction techniques—TV, visitors, music, activity. Avoid overfatigue.
Avoid social isolation and sensory overload.
Teach or reinforce relaxation and rhythmic breathing techniques—use positive visual imagery if patient is receptive.
Encourage patient to be active during pain-free intervals.
Provide for uninterrupted nighttime sleep if possible.
    Schedule needed medications and treatments to avoid awakening patient.
    Time analgesics to support needed sleep.
Apply cutaneous stimulation if appropriate. Teach patient techniques for safe use of heat and cold at home.
Promote optimal nutrition.
    Monitor weight.

Offer small frequent meals attractively served.

Administer analgesics and adjuncts as prescribed.

Monitor vital signs.

Assess level of consciousness and maintain patient safety.

Prevent constipation through diet modification or use of stool softeners.

Administer an adequate dose—assess for effectiveness of drug.

Start with a high dose and work back slowly as control is established.

Assess for signs of tolerance with prolonged administration: increased complaints of pain, shorter duration of relief, anxiety, preoccupation with medication schedule.

Offer analgesics for acute pain around the clock rather than as needed.

Follow equianalgesic tables when converting from parenteral to other forms of administration.

Reassure patient concerning issue of addiction.

Explore the use of adjuncts with physician if pain control remains inadequate.

Encourage patient to seek assistance and support from pain clinics, counseling, and religious beliefs as appropriate.

EVALUATION

Patient is pain-free or experiencing only manageable levels of pain.

Patient has resumed normal activity pattern.

Patient experiences restful sleep at night.

Patient has a normal pattern of bowel elimination.

Patient is knowledgeable about the management of pain and uses a variety of appropriate strategies.

Patient feels in control of the pain management protocol.

BIBLIOGRAPHY

Barbour LA, McGuire DB, and Kirchhoff KT: Nonanalgesic methods of pain control used by cancer outpatients, Oncol Nurs Forum **13**(6):56-60, 1986.

Coyle N: Analgesics and pain, Nurs Clin North Am **22**:727-741, 1987.

Geach B: Pain and coping, Image **19**(1):12-15, 1987.

Graffam S and Johnson A: A comparison of two relaxation strategies for the relief of pain and its distress, J Pain Symptom Manage **2**(4):229-231, 1987.

Harrison M and Cotanch PH: Pain: advances and issues in critical care, Nurs Clin North Am **22**:691-697, 1987.

Kanner RM: Are the people who need analgesics getting them?, Am J Nurs **86**:589, 1986.

Kleiman RL and others: PCA vs. regular IM injections for severe post-op pain, Am J Nurs **87**:1491-1492, 1987.

Lamb S and Barbaro NM: Neurosurgical approaches to the management of chronic pain syndromes, Orthop Nurs **6**(1):23-29, 1987.

Lisson EL: Ethical issues related to pain control, Nurs Clin North Am **22**:649-659, 1987.

McCaffery M: A practical "postable" chart of equianalgesic doses, Nursing 87, **17**(8):56-57, 1987.

McCaffery M: Giving meperidine for pain: should it be so mechanical?, Nursing 87, **17**(4):60-64, 1987.

McCaffery M and Beebe A: Pain: clinical manual for nursing practice, St Louis, 1989, The CV Mosby Co.

Miller TW and Jay LL: Cognitive-behavioral and pharmaceutical approaches to sensory pain management, Top Clin Nurs **6**(4):34-43, 1985.

Paice JA: New delivery systems in pain management, Nurs Clin North Am **22**:715-725, 1987.

Relieving pain: an analgesic guide: principles of analgesic use, Am J Nurs **88**:815-826, 1988.

Vandenbosch TM: How to use a pain flow-sheet effectively, Nursing 88, **18**(8):50-51, 1988.

Watt-Watson JH: Nurses knowledge of pain issues: a survey, J Pain Symptom Manage **2**(4):207, 1987.

Watt-Watson JH: What do we need to know about pain? Assessing pain and giving narcotics, Am J Nurs **87**:1217-1218, 1987.

Whipple B: Methods of pain control: review of research and literature, Image **19**(3):142-146, 1987.

Wright SM: The use of therapeutic touch in the management of pain, Nurs Clin North Am **22**:705-713, 1987.

Nursing Diagnoses

Activity intolerance
Altered family processes
Altered growth and development
Altered health maintenance
Altered nutrition: less than body requirements
Altered nutrition: more than body requirements
Altered nutrition: potential for more than body requirements
Altered oral mucous membranes
Altered parenting
Altered patterns of urinary elimination
Altered protection
Altered role performance
Altered sexuality patterns
Altered thought processes
Altered (specify type) tissue perfusion (renal, cerebral, cardiopulmonary, gastrointestinal, peripheral)
Anticipatory grieving
Anxiety
Bathing/hygiene self-care deficit
Body image disturbance
Bowel incontinence
Chronic pain
Colonic constipation
Constipation
Decisional conflict (specify)
Decreased cardiac output
Defensive coping
Diarrhea
Diversional activity deficit
Dressing/grooming self-care deficit
Dysfunctional grieving
Dysreflexia
Effective breastfeeding
Family coping: potential for growth
Fatigue
Fear
Feeding self-care deficit

Fluid volume deficit (1)
Fluid volume deficit (2)
Fluid volume excess
Functional incontinence
Health-seeking behaviors (specify)
Hopelessness
Hyperthermia
Hypothermia
Impaired adjustment
Impaired gas exchange
Impaired home maintenance management
Impaired physical mobility
Impaired skin integrity
Impaired social interaction
Impaired swallowing
Impaired tissue integrity
Impaired verbal communication
Ineffective airway clearance
Ineffective breastfeeding
Ineffective breathing pattern
Ineffective denial
Ineffective family coping: compromised
Ineffective family coping: disabling
Ineffective individual coping
Ineffective thermoregulation
Knowledge deficit (specify)
Noncompliance (specify)
Pain
Parental role conflict
Perceived constipation
Personal identity disturbance
Post-trauma response
Potential activity intolerance
Potential altered body temperature
Potential altered parenting
Potential fluid volume deficit
Potential for aspiration
Potential for disuse syndrome

From Kim, MJ, McFarland, GK, and McLane, AM: Pocket guide to nursing diagnoses, ed 4, St Louis, 1991, The CV Mosby Co.

Potential for infection
Potential for injury
Potential for poisoning
Potential for suffocation
Potential for trauma
Potential for violence: self-directed or directed at others
Potential impaired skin integrity
Powerlessness
Rape-trauma syndrome
Rape-trauma syndrome: compound reaction
Rape-trauma syndrome: silent reaction
Reflex incontinence
Self-esteem disturbance

Chronic low self-esteem
Situational low self-esteem
Sensory/perceptual alterations (specify) (visual, auditory, kinesthetic, gustatory, tactile, olfactory)
Sexual dysfunction
Sleep pattern disturbance
Social isolation
Spiritual distress (distress of the human spirit)
Stress incontinence
Toileting self-care deficit
Total incontinence
Unilateral neglect
Urge incontinence
Urinary retention

Normal Laboratory Values

Blood, plasma or serum values

Test	Reference Range	
	Conventional Values	**SI Units***
Acetoacetate plus acetone	0.30-2.0 mg/dl	3-20 mg/L
Acetone	Negative	Negative
Acid phosphatase	Adults: 0.10-0.63 U/ml (Bessey-Lowry) 0.5-2.0 U/ml (Bodansky) 1.0-4.0 U/ml (King-Armstrong) Children: 6.4-15.2 U/L	28-175 nmol/s/L
Activated partial thromboplastin time (APTT)	30-40 sec	30-40 sec
Adrenocorticotropic hormone (ACTH)	6 AM 15-100 pg/ml 6 PM <50 pg/ml	10-80 ng/L <50 ng/L
Alanine aminotransferase (ALT)	5-35 IU/L	5-35 U/L
Albumin	3.2-4.5 g/dl	35-55 g/L
Alcohol	Negative	Negative
Aldolase	Adults: 3.0-8.2 Sibley-Lehninger units/dl Children: approximately 2 × adult values Newborns: approximately 4 × adult values	22-59 mU/L at 37° C
Aldosterone	Peripheral blood: Supine: 7.4 ± 4.2 ng/dl Upright: 1-21 ng/dl Adrenal vein: 200-800 ng/dl	0.08-0.3 nmol/L 0.14-0.8 nmol/L
Alkaline phosphatase	Adults: 30-85 ImU/ml Children and adolescents: <2 yr: 85-235 ImU/ml 2-8 yr: 65-210 ImU/ml 9-15 yr: 60-300 ImU/ml (active bone growth) 16-21 yr: 30-200 ImU/ml	
Alpha-aminonitrogen	3-6 mg/dl	2.1-3.9 mmol/L
Alpha-1-antitrypsin	>250 mg/dl	
Alpha fetoprotein (AFP)	<25 ng/ml	
Ammonia	Adults: 15-110 µg/dl Children: 40-80 µg/dl Newborns: 90-150 µg/dl	47-65 µmol/L
Amylase	56-190 IU/L 80-150 Somogyi units/ml	25-125 U/L

*The use of the System of International Units (SI) was recommended at the 30th World Health Assembly in 1977 to implement an international language of measurement. Because this system is being adopted by many laboratories, many of the common values are expressed in both conventional and SI units. SI units are calculated by multiplying the conventional unit by a number factor. The SI measurement system uses *moles* as the basic unit for the amount of a substance, *kilograms* for its mass, and *meter* for its length.

Continued.

Blood, plasma or serum values—cont'd

	Reference Range	
Test	Conventional Values	SI Units
Antiotensin-converting enzyme (ACE)	23-57 U/ml	
Antinuclear antibodies (ANA)	Negative	

Antistreptolysin O (ASO)	Adults: ≤160 Todd units/ml
	Children:
	  Newborns: similar to mother's value
	  6 mo-2 yr: ≤50 Todd unit/ml
	  2-4 yr: ≤160 Todd units/ml
	  5-12 yr: ≤200 Todd units/ml	

Antithyroid microsomal antibody	Titer <1:100	
Antithyroglobulin antibody	Titer <1:100	
Ascorbic acid (vitamin C)	0.6-1.6 mg/dl	23-57 μmol/L
Aspartate aminotransferase (AST, SGOT)	12-36 U/ml 5-40 IU/L	0.10-0.30 μmol/s/L 5-40 U/L
Australian antigen (hepatitis-associated antigen, HAA)	Negative	Negative
Barbiturates	Negative	Negative
Base excess	Men: −3.3 to +1.2 Women: −2.4 to +2.3	0 ± 2 mmol/L 0 ± 2 mmol/L
Bicarbonate (HCO_3^-)	22-26 mEq/L	22-26 mmol/L
Bilirubin		
Direct (conjugated)	0.1-0.3 mg/dl	1.7-5.1 μmol/L
Indirect (unconjugated)	0.2-0.8 mg/dl	3.4-12.0 μmol/L
Total	Adults and children: 0.1-1.0 mg/dl Newborns:1-12 mg/dl	5.1-17.0 μmol/L
Bleeding time (Ivy method)	1-9 min	
Blood count (see Complete blood count)		
Blood gases (arterial)		
pH	7.35-7.45	
Pco_2	35-45 mm Hg	4.7-6.0 kPa
HCO_3^-	22-26 mEq/L	21-28 nmol/L
Po_2	80-100 mm Hg	11-13 kPa
O_2 saturation	95%-100%	
Blood urea nitrogen (BUN)	5-20 mg/dl	3.6-7.1 mmol/L
Bromide	Up to 5 mg/dl	0-63 mmol/L
Bromosulfonphthalein (BSP)	<5% retention after 45 min	
CA 15-3	<22 U/ml	
CA-125	0-35 U/ml	
CA 19-9	<37 U/ml	
C-reactive protein (CRP)	<6 μg/ml	
Calcitonin	<50 pg/ml	<50 pmol/L
Calcium (Ca)	9.0-10.5 mg/dl (total) 3.9-4.6 mg/dl (ionized)	2.25-2.75 mmol/L 1.05-1.30 mmol/L
Carbon dioxide (CO_2) content	23-30 mEq/L	21-30 mmol/L
Carboxyhemoglobin (COHb)	3% of total hemoglobin	
Carcinoembryonic antigen (CEA)	<2 ng/ml	0-2.5 μg/L
Carotene	50-200 μg/dl	0.74-3.72 μmol/L
Chloride (ClI)	90-110 mEq/L	98-106 mmol/L
Cholesterol	150-250 mg/dl	3.90-6.50 mmol/L
Clot retraction	50%-100% clot retraction in 1-2 hr, complete retraction within 24 hr	
Complement	C_3: 70-176 mg/dl C_4: 16-45 mg/dl	0.55-1.20 g/L 0.20-0.50 g/L
Complete blood count (CBC)		
Red blood cell (RBC) count	Men: 4.7-6.1 million/mm³ Women: 4.2-5.4 million/mm³ Infants and children: 3.8-5.5 million/mm³ Newborns: 4.8-7.1 million/mm³	

Blood, plasma or serum values—cont'd

Test	Reference Range	
	Conventional Values	**SI Units**
Hemoglobin Hgb)	Men: 14-18 g/dl	8.7-11.2 mmol/L
	Women: 12-16 g/dl (pregnancy: >11 g/dl)	7.4-9.9 mmol/L
	Children: 11-16 g/dl	1.74-2.56 mmol/L
	Infants: 10-15 g/dl	
	Newborns: 14-24 g/dl	2.56-3.02 mmol/L
Hematocrit (Hct)	Men: 42%-52%	
	Women: 37%-47% (pregnancy: >33%)	
	Children: 31%-43%	
	Infants: 30%-40%	
	Newborns: 44%-64%	
Mean corpuscular volume (MCV)	Adults and children: 80-95 μ^3	80-95 fL
	Newborns: 96-108 μ^3	
Mean corpuscular hemoglobin (MCH)	Adults and children: 27-31 pg	0.42-0.48 fmol
	Newborns: 32-34 pg	
Mean corpuscular hemoglobin concentration (MCHC)	Adults and children: 32-36 g/dl	0.32-0.36
	Newborns: 32-33 g/dl	
White blood cell count (WBC)	Adults and children >2 yr: 5000-10,000/cm^3	
	Children ≤2 yr: 6200-17,000/mm^3	
	Newborns: 9000-30,000/mm^3	
Differential count		
Neutrophils	55%-70%	
Lymphocytes	20%-40%	
Monocytes	2%-8%	
Eosinophils	1%-4%	
Basophils	0.5%-1%	
Platelet count	150,000-400,000/mm^3	
Coombs' test		
Direct	Negative	Negative
Indirect	Negative	Negative
Copper (Cu)	70-140 μg/dl	11.0-24.3 μmol/L
Cortisol	6-28 μg/dl (AM)	170-635 nmol/L
	2-12 μg/dl (PM)	82-413 nmol/L
CPK isoenzyme (MB)	<5% total	
Creatinine	0.7-1.5 mg/dl	<133 μmol/L
Creatinine clearance	Men: 95-105 ml/min	<133 μmol/L
	Women: 95-125 ml/min	
Creatinine phosphokinase (CPK)	5-75 mU/ml	12-80 units/L
Cryoglobulin	Negative	Negative
Differential (WBC) count		
Neutrophils	55%-70%	
Lymphocytes	20%-40%	
Monocytes	2%-8%	
Eosinophils	1%-4%	
Basophils	0.5%-1%	
Digoxin	Therapeutic levels: 0.5-2.0 ng/ml	40-79 μmol/L
	Toxic level: >2.4 ng/ml	>119 μmol/L
Erythrocyte count (see Complete blood count)		
Erythrocyte sedimentation rate (ESR)	Men: up to 15 mm/hr	
	Women: up to 20 mm/hr	
	Children: up to 10 mm/hr	
Ethanol	80-200 mg/dl (mild to moderate intoxication)	17-43 mmol/L
	250-400 mg/dl (marked intoxication)	54-87 mmol/L
	>400 mg/dl (severe intoxication)	>87 mmol/L
Euglobulin lysis test	90 min-6 hr	
Fats	Up to 200 mg/dl	
Ferritin	15-200 ng/ml	15-200 μg/L
Fibrin degradation products (FDP)	<10 μg/ml	

Continued.

Blood, plasma or serum values—cont'd

Test	Reference Range	
	Conventional Values	**SI Units**
Fibrinogen (factor I)	200-400 mg/dl	5.9-11.7 µmol/L
Fibrinolysis/euglobulin lysis test	90 min-6 hr	
Fluorescent treponemal antibody (FTA)	Negative	Negative
Fluoride	<0.05 mg/dl	<0.027 mmol/L
Folic acid (Folate)	5-20 µg/ml	14-34 mmol/L
Follicle-stimulating hormone (FSH)	Men: 0.1-15.0 ImU/ml	
	Women: 6-30 ImU/ml	
	Children: 0.1-12.0 ImU/ml	
	Castrate and postmenopausal: 30-200 ImU/ml	
Free thyroxine index (FTI)	0.9-2.3 ng/dl	
Galactose-1-phosphate uridyl transferase	18.5-28.5 U/g hemoglobin	
Gammaglobulin	0.5-1.6 g/dl	
Gamma-glutamyl transpeptidase (GGTP)	Men: 8-38 U/L	5-40 U/L 37° C
	Women: <45 yr: 5-27 U/L	
Gastrin	40-150 pg/ml	40-150 ng/L
Glucagon	50-200 pg/ml	14-56 pmol/L
Glucose, fasting (FBS)	Adults: 70-115 mg/dl	3.89-6.38 mmol/L
	Children: 60-100 mg/dl	
	Newborns: 30-80 mg/dl	
Glucose, 2-hr postprandial (2-hr PPG)	<140 mg/dl	
Glucose-6-phosphate dehydrogenase (G-6-PD)	8.6-18.6 IU/g of hemoglobin	
Glucose tolerance test (GTT)	Fasting: 70-115 mg/dl	
	30 min: <200 mg/dl	
	1 hr: <200 mg/dl	
	2 hr: <140 mg/dl	
	3 hr: 70-115 mg/dl	
	4 hr: 70-115 mg/dl	
Glycosylated hemoglobin	Adults: 2.2%-4.8%	
	Children: 1.8%-4.0%	
	Good diabetic control: 2.5%-6%	
	Fair diabetic control: 6.1%-8%	
	Poor diabetic control: >8%	
Growth hormone	<10 ng/ml	<10 µg/L
Haptoglobin	100-150 mg/dl	16-31 µmol/L
Hematocrit (Hct)	Men: 42%-52%	
	Women: 37%-47% (pregnancy: >33%)	
	Children: 31%-43%	
	Infants: 30%-40%	
	Newborns: 44%-64%	
Hemoglobin (HgB)	Men: 14-18 g/dl	8.7-11.2 mmol/L
	Women: 12-16 g/dl (pregnancy: >11 g/dl)	7.4-9.9 mmol/L
	Children: 11-16 g/dl	
	Infants: 10-15 g/dl	
	Newborns: 14-24 g/dl	
Hemoglobin electrophoresis	Hgb A$_1$: 95%-98%	
	Hgb A$_2$: 2%-3%	
	Hgb F: 0.8%-2%	
	Hgb S: 0	
	Hgb C: 0	
Hepatitis B surface antigen (HB$_s$AG)	Nonreactive	Nonreactive
Heterophil antibody	Negative	Negative
HLA-B27	None	None
Human chorionic gonadotropin (HCG)	Negative	Negative

Blood, plasma or serum values—cont'd

Test	Conventional Values	SI Units
	Reference Range	
Human placental lactogen (HPL)	Rise during pregnancy	
5-Hydroxyindoleacetic acid (5-HIAA)	2.8-8.0 mg/24 hr	
Immunoglobulin quantification	IgG: 550-1900 mg/dl	5.5-19.0 g/L
	IgA: 60-333 mg/dl	0.6-3.3 g/L
	IgM: 45-145 mg/dl	0.45-1.5 g/L
Insulin	4-20 μU/ml	36-179 pmol/L
Iron (Fe)	60-190 μg/dl	13-31 μmol/L
Iron-binding capacity, total (TIBC)	250-420 μg/dl	45-73 μmol/L
Iron(transferrin) saturation	30%-40%	
Ketone bodies	Negative	Negative
Lactic acid	0.6-1.8 mEq/L	
Lactic dehydrogenase (LDH)	90-200 ImU/ml	0.4-1.7 μmol/s/L
LDH isoenzymes	LDH-1: 17%-27%	
	LDH-2: 28%-38%	
	LDH-3: 19%-27%	
	LDH-4: 5%-16%	
	LDH-5: 6%-16%	
Lead	120 μg/dl or less	<1.0 μmol/L
Leucine aminopeptidase (LAP)	Men: 80-200 U/ml	
	Women: 75-185 U/ml	
Leukocyte count (see Complete blood count)		
Lipase	Up to 1.5 units/ml	0.417 U/L
Lipids		
Total	400-1000 mg/dl	4-8 g/L
Cholesterol	150-250 mg/dl	3.9-6.5 mmol/L
Triglycerides	40-150 mg/dl	0.4-1.5 g/L
Phospholipids	150-380 mg/dl	1.9-3.9 mmol/L
Long-acting thyroid stimulating hormone (LATS)	Negative	Negative
Magnesium (Mg)	1.6-3.0 mEq/L	0.8-1.3 mm/L
Methanol	Negative	Negative
Mononucleosis spot test	Negative	Negative
Nitrogen, nonprotein	15-35 mg/dl	10.7-25.0 mmol/L
Nuclear antibody (ANA)	Negative	Negative
5'-Nucleotidase	Up to 1.6 units	27-233 nmol/s/L
Osmolality	275-300 mOsm/kg	
Oxygen saturation (arterial)	95%-100%	0.95-1.00 of capacity
Parathormone (PTH)	<2000 pg/ml	
Partial thromboplastin time, activated (APTT)	30-40 sec	
Pco₂	35-45 mm Hg	
pH	7.35-7.45	7.35-7.45
Phenylalanine	Up to 2 mg/dl	<0.18 mmol/L
Phenylketonuria (PKU)	Negative	Negative
Phenytoin (Dilantin)	Therapeutic level: 10-20 μg/ml	
Phosphatase (acid)	0.10-0.63 U/ml (Bessey-Lowry)	0.11-0.60 U/L
	0.5-2.0 U/ml (Bodansky)	
	1.0-4.0 U/ml (King-Armstrong)	
Phosphatase (alkaline)	Adults: 30-85 ImU/ml	20-90 units/L
	Children and adolescents:	
	<2 yr: 85-235 ImU/ml	
	2-8 yr: 65-210 ImU/ml	
	9-15 yr: 60-300 ImU/ml	
	(active bone growth)	
	16-21 yr: 30-200 ImU/ml	
Phospholipids (see Lipids)		
Phosphorus (P, PO₄)	Adults: 2.5-4.5 mg/dl	0.78-1.52 mmol/L
	Children: 3.5-5.8 mg/dl	1.29-2.26 mmol/L

Continued.

Blood, plasma or serum values—cont'd

Test	Reference Range	
	Conventional Values	SI Units
Platelet count	150,000-400,000/mm^3	
Po$_2$	80-100 mm Hg	
Potassium (K)	3.5-5.0 mEq/L	3.5-5.0 mmol/L
Progesterone	Men, prepubertal girls, and postmeno-pausal women: <2 ng/ml	6 nmol/L
	Women, luteal: peak >5 ng/ml	>16 nmol/L
Prolactin	2-15 ng/ml	2-15 μg/L
Protein (total)	6-8 g/dl	55-80 g/L
Albumin	3.2-4.5 g/dl	35-55 g/L
Globulin	2.3-3.4 g/dl	20-35 g/L
Prothrombin time (PT)	11.0-12.5 sec	11.0-12.5 sec
Pyruvate	0.3-0.9 mg/dl	34-103 μmol/L
Red blood cell count (see Complete blood count)		
Red blood cell indexes (see Complete blood count)		
Renin		
Reticulocyte count	Adults and children: 0.5%-2% of total erythrocytes	
	Infants: 0.5%-3.1% of total erythrocytes	
	Newborns: 2.5%-6.5% of total erythrocytes	
Rheumatoid factor	Negative	Negative
Salicylates	Negative	
	Therapeutic: 20-25 mg/dl (to age 10: 25-30 mg/dl)	1.4-1.8 mmol/L
	Toxic: >30 mg/dl (after age 60: >20 mg/dl)	>2.2 mmol/L
Schilling test (vitamin B$_{12}$ absorption)	8%-40% excretion/24 hr	
Serologic test for syphilis (STS)	Negative (nonreactive)	
Serum glutamic oxaloacetic transaminase (SGOT, AST)	12-36 U/ml 5-40 IU/L	0.10-0.30 μmol/s/L
Serum glutamic-pyruvic transaminase (SGPT, ALT)	5-35 IU/L	0.05-0.43 μgmol/s/L
Sickle cell	Negative	
Sodium (Na$^+$)	136-145 mEq/L	136-145 mmol/L
Sugar (see glucose)		
Syphilis (see Serologic test for, Fluorescent treponemal antibody, Venereal Disease Research Laboratory)		
Testosterone	Men: 300-1200 ng/dl	10-42 nmol/L
	Women: 30-95 ng/dl	1.1-3.3 nmol/L
	Prepubertal boys and girls: 5-20 ng/dl	0.165-0.70 nmol/L
Thymol flocculation	Up to 5 units	
Thyroglobulin antibody (see Antithyroglobulin antibody)		
Thyroid-stimulating hormone (TSH)	1-4 μU/ml	5 mU/L
	Neonates: <25 μIU/ml by 3 days	
Thyroxine (T$_4$)	Murphy-Pattee:	50-154 nmol/L
	neonates: 10.1-20.1 μg/dl	
	1-6 yr: 5.6-12.6 μg/dl	
	6-10 yr: 4.9-11.7 μg/dl	
	>10 yr: 4-11 μg/dl	
	Radioimmunoassay: 5-10 μg/dl	
Thyroxine-binding globulin (TBG)	12-28 μg/ml	129-335 nmol/L
Transaminase (see Serum glutamic-oxaloacetic transaminase, Serum glutamic pyruvic transaminase)		
Triglycerides	40-150 mg/dl	0.4-1.5 g/L

Blood, plasma or serum values—cont'd

Test	Reference Range	
	Conventional Values	SI Units
Triiodothyronine (T_3)	110-230 ng/dl	1.2-1.5 nmol/L
Triiodothyronine (T_3) resin uptake	25%-35%	
Tubular phosphate reabsorption (TPR)	80%-90%	
Urea nitrogen (see Blood urea nitrogen)		
Uric acid	Men: 2.1-8.5 mg/dl	0.15-0.48 mmol/L
	Women: 2.0-6.6 mg/dl	0.09-0.36 mmol/L
	Children: 2.5-5.5 mg/dl	
Venereal Disease Research Laboratory (VDRL)	Negative	Negative
Vitamin A	20-100 g/dl	0.7-3.5 μmol/L
Vitamin B_{12}	200-600 pg/ml	148-443 pmol/L
Vitamin C	0.6-1.6 mg/dl	23-57 μmol/L
Whole blood clot retraction (see Clot retraction		
Zinc	50-150 μg/dl	

Urine values

Test	Reference Range	
	Conventional Values	SI Units
Acetone plus acetoacetate (ketone bodies)	Negative	Negative
Addis count (12-hr)	Adults:	Negative
	WBCs and epithelial cells: 1.8 million/ 12 hr	
	RBCs: 500,000/12 hr	
	Hyaline casts: Up to 5000/12 hr	
	Children:	
	WBCs: <1 million/12 hr	
	RBCs: <250,000/12 hr	
	Casts: >5000/12 hr	
	Protein: <20 mg/12 hr	
Albumin	Random: ≤8 mg/dl	Negative
	24 hr: 10 100 mg/24 hr	10 100 mg/24 hr
Aldosterone	2-16 μg/24 hr	5.5-72 nmol/24 hr
Alpha-aminonitrogen	0.4-1.0 g/24 hr	28-71 nmol/24 hr
Amino acid	50-200 mg/24 hr	
Ammonia (24-hr)	30-50 mEq/24 hr	30-50 nmol/24 hr
	500-1200 mg/24 hr	
Amylase	≤5000 Somogyi units/24 hr	6.5-48.1 U/hr
	3-35 IU/hr	
Arsenic (24 hr)	<50 μg/L	<0.65 mol/L
Ascorbic acid (vitamin C)	Random: 1-7 ng/dl	0.06-0.40 mmol/L
	24-hr: >50 mg/24 hr	>0.29 mmol/24 hr
Bacteria	None	None
Bence Jones protein	Negative	Negative
Bilirubin	Negative	Negative
Blood or hemoglobin	Negative	Negative
Borate (24-hr)	<2 mg/L	<32 μmol/L
Calcium	Random: 1 + turbidity	1 + turbidity
	24-hr: 1-300 mg (diet dependent)	

Continued.

Urine values-cont'd

Test	Conventional Values	SI Units
		Reference Range
Catecholamines (24-hr)	Epinephrine: 5-40 µg/24 hr	<55 nmol/24 hr
	Norepinephrine: 10-80 µg/24 hr	<590 nmol/24 hr
	Metanephrine: 24-96 µg/24 hr	0.5-8.1 µmol/24 hr
	Normetanephrine: 75-375 µg/24 hr	
Chloride (24-hr)	140-250 mEq/24 hr	140-250 mmol/24 hr
Color	Amber-yellow	Amber-yellow
Concentration test (Fishberg test)	Specific gravity: >1.025	>1.025
	Osmolality: 850 mOsm/L	>850 mOsm/L
Copper (Cu) (24-hr)	Up to 25 µg/24 hr	0-0.4 µmol/24 hr
Coproporphyrin (24-hr)	100-300 µg/24 hr	150-460 nmol/24 hr
Creatine	Adults: <100 mg/24 hr of <6% creatinine	
	Pregnant women: ≤12%	
	Infants <1 yr: equal to creatinine	
	Older children: ≤30% of creatinine	
Creatinine (24-hr)	15-25 mg/kg body wt/24 hr	0.13-0.22 nmol/kg body wt/24 hr
Creatinine clearance (24-hr)	Men: 90-140 ml/min	90-140 ml/min
	Women: 85-125 ml/min	85-125 ml/min
Crystals	Negative	Negative
Cystine or cysteine	Negative	Negative
Delta-aminolevulinic acid (ΔALA)	1-7 mg/24 hr	10-53 µmol/24 hr
Epinephrine (24-hr)	5-40 µg/24 hr	
Epithelial cells and casts	Occasional	Occasional
Estriol (24-hr)	>12 mg/24 hr	
Fat	Negative	Negative
Fluoride (24-hr)	<1 mg/24 hr	0.053 mmol/24 hr
Follicle-stimulating hormone (FSH) (24-hr)	Men: 2-12 IU/24 hr	
	Women:	
	During menses: 8-60 IU/24 hr	
	During ovulation: 30-60 IU/24 hr	
	During menopause: >50 IU/24 hr	
Glucose	Negative	Negative
Granular casts	Occasional	Occasional
Hemoglobin and myoglobin	Negative	Negative
Homogentisic acid	Negative	Negative
Human chorionic gonadotropin (HCG)	Negative	Negative
Hyaline casts	Occasional	Occasional
17-Hydroxycorticosteroids (17-OCHS) (24-hr)	Men: 5.5-15.0 mg/24 hr	8.3-25 µmol/24 hr
	Women: 5.0-13.5 mg/24 hr	5.5-22 µmol/24 hr
	Children: lower than adult values	
5-Hydroxyindoleacetic acid (5-HIAA, serotonin) (24-hr)	Men: 2-9 mg/24 hr	10-47 µmol/24 hr
	Women: lower than men	
Ketones (see Acetone plus acetoacetate)		
17-Ketosteroids (17-KS) (24-hr)	Men: 8-15 mg/24 hr	21-62 µmol/24 hr
	Women: 6-12 mg/24 hr	14-45 µmol/24 hr
	Children:	
	12-15 yr: 5-12 mg/24 hr	
	<12 yr: <5 mg/24 hr	
Lactose (24-hr)	14-40 mg/24 hr	41-116 µm
Lead	<0.08 g/ml or <120 g/24 hr	0.39 µmol/L
Leucine aminopeptidase (LAP)	2-18 U/24 hr	
Magnesium (24-hr)	6.8-8.5 mEq/24 hr	3.0-4.3 mmol/24 hr
Melanin	Negative	Negative
Odor	Aromatic	Aromatic
Osmolality	500-800 mOsm/L	38-1400 mmol/kg water
pH	4.6-8.0	4.6-8.0

Urine values—cont'd

Test	Reference Range	
	Conventional Values	SI Units
Phenolsulfonphthalein (PSP)	15 min: at least 25%	At least 0.25
	30 min: at least 40%	At least 0.40
	120 min: at least 60%	At least 0.60
Phenylketonuria (PKU)	Negative	Negative
Phenylpyruvic acid	Negative	Negative
Phosphorus (24-hr)	0.9-1.3 g/24 hr	29-42 mmol/24 hr
Porphobilinogen	Random: negative	Negative
	24-hr: up to 2 mg/24 hr	
Porphyrin (24-hr)	50-300 mg/24 hr	
Potassium (K^+) (24 hr)	25-100 mEq/24 hr	25-100 nmol/24 hr
Pregnancy Test	Positive in normal pregnancy or with tumors producing HCG	Positive in normal pregnancy or with tumors producing HCG
Preganediol	After ovulation: >1 mg/24 hr	
Protein (albumin)	Random: ≤8 mg/dl	
	10-100 mg/24 hr	>0.05 g/24 hr
Sodium (Na^+) (24-hr)	100-260 mEq/24 hr	100-260 nmol/24 hr
Specific gravity	1.010-1.025	1.010-1.025
Steroids (see 17-Hydroxycortico-steroids and 17-Ketosteroids)		
Sugar (see Glucose)		
Titratable acidity (24-hr)	20-50 mEq/24 hr	20-50 mmol/24 hr
Turbidity	Clear	Clear
Urea nitrogen (24-hr)	6-17 g/24 hr	0.21-0.60 mol/24 hr
Uric acid (24-hr)	250-750 mg/24 hr	1.48-4.43 mmol/24 hr
Urobilinogen	0.1-1.0 Ehrlich U/dl	0.1-1.0 Ehrlich U/dl
Uroporphyrin	Negative	Negative
Vanillylmandelic acid (VMA) (24-hr)	1-9 mg/24 hr	<40 μmol/24 hr
Zinc (24-hr)	0.20-0.75 mg/24 hr	

Special endocrine tests

Test	Reference Range	
	Conventional Values	SI Units
Steroid Hormones		
Aldosterone	Excretion: 5-19 μg/24 hr	14-53 nmol/24 hr
Fasting, at rest, 210 mEq sodium diet	Supine: 48 ± 29 pg/ml	133 ± 80 pmol/L
	Upright: (2 hr) 65 ± 23 pg/ml	180 ± 64 pmol/L
Fasting, at rest, 110 mEq sodium diet	Supine: 107 ± 435 pg/ml	279 ± 125 pmol/L
	Upright: (2 hr) 239 ± 123 pg/ml	663 ± 341 pmol/L
Fasting, at rest, 10 mEq sodium diet	Supine: 175 ± 75 pg/ml	485 ± 208 pmol/L
	Upright: (2 hr) 532 ± 228 pg/ml	1476 ± 632 pmol/L
Cortisol		
Fasting	8 AM: 5-25 μg/dl	0.14-0.69 μmol/L
At rest	8 PM: Below 10 μg/dl	0-0.28 μmol/L
20 U ACTH	4 h ACTH test: 30-45 μg/dl	0.83-1.24 μmol/L
Dexamethasone at midnight	Overnight suppression test: Below 5 μg/dl	<0.14 nmol/L
	Excretion: 20-70 μg/24 hr	55-193 nmol/24 hr
11-Deoxycortisol	Responsive: Over 7.5 μg/dl (after metrapone)	>0.22 μmol/L
Testosterone	Adult male: 300-1100 ng/dl	10.4-38.1 nmol/L
	Adolescent male: over 100 ng/dl	>3.5 nmol/L
	Females: 25-90 ng/dl	0.87-3.12 nmol/L
Unbound testosterone	Adult male: 3.06-24.0 ng/dl	106-832 pmol/L
	Adult female: 0.09-1.28 ng/dl	3.1-44.4 pmol/L

Continued.

Cerebrospinal fluid values

Test	Reference Range	
	Conventional Values	**SI Units**
Polypeptide Hormones		
Adrenocorticotropin (ACTH)	15-70 pg/ml	3.3-15.4 pmol/L
Calcitonin	Undetectable in normals	0
	>100 pg/ml in medullary carcinoma	>29.3 pmol/L
Growth hormone		
Fasting, at rest	Below 5 ng/ml	<233 pmol/L
After exercise	Children: over 10 ng/ml	>465 pmol/L
	Male: Below 5 ng/ml	<233 pmol/L
	Female: Up to 30 ng/ml	0-1395 pmol/L
After glucose	Male: Below 5 ng/ml	<233 pmol/L
	Female: Below 10 ng/ml	0-465 pmol/L
Insulin		
Fasting	6-26 μU/ml	43-187 pmol/L
During hypoglycemia	Below 20 μU/ml	<144 pmol/L
After glucose	Up to 150 μU/ml	0-1078 pmol/L
Luteinizing hormone	Male: 6-18 mU/ml	6-18 u/L
Pre- or postovulatory	Female: 5-22 mU/ml	5-22 u/L
Midcycle peak	30-250 mU/ml	30-250 u/L
Parathyroid hormone	<10 μl equiv/ml	< 10 ml equiv/ml
Prolactin	2-15 ng/ml	0.08-6.0 nmol/L
Renin activity		
Normal diet	Supine: 1.1 ± 0.8 ng/ml/hr	0.9 ± 0.6 (nmol/L)hr
	Upright: 1.9 ± 1.7 ng/ml/hr	1.5 ± 1.3 (nmol/L)hr
Low-sodium diet	Supine: 2.7 ± 1.8 ng/ml/hr	2.1 ± 1.4 (nmol/L)hr
	Upright: 6.6 ± 2.5 ng/ml/hr	5.1 ± 1.9 (nmol/L)hr
Low-sodium diet	Diuretics: 10.0 ± 3.7 ng/ml/hr	7.7 ± 2.9 (nmol/L)hr
Thyroid Hormones		
Thryoid-stimulating-hormone (TSH)	0.5-3.5 μU/ml	0.5-3.5 mU/L
Thyroxine-binding globulin capacity	15-25 μg T_4/dl	193-322 nmol/L
Total tri-iodothyronine by radioimmunoassay (T_3)	70-190 ng/dl	1.08-2.92 nmol/L
Total thyroxine by RIA (T_4)	4-12 μg/dl	52-154 nmol/L
T_3 resin uptake	25%-35%	0.25-0.35
Free thyroxine index (FT_4I)	1-4 ng/dl	12.8-51.2 pmol/L
Bilirubin	0	0 μmol/L
Chloride	120-130 mEq/L	
	(20 mEq/L higher than serum)	
Albumin	Mean: 29.5 mg/dl	0.295 g/L
	± 112 SD: 11-48 mg/dl	± 112 SD: 0.11-0.48 g/L
IgG	Mean: 4.3 mg/dl	0.043 g/L
	± 112 SD: 0-8.6 mg/dl	± 112 SD: 0-0.086
Glucose	50-75 mg/dl	2.8-4.2 mmol/L
	(30%-50% less than blood)	
Pressure (initial)	70-180 mm of water	70-80 arb. u.
Protein:		
Lumbar	15-45 mg/dl	0.15-0.45 g/L
Cisternal	15-25 mg/dl	0.15-0.25 g/L
Ventricular	5-15 mg/dl	0.05-0.15 g/L

Hematologic values

Test	Reference Range	
	Conventional Values	**SI Units**
Coagulation factors:		
Factor I (fibrinogen)	0.15%-0.35 g/dl	4.0-10.0 μmol/L
Factor II (prothrombin)	60%-140%	0.60-1.40
Factor V(accelerator globulin)	60%-140%	0.60-1.40
Factor VII-X (proconvertin-Stuart)	70%-130%	0.70-1.30
Factor X (Stuart factor)	70%-130%	0.70-1.30
Factor VIII (antihemophilic globu-lin)	50%-200%	0.50-2.0
Factor IX (plasma thromboplastic cofactor)	60%-140%	0.60-1.40
Factor XI (plasma thromboplastic antecedent)	60%-140%	0.60-1.40
Factor XII (Hageman factor)	60%-140%	0.60-1.40
Coagulation screening tests:		
Bleeding time (Simplate)	3-9 min	180-540 sec
Prothrombin time	Less than 2-sec deviation from control	Less than 2-sec deviation from control
Partial thromboplastin time (acti-vated)	25-37 sec	25-37 sec
Whole-blood clot lysis	No clot lysis in 24 hr	0/d
Fibrinolytic studies:		
Euglobin lysis	No lysis in 2 hr	0 (in 2 hr)
Fibrinogen split products:	Negative reaction at greater than 1:4 dilu-tion	0 (at >1:4 dilution)
Thrombin time	Control ± 5 sec	Control ± 5 sec
"Complete" blood count:		
Hematocrit	Male: 45%-52%	Male: 0.42-0.52
	Female: 37%-48%	Female: 0.37-0.48
Hemoglobin	Male: 13-18 g/10 ml	Male: 8.1-11.2 mmol/L
	Female: 12-16 g/dl	Female: 7.4-9.9 mmol/L
Leukocyte count	4300-10,800/mm^3	4.3-10.8 × 10^9/L
Erythrocyte count	4.2-5.9 million/mm^3	4.2-5.9 × 10^{12}/L
Mean corpuscular volume (MCV)	80-94 μm^3	80-94 fL
Mean corpuscular hemoglobin (MCH)	27-32 pg	1.7-2.0 fmol
Mean corpuscular hemoglobin concentration (MCHC)	32%-36%	19-22.8 mmol/L
Erythrocyte sedimentation rate (Westergren method)	Male: 1-13 mm/hr	Male: 1-13 mm/hr
	Female: 1-20 mm/hr	Female: 1-20 mm/hr
Erythrocyte enzymes		
Glucose-6-phosphate dehydroge-nase	5-15 U/gHb	5-15 U/g
Pyruvate kinase	13-17 U/gHb	13-17 U/g
Ferritin (serum)		
Iron deficiency	0-20 ng/ml	0-20 μg/L
Iron excess	Greater than 400 ng/L	>400 μg/L
Folic acid		
Normal	Greater than 1.9 ng/ml	>4.3 mmol/L
Borderline	1.0-1.9 ng/ml	2.3-4.3 mmol/L
Haptoglobin	100-300 mg/dl	1.0-3.0 g/L
Hemoglobin studies:		
Electrophoresis for A$_2$ hemoglobin	1.5%-3.5%	0.015-0.035
Hemoglobin F (fetal hemoglobin)	Less than 2%	<0.02
Hemoglobin, met- and sulf-	0	0
Serum hemoglobin	2-3 mg/dl	1.2-1.9 μmol/L
Thermolabile hemoglobin	0	0
L.E. (lupus erythematosus) prepara-tion:		
Heparin as anticoagulant	0	0
Defibrinated blood	0	0

Continued.

Hematologic values—cont'd

Test	Reference Range	
	Conventional Values	**SI Units**
Leukocyte alkaline phosphatase:		
Quantitative method	15-40 mg of phosphorus liberated/hr/10^{10} cells	15-40 mg/hr
Qualitative method	Males: 33-188 U	33-188 U
	Females (off contraceptive pill): 30-160 U	30-160 U
Muramidase	Serum, 3-7 μg/ml	3-7 mg/L
	Urine, 0-2 μg/ml	0-2 mg/L
Osmotic fragility of erythrocytes	Increased if hemolysis occurs in over 0.5% NaCl; decreased if hemolysis is incomplete in 0.3% NaCl	
Peroxide hemolysis	Less than 10%	<0.10
Platelet count	150,000-350,000/mm^3	150-350 × 10^9/L
Platelet function test:		
Clot retraction	50%-100%/2 hr	0.50-1.00/2 hr
Platelet aggregation	Full response to ADP, epinephrine, and collagen	1.0
Platelet factor 3	33-57 sec	33-57 sec
Reticulocyte count	0.5%-1.5% red cells	0.005-0.15
Vitamin B$_{12}$	90-280 pg/ml (borderline: 70-90)	66-207 pmol/L (borderline: 52-66)

Miscellaneous values

Test	Reference Range	
	Conventional Values	**SI Units**
Autoantibodies in serum		
Thyroid colloid and microsomal antigens	Absent	
Stomach parietal cells	Absent	
Smooth muscle	Absent	
Kidney mitochondria	Absent	
Rabbit renal collecting ducts	Absent	
Cytoplasma of ova, theca cells, testicular interstitial cells	Absent	
Skeletal muscle	Absent	
Adrenal gland	Absent	
Carcinoembryonic antigen (CEA) in blood	0-2.5 ng/ml, 97% healthy nonsmokers	0-2.5 μg/L, 97% healthy nonsmokers
Cryoprecipitable proteins in blood	0	0 arb. unit
Digitoxin in serum	17 ± 6 ng/ml	22 ± 7.8 nmol/L
Digoxin in serum		
0.25 mg/24 hr	1.2 ± 0.4 ng/ml	1.54 ± 0.5 nmol/L
0.5 mg/24 hr	1.5 ± 0.4 ng/ml	1.92 ± 0.5 nmol/L
Duodenal drainage:		
pH	5.5-7.5	5.5-7.5
Amylase	Over 1200 U/total sample	>1.2 arb. u
Trypsin	Values from 35% to 160% "normal"	0.35-1.60
Viscosity	3 min or less	180 sec or less
Gastric analysis	Basal:	
	Females 2.0 ± 1.8 mEq/h	0.6 ± 0.5
	Males 3.0 ± 2.0 mEq/h	0.8 ± 0.6 μmol/sec
	Maximal: (after histalog or gastrin)	
	Females 16 ± 5 mEq/h	4.4 ± 1.4 μmol/sec
	Males 23 ± 5 mEq/h	6.4 ± 1.4 μmol/sec
Gastrin-l in blood	0.200 pg/ml	0-95 pmol/L

Miscellaneous values—cont'd

	Reference Range	
Test	**Conventional Values**	**SI Units**
Immunologic tests		
Alpha-feto-globulin	Abnormal if present	
Alpha 1-antitrypsin	200-400 mg/dl	2.0-4.0 g/L
Antinuclear antibodies	Positive if detected with serum diluted 1:10	
Anti-DNA antibodies	Less than 15 U/ml	
Complement, total hemolytic	150-250 U/ml	
C3	Range 55-120 ng/dl	0.55-1.2 g/L
C4	Range 20-50 mg/dl	0.2-0.5 g/L
Immunoglobulins in blood:		
IgG	1140 mg/dl; range 540-1663	11.4 g/L 5.5-16.6 g/L
IgA	214 mg/dl; range 66-344	2.14 g/L 0.66-3.44 g/L
IgM	168 mg/dl; range 39-290	1.68 g/L 0.39-2.9 g/L
Viscosity	1.4-1.8 expressed as relative viscosity of serum compared with water	
Iontophoresis	Children: 0-40 mEq sodium/L	0-40 mmol/L
	Adults: 0-60 mEq sodium/L	0-60 mmol/L
Propranolol (includes bioactive 4-OH metabolite) in serum 4 hr after last dose	100-300 ng/ml	386-1158 nmol/L
Stool fat	Less than 5 g in 24 hr or less than 4% of measured fat intake in 3-day period	< 5/24 hr
Stool nitrogen	Less than 2 g/24 hr or 10% of urinary nitrogen	<2 g/24 hr
Synovial fluid:		
Glucose	Not less than 20 mg/dl lower than simultaneously drawn blood sugar	See blood glucose mmol/L

Mucin	Type 1 or 2
	Grades as:
	    Type 1—tight clump
	    Type 2—soft clump
	    Type 3—soft clump that breaks up
	    Type 4—cloudy, no clump
		1-2 arb. u

D-Xylose absorption	5-8 g/5 hr in urine 40 mg/dl in blood 2 hr after ingestion of 25 g of D-xylose	33-53 mmol 2.7 mmol/L

Abbreviations in Common Usage

ā	Before		CSF	Cerebrospinal fluid
aa	Of each		CT	Computed tomography
ac	Before meals		CVA	Cerebrovascular accident
ad lib	As desired		CVA	Costovertebral angle
A/G ratio	Albumin/globulin ratio		CVP	Central venous pressure
AK	Above knee		Cx	Cervix
aPTT	Activated partial thromboplastin time		Cysto	Cystoscopy
A/R pulse	Apical/radial pulse		D/C	Discontinue
ARDS	Adult respiratory distress syndrome		D & C	Dilation and curettage
ARV	Aortic valve replacement		Diff	Differential white blood cell count
ASCVD	Arteriosclerotic cardiovascular disease		DIP	Distal interphalangeal joint
ASHD	Arteriosclerotic heart disease		DJD	Degenerative joint disease
BaE	Barium enema		DM	Diabetes mellitus
BFT	Biofeedback therapy		DOA	Dead on arrival
b.i.d.	Twice daily		DOE	Dyspnea on exertion
BK	Below knee		DPT	Diphtheria, pertussis, tetanus toxoid
BMR	Basal metabolism rate		Dx	Diagnosis
BPH	Benign prostatic hypertrophy		ECG	Electrocardiogram
B.R.P.	Bathroom privileges		EEG	Electroencephalogram
BS	Bowel sounds		EENT	Eye, ear, nose, and throat
BSP	Bromsulphalein		EMG	Electromyogram
BUN	Blood urea nitrogen		ENT	Ear, nose, and throat
Bx	Biopsy		ESR	Erythrocyte sedimentation rate
c̄	With		FB	Foreign body
CA	Cancer		FBS	Fasting blood sugar
CABG	Coronary artery bypass graft		FH	Family history
CAD	Coronary artery disease		FUO	Fever of unknown origin
CBC	Complete blood count		FWB	Full weight bearing
cc	Chief complaint		Fx	Fracture
CCK	Cholecystokinin		GI	Gastrointestinal
C.D.	Constant drainage		gtt	Drops
CDC	Centers for Disease Control		GTT	Glucose tolerance test
CHF	Congestive heart failure		GU	Genitourinary
CNS	Central nervous system		h	Hour
c/o	Complained of		HAV	Hepatitis A virus
COPD	Chronic obstructive pulmonary disease		HBV	Hepatitis B virus
CPK	Creatine phosphokinase		Hct	Hematocrit
CPR	Cardiopulmonary resuscitation		HCTZ	Hydrochlorothiazide
C & S	Culture and sensitivies		HCVD	Hypertensive cardiovascular disease

HDL	High-density lipoproteins	NPN	Nonprotein nitrogen
Hgb	Hemoglobin	N.P.O.	Nothing by mouth
HMO	Health maintenance organization	NVD	Neck vein distention
HNP	Herniated nucleus pulposus	NWB	Non−weight bearing
HPI	History of present illness	OD	Overdose
HTN	Hypertension	O.D.	Right eye
h.s.	At bedtime	OOB	Out of bed
Hwb	Hot water bottle	O.R.	Operating room
hx	History	ORIF	Open reduction internal fixation
IABP	Intraaortic balloon counterpulsation	O.S.	Left eye
ICP	Intracranial pressure	O.T.	Occupational therapy
ICS	Intercostal space	O.U.	Both eyes
ICU	Intensive care unit	p̄	After
IDDM	Insulin-dependent diabetes mellitus	P & A	Percussion and auscultation
IHSS	Idiopathic hypertrophic subaortic stenosis	PAEDP	Pulmonary artery end-diastolic pressure
IM	Intramuscular	PAP	Papanicolaou smear
IMB	Intermenstrual bleeding	PAP	Pulmonary artery pressure
I & O	Intake and output	PBI	Protein bound iodine
IPPB	Intermittent positive pressure breathing	p.c.	After meals
		PCWP	Pulmonary capillary wedge pressure
ITP	Idiopathic thrombocytopenic purpura	P.D.	Postural drainage
IV	Intravenous	PEEP	Positive end expiratory pressure
IVC	Intravenous cholangiogram	PERRLA	Pupils equal, round, reactive to light and accommodation
IVP	Intravenous pyelogram		
LBP	Low back pain	PFT	Pulmonary function test
LDH	Lactic dehydrogenase	Ph	Post history
LDL	Low density lipoproteins	PI	Present illness
L.E. prep	Lupus erythematosus prep	PIP	Proximal interphalangeal joint
LLL	Left lower lobe	Plt	Platelet
LLQ	Left lower quadrant	PMI	Point of maximal impulse
LMD	Local medical doctor	PMNs	Polymorphonuclear leukocytes
LMP	Last menstrual period	PMP	Past menstrual period
LMP	Local medical physician	PND	Paroxysmal nocturnal dyspnea
LOC	Level of consciousness	PNS	Peripheral nervous system
LP	Lumbar puncture	p.o.	By mouth
LVEDP	Left ventricular end-diastolic pressure	POD	Postoperative day
L & W	Living and well	PPD	Postpartum day
lytes	Electrolytes	PPD	Purified protein derivative
ⓜ	Murmur	prn	According to necessity
MCH	Mean corpuscular hemoglobin	Pro time	Prothrombin time
MCHC	Mean corpuscular hemoglobin concentration	PSP	Phenosulphonphthalein
		PSRO	Professional standards review organization
MCP	Metacarpophalangeal joint	PT	Prothrombin time
MCV	Mean corpuscular volume	P.T.	Physical therapy
MGW	Magnesium, glycerin, and water enema	PTA	Prior to admission
MST	Mean survival time	PTT	Partial thromboplastin time
MTP	Metatarsalphalangeal joint	PVC	Premature ventricular contraction
MVR	Mitral valve replacement	PWB	Partial weight bearing
MWB	Minimal weight bearing	PZI	Protamine zinc insulin
NAD	No acute distress	qd	Every day
NIDDM	Noninsulin dependent diabetes mellitus	qh	Every hour
		qhs	At bedtime
NMR	Nuclear magnetic resonance	qid	Four times a day
NPH	Nonprotein Hadedorn (insulin)	qns	Quantity not sufficient

qod	Every other day
qoh	Every other hour
qpr	At earliest convenience
qs	As much as necessary (quantity sufficient)
RBC	Red blood cells
RLL	Right lower lobe
RLQ	Right lower quandrant
R/O	Rule out
ROS	Review of symptoms
RSR	Regular sinus rhythm
Rx	Treatment
$\bar{s}$	Without
SBE	Subacute bacterial endocarditis
sc	Subcutaneous
Sed rate	Sedimentation rate
SGOT	Serum glutamic oxidase transaminase
SGPT	Serum glutamic pyruvate transaminase
SLE	Systemic lupus erythematosus
SLR	Straight leg raising
SOB	Short of breath
s.o.s.	Administer once if necessary
S/P	Status post (occurred in past)
SR	Systems review
SSE	Soapsuds enema
stat	At once
STD	Sexually transmitted disease
STS	Serologic test for syphilis
T_3	Triiodothyronine
T_4	Thyroxine
tab	Tablet

TBC	Tuberculosis
TBG	Thyroxine binding globulin
TENS	Transcutaneous electrical nerve stimulator
THA	Total hip arthroplasty
THR	Total hip replacement
TIA	Transient ischemic attacks
t.i.d.	Three times a day
TKA	Total knee arthroplasty
TKR	Total knee replacement
TM	Tympanic membrane
TP	Total protein
TPN	Total parenteral nutrition (hyperalimentation)
TSP	Total serum protein
TSS	Toxic shock syndrome
TURP	Transurethral resection of prostate
Tx	Traction
ung	Ointment
URI	Upper respiratory infection
US	Ultrasound
UTI	Urinary tract infection
UV	Ultraviolet
VC	Vital capacity
VDRL	Venereal Disease Research Laboratory Test
VNA	Visiting nurse association
VS	Vital signs
wa	While awake
WBC	White blood count
WNL	Within normal limits

Recommended Daily Dietary Allowances, Revised 1989

Median heights and weights and recommended energy intake

Category	Age (yr) or Condition	Weight (kg)	Weight (lb)	Height (cm)	Height (in)	REE* (kcal/day)	Average Energy Allowance (kcal)† Multiples of REE	Per kg	Per day‡
Infants	0.0-0.5	6	13	60	24	320		108	650
	0.5-1.0	9	20	71	28	500		98	850
Children	1-3	13	29	90	35	740		102	1300
	4-6	20	44	112	44	950		90	1800
	7-10	28	62	132	52	1130		70	2000
Males	11-14	45	99	157	62	1440	1.70	55	2500
	15-18	66	145	176	69	1760	1.67	45	3000
	19-24	72	160	177	70	1780	1.67	40	2900
	25-50	79	174	176	70	1800	1.60	37	2900
	51+	77	170	173	68	1530	1.50	30	2300
Females	11-14	46	101	157	62	1310	1.67	47	2200
	15-18	55	120	163	64	1370	1.60	40	2200
	19-24	58	128	164	65	1350	1.60	38	2200
	25-50	63	138	163	64	1380	1.55	36	2200
	51+	65	143	160	63	1280	1.50	30	1900
Pregnant	1st trimester								
	2nd trimester								+0
	3rd trimester								+300
Lactating	1st 6 months								+500
	2nd 6 months								+500

From Recommended Dietary Allowances, Revised 1989. Food and Nutrition Board National Academy of Sciences–National Research Council, Washington, D.C.

The data in this table have been assembled from the observed median heights and weights of children together with desirable weights for adults for the mean heights of men (70 in) and women (64 in) between the ages of 18 and 34 years as surveyed in the U.S. population (HEW/NCHS data).

The energy allowances for the young adults are for men and women doing light work. The allowances for the two older age groups represent mean energy needs over these age spans, allowing for a 2% decrease in basal (resting) metabolic rate per decade and a reduction in activity of 200 kcal per day for men and women between 51 and 75 years, 500 kcal for men over 75 years, and 400 kcal for women over 75. The customary range of daily energy output is shown for adults in parentheses and is based on a variation in energy needs of ±400 kcal at any one age, emphasizing the wide range of energy intakes appropriate for any group of people.

Energy allowances for children through age 18 are based on median energy intakes of children these ages followed in longitudinal growth studies. The values in parentheses are 10th and 90th percentiles of energy intake, to indicate the range of energy consumption among children of these ages.

*Resting energy expenditure.

†In the range of light to moderate activity, the coefficient of variation is ±20%.

‡Figure is rounded.

Daily dietary guide—the basic four food groups

Food Group	Main Nutrients	Daily Amounts*
Milk		
Milk, cheese, ice cream, or other products made with whole or skimmed milk	Calcium Protein Riboflavin	Children under 9: 2-3 cups Children 9-12: 3 or more cups Teenagers: 4 or more cups Adults: 2 or more cups Pregnant women: 3 or more cups Nursing mothers: 4 or more cups (1 cup = 8 oz fluid milk or designated milk equivalent†)
Meats		

Beef, veal, lamb, pork, poultry, fish, eggs	Protein
	Iron
	Thiamin
		2 or more servings
		Count as 1 serving
		  2-3 oz of lean, boneless, cooked meat, poultry, or fish
		  2 eggs

Alternates: dry beans, dry peas, nuts, peanut butter	Niacin Riboflavin	1 cup cooked dry beans or peas 4 tbsp peanut butter
Vegetables and fruits		4 or more servings Count as 1 serving ½ cup of vegetable or fruit or a portion such as 1 medium apple, banana, orange, potato, or ½ a medium grapefruit, melon Include
	Vitamin A	A dark-green or deep-yellow vegetable or fruit rich in vitamin A at least every other day
	Vitamin C (ascorbic acid) Smaller amounts of other vitamins and minerals	A citrus fruit or other fruit or vegetable rich in vitamin C daily Other vegetables and fruits including potatoes
Bread and cereals		4 or more servings of whole grain, enriched or restored Count as 1 serving
	Thiamin Niacin Riboflavin Iron Protein	1 slice of bread 1 oz (1 cup) ready-to-eat cereal, flake or puff varieties ½-¾ cup cooked cereal ½-¾ cup cooked pastas (macaroni, spaghetti, noodles) Crackers: 5 saltines, 2 squares graham crackers

*Use additional amounts of these foods or added butter, margarine, oils, sugars, etc., as desired or needed.
†Milk equivalents: 1 oz cheddar cheese, 3 servings cottage cheese, 1 cup fluid skimmed milk, 1 cup buttermilk, ½ cup dry skimmed milk powder, 1 cup ice milk, 1⅔ cups ice cream, ½ cup evaporated milk.

Recommended dietary allowances,[a] revised 1989

Category	Age (yr) or Condition	Weight[b] (kg)	Weight[b] (lb)	Height[b] (cm)	Height[b] (in)	Protein (g)	Fat-Soluble Vitamins Vitamin A (µg RE)[c]	Vitamin D (µg RE)[d]	Vitamin E (mg α-TE)[e]	Vitamin K (µg)
Infants	0.0-0.5	6	13	60	24	13	375	7.5	3	5
	0.5-1.0	9	20	71	28	14	375	10	4	10
Children	1-3	13	29	90	35	16	400	10	6	15
	4-6	20	44	112	44	24	500	10	7	20
	7-10	28	62	132	52	28	700	10	7	30
Males	11-14	45	99	157	62	45	1000	10	10	45
	15-18	66	145	176	69	59	2000	10	10	65
	19-24	72	160	177	70	58	1000	10	10	70
	25-50	79	174	176	70	63	1000	5	10	80
	51+	77	170	173	68	63	1000	5	10	80
Females	11-14	46	101	157	62	46	800	10	8	45
	15-18	55	120	163	64	44	800	10	8	55
	19-24	58	128	164	65	46	800	10	8	60
	25-50	63	138	163	64	50	800	5	8	65
	51+	65	143	160	63	50	800	5	8	65
	Pregnant					60	800	10	10	65
	Lactating									
	1st 6 mo					65	1300	10	12	65
	2nd 6 mo					62	1200	10	11	65

Category	Age (yr) or Condition	Weight (kg)	Weight (lb)	Height (cm)	Height (in)	Water-Soluble Vitamins Vitamin C (mg)	Thiamin (mg)	Riboflavin (mg)	Niacin (mg NE)[f]	Vitamin B$_6$ (mg)	Folate (µg)	Vitamin B$_{12}$ (µg)
Infants	0.0-0.5	6	13	60	24	30	0.3	0.4	5	0.3	25	0.3
	0.5-1.0	9	20	71	28	35	0.4	0.5	6	0.6	35	0.5
Children	1-3	13	29	90	35	40	0.7	0.8	9	1.0	50	0.7
	4-6	20	44	112	44	45	0.9	1.1	12	1.1	75	1.0
	7-10	28	62	132	52	45	1.0	1.2	13	1.4	100	1.4
Males	11-14	45	99	157	62	50	1.3	1.5	17	1.7	150	2.0
	15-18	66	145	176	69	60	1.5	1.8	20	2.0	200	2.0
	19-24	72	160	177	70	60	1.5	1.7	19	2.0	200	2.0
	25-50	79	174	176	70	60	1.5	1.7	19	2.0	200	2.0
	51+	77	170	173	68	60	1.2	1.4	15	2.0	200	2.0
Females	11-14	46	101	147	62	50	1.1	1.3	15	1.4	150	2.0
	15-18	55	120	163	64	60	1.1	1.3	15	1.5	180	2.0
	19-24	58	128	164	65	60	1.1	1.3	15	1.6	180	2.0
	25-50	63	138	163	64	60	1.1	1.3	15	1.6	180	2.0
	51+	65	143	160	63	60	1.0	1.2	13	1.6	180	2.0
	Pregnant					70	1.5	1.6	17	2.2	400	2.2
	Lactating											
	1st 6 mo					95	1.6	1.8	20	2.1	280	2.6
	2nd 6 mo					90	1.6	1.7	20	2.1	260	2.6

Modified from Food and Nutrition Board, National Academy of Sciences–National Research Council.

[a]The allowances, expressed as average daily intakes over time, are intended to provide for individual variations among most normal persons as they live in the United States under usual environmental stresses. Diets should be based on a variety of common foods in order to provide other nutrients for which human requirements have been less well defined.

[b]Weights and heights of Reference Adults are actual medians for the U.S. population of the designated age, as reported by NHANES II. The use of these figures does not imply that the height-to-weight ratios are ideal.

[c]Retinol equivalents; 1 retinol equivalent = 1 µg retinol or 6 µg β-carotene.

[d]As cholecalciferol; 10 µg cholecalciferol = 400 IU of vitamin D.

[e]α-Tocopherol equivalents. 1 mg d-α tocopherol = 1 α-TE.

[f]1 NE (niacin equivalent) is equal to 1 mg of niacin or 60 mg of dietary tryptophan.

Continued.

Recommended dietary allowances, revised 1989—cont'd

Category	Age (yr) or Condition	Weight(b) (kg)	(lb)	Height(b) (cm)	(in)	Minerals Calcium (mg)	Phosphorus (mg)	Magnesium (mg)	Iron (mg)	Zinc (mg)	Iodine (µg)	Selenium (µg)
Infants	0.0-0.5	6	13	60	24	400	300	40	6	5	40	10
	0.5-1.0	9	20	71	28	600	500	60	10	5	50	15
Children	1-3	13	29	90	35	800	800	80	10	10	70	20
	4-6	20	44	112	44	800	800	120	10	10	90	20
	7-10	28	62	132	52	800	800	170	10	10	120	30
Males	11-14	45	99	157	62	1200	1200	270	12	15	150	40
	15-18	66	145	176	69	1200	1200	400	12	15	150	50
	19-24	72	160	177	70	1200	1200	350	10	15	150	70
	25-50	79	174	176	70	800	800	350	10	15	150	70
	51+	77	170	173	68	800	800	350	10	15	150	70
Females	11-14	46	101	157	62	1200	1200	280	15	12	150	45
	15-18	55	120	163	64	1200	1200	300	15	12	150	50
	19-24	58	128	164	65	1200	1200	280	15	12	150	55
	25-50	63	138	163	64	800	800	280	15	12	150	55
	51+	65	143	160	63	800	800	280	10	12	150	55
	Pregnant					1200	1200	320	30	15	175	65
	Lactating											
	1st 6 mo					1200	1200	355	15	19	200	75
	2nd 6 mo					1200	1200	340	15	16	200	75

Recommended daily dietary allowances of some selected nutrients for pregnancy and lactation (National Research Council, 1989 revision)

Nutrients	Nonpregnant girl 12-14 yr 47 kg (103 lb)	Nonpregnant girl 14-18 yr 55 kg (120 lb)	Nonpregnant woman 25 yr 58 kg (128 lb)	Pregnancy Added need	Pregnancy Girl 12-14 yr	Pregnancy Girl 14-18 yr	Pregnancy Woman 25 yr	Lactation (850 ml daily) Added need	Lactation Girl 12-14 yr	Lactation Girl 14-18 yr	Lactation Woman 25 yr
Kilocalories	2200	2200	2200	300	2500	2500	2500	500	2700	2700	2700
Protein (g)	46	46	50	10-15	60	60	60	15	65	68	65
Calcium (g)	1.2	1.2	0.8	0.4	1.6	1.6	1.2	0.4	1.6	1.6	1.2
Iron (mg)	15	15	15	15	30	30	30	0	15	15	15
Vitamin A (RE)*	800	800	800	0	800	800	800	500	1300	1300	1300
Thiamin (mg)	1.1	1.1	1.1	0.4	1.5	1.5	1.5	0.5	1.6	1.6	1.6
Riboflavin (mg)	1.3	1.3	1.3	0.3	1.6	1.6	1.6	0.5	1.8	1.8	1.8
Niacin equivalent and tryptophan (mg)	15	15	15	2	17	17	17	5	20	20	20
Ascorbic acid (mg)	50	60	60	10	60	70	70	35	95	95	95
Vitamin D (µg)†	10	10	5	5	15	15	10	5	15	15	10

*Retinol equivalents.
†Cholecalciferol; 10 µg equals 400 IU vitamin D.

Estimated safe and adequate daily dietary intakes of selected vitamins and minerals*

Category	Age (yr)	Vitamins		Trace Elements†				
		Biotin (µg)	Pantothenic Acid (mg)	Copper (mg)	Manganese (mg)	Fluoride (mg)	Chromium (µg)	Molybedenum (µg)
Infants	0-0.5	10	2	0.4-0.6	0.3-0.6	0.1-0.5	10-10	15-30
	0.5-1	15	3	0.6-0.7	0.6-1.0	0.2-1.0	20-60	20-40
Children and adolescents	1-3	20	3	0.7-1.0	1.0-1.5	0.5-1.5	20-80	25-50
	4-6	25	3-4	1.0-1.5	1.5-2.0	1.0-2.5	30-120	30-75
	7-10	30	4-5	1.0-2.0	2.0-3.0	1.5-2.5	50-200	50-150
	11+	30-100	4-7	1.5-2.5	2.0-5.0	1.5-2.5	50-200	75-250
Adults		30-100	4-7	1.5-3.0	2.0-5.0	1.5-4.0	50-200	75-250

From Food and Nutrition Board, National Academy of Sciences–National Research Council, 1989.
*Because there is less information on which to base allowances, these figures are not given in the main table of RDA and are provided here in the form of ranges of recommended intakes.
†Since the toxic levels for many trace elements may be only several times usual intakes, the upper levels for the trace elements given in this table should not be habitually exceeded.

Estimated sodium, chloride, and potassium minimum requirements of healthy persons*

Age	Weight (kg)*	Sodium (mg)*,†	Chloride (mg)*,†	Potassium (mg)‡
Months				
0-5	4.5	120	180	500
6-11	8.9	200	300	700
Years				
1	11.0	225	350	1,000
2-5	16.0	300	500	1,400
6-9	25.0	400	600	1,600
10-18	50.0	500	750	2,000
>18§	70.0	500	750	2,000

From Food and Nutrition Board, National Academy of Sciences–National Research Council, 1989.
*No allowance has been included for large, prolonged losses from the skin through sweat.
†There is no evidence that higher intakes confer any health benefit.
‡Desirable intakes of potassium may considerably exceed these values (~3.500 mg for adults).
§No allowance included for growth. Values for those below 18 years assume a growth rate at the 50th percentile reported by the National Center for Health Statistics and averaged for males and females.

Signs of Malnutrition

Physical signs indicative or suggestive of malnutrition

Body Area	Normal Appearance	Signs Associated with Malnutrition
Hair	Shiny, firm, not easily plucked	Lack of natural shine; hair dull and dry, thin and sparse; hair fine, silky, and straight; color changes (flag sign); can be easily plucked
Face	Skin color uniform; smooth, pink, healthy appearance; not swollen	Skin color loss (depigmentation); skin dark over cheeks and under eyes (malar and supraorbital pigmentation); lumpiness or flakiness of skin of nose and mouth; swollen face; enlarged parotid glands; scaling of skin around nostrils (nasolabial seborrhea)
Eyes	Bright, clear, shiny; no sores at corners of eyelids; membranes a healthy pink and moist; no prominent blood vessels or mound of tissue or sclera	Eye membranes are pale (pale conjunctivae); redness of membranes (conjunctival injection), Bitot's spots; redness and fissuring of eyelid corners (angular palpebritis); dryness of eye membranes (conjunctival xerosis); cornea has dull appearance (corneal xerosis); cornea soft (keratomalacia); scar on cornea; ring of fine blood vessels around cornea (circumcorneal injection)
Lips	Smooth, not chapped or swollen	Redness and swelling of mouth or lips (cheilosis), especially at corners of mouth (angular fissures and scars)
Tongue	Deep red in appearance; not swollen or smooth	Swelling; scarlet and raw tongue; magenta (purplish color) tongue; smooth tongue; swollen sores; hyperemic and hypertrophic papillae; atrophic papillae
Teeth	No cavities; no pain; bright	May be missing or erupting abnormally; gray or black spots (fluorosis); cavities (caries)
Gums	Healthy; red; do not bleed; not swollen	"Spongy" and bleed easily; recession of gums
Glands	Face not swollen	Thyroid enlargement (front of neck); parotid enlargement (cheeks become swollen)
Skin	No signs of rashes, swellings, dark or light spots	Dryness of skin (xerosis); sandpaper feel of skin (follicular hyperkeratosis); flakiness of skin; skin swollen and dark; red swollen pigmentation of exposed areas (pellagrous dermatosis); excessive lightness or darkness of skin (dyspigmentation); black and blue marks from skin bleeding (petechiae); lack of fat under skin
Nails	Firm, pink	Nails are spoon shaped (koilonychia); brittle, ridged nails
Muscular and skeletal systems	Good muscle tone, some fat under skin; can walk or run without pain	Muscles have "wasted" appearance; baby's skull bones are thin and soft (craniotabes); round swelling of front and side of head (frontal and parietal bossing); swelling of ends of bones (epiphyseal enlargement); small bumps on both sides of chest wall (on ribs), beading of ribs; baby's soft spot on head does not harden at proper time (persistently open anterior fontanelle); knock-knees or bowlegs; bleeding into muscle (musculoskeletal hemorrhages); person cannot get up or walk properly

*From Christakis, G: Am J Public Health 63(suppl):1-82, 1973.

Physical signs indicative or suggestive of malnutrition — cont'd

Body area	Normal appearance	Signs associated with malnutrition
Internal systems		
Cardiovascular	Normal heart rate and rhythm; no murmurs or abnormal rhythms; normal blood pressure for age	Rapid heart rate (above 100, tachycardia); enlarged heart; abnormal rhythm; elevated blood pressure
Gastrointestinal	No palpable organs or masses (in children, however, liver edge may be palpable)	Liver enlargement; enlargement of spleen (usually indicates other associated diseases)
Nervous	Psychologic stability; normal reflexes	Mental irritability and confusion; burning and tingling of hands and feet (paresthesia); loss of position and vibratory sense; weakness and tenderness of muscles (may result in inability to walk); decrease and loss of ankle and knee reflexes

Index